In Search of Gentle Death

The Fight for Your Right to Die with Dignity

Richard N. Côté

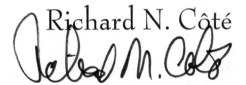

CORINTHIAN
BOOKS

Mt. Pleasant, South Carolina

Publisher's Cataloging-in-Publication Data
(*Provided by Quality Books, Inc.*)

Côté, Richard N., 1945-
  In search of gentle death: the fight for your right to die with dignity / Richard N. Côté. — 1st ed.
  p. cm.
  Includes bibliographical references and index.
  LCCN 2011900559
  ISBN-13: 9781929175369 (trade hardcover edition)
  ISBN-13: 9781929175437 (eBook edition)
  ISBN-13: 9781929175505 (PDF on CD edition)

  1. Right to die. 2. Death. 3. Assisted suicide.
I. Title.

R726.C68 2012   179.7
                           QBI11-600128
BISAC categories:
SOC036000 / Social sciences (death and dying)
MED 050000 / Medical ethics
MED 042000 / Medicine – terminal care

Hardcover edition, first printing, April 2012
eBook version 1.0 (Kindle and ePub), April 2012

This book is dedicated to Georgene "Gigi" Sandberg (1926-2009), a daring pioneer and caring member of the Hemlock Society USA, who first saw my work in its germination stage and enabled it to grow and flower.

Contents

More Advance Reviews

"Côté's history of the international Death With Dignity Movement combines a monumental amount of research with a writing style that will appeal to anyone interested in end-of-life issues and the pursuit of a 'good death.' Insider information and personal revelations about individuals not previously reported make this a *must read.* — Richard MacDonald, M.D., former medical director Hemlock Society USA.

"A well-written, engrossing look at the international right-to-die movement. Côté has done extensive research and knows the leaders in every country where there is a struggle for the right to receive legal assisted dying. — Faye E. Girsh, Ed.D., past president Hemlock Society USA; president (2012—) World Federation of Right to Die Societies.

"We are all unique individuals, which makes it unsurprising that there are many contrasting views on assisted dying. Richard Côté's extremely well-researched book, based on extensive personal interviews, expertly draws out these nuances as they have evolved in Australia and New Zealand." —Rodney Syme, M.D., author, *A Good Death*; vice-president Death With Dignity-Victoria, Australia.

"Our movement, as is any concerted human endeavor, is a patchwork quilt of personality and diversity in approach to achieve an end. Côté has masterfully brought a sense of cohesion to the portrayal of this effort." — Theodore Goodwin, cofounder of the Final Exit Network and former president of the board of directors of the World Federation of Right to Die Societies.

"This fascinating book is the first to describe in gripping detail the long worldwide fight for choice at the end of life. A well-written, must-read for all who support the death-with-dignity cause. — Elizabeth "Libby" Wilson, M.D., founder of Friends-at-the-End (FATE), Glasgow, Scotland.

"Dr. Jack Kevorkian's uncompromising position on physician-assisted suicide and his struggles to implement societal change are well-documented and impartially presented through Côté's extensive research and balanced presentation." — Neal Nicol, professional colleague of Dr. Jack Kevorkian.

"Never before Côté has anyone documented in such depth and detail the fight for the right to die with dignity in Canada and the men and women who have made it possible." — Ruth von Fuchs, president the Right to Die Society of Canada.

Foreword

A book such as this one has not been published before because the euthanasia movement has exploded worldwide since 1990. Death-with-dignity laws have been passed in Australia, the Netherlands, Belgium, Luxembourg, and the U.S. states of Oregon and Washington. Assisted suicide has been legalized in Switzerland and decriminalized in Colombia and the state of Montana. But who are the dedicated individuals behind the new and forceful campaigns for choices in dying?

Whilst I did not start the right-to-die movement, which began in a small way in the 1930s, I am credited with kick-starting the modern version in America in the 1980s with the controversial Hemlock Society with its innovative how-to books and unusual legislative campaigns.

The progress of choice in dying in the last twenty years has been phenomenal and continues to accelerate, thanks to the many fine people who stepped forward to give their talents and labor to this noble cause. This book records their struggles against antiquated laws, bigotry, medical pedantry, political nervousness, and—most of all—unrelenting religious opposition. There were many casualties along the way as some found that they could not bear the strain of fierce controversy, media attacks, and public vilification, which this hot-button subject attracts.

Many people joined this campaign because of a harrowing personal experience in the death of a loved one or close friend. But others joined because their philosophy of life and ethics demanded that there be freedom of choice both in a woman's right to an abortion and chosen dying.

My first wife, Jean, witnessed her mother die of lung cancer in appalling pain and distress because nobody had prepared, medically and psychologically, for the end. Jean came away traumatized. Thus, when she was herself dying from breast cancer, she planned nearly a year ahead for an accelerated death on her own terms. And implemented it. My subsequent memoir, *Jean's Way*, over the next thirty-odd years slowly helped point the way to a more compassionate understanding of the feelings and rights of the dying.

Jean's plan to ask me for assistance, a doctor to provide lethal drugs, and then to wait until the end is near, is in fact the practical basis of the Oregon and Washington physician-assisted suicide laws, the first in North America. More campaigns are underway.

From the start, back in the 1980s, those of us who were pushing for the right to die in a manner and at a time of our own choosing knew that we needed support from the medical profession. After all, doctors alone have legal access to serious drugs as well as being experienced judges of the dying process. For a long time, we reached out for such backing; yet it was slow in coming. When medical support did come it was mostly from retired physicians. Still, as significant public support became apparent, courageous doctors like Timothy Quill, Richard MacDonald, Elizabeth "Libby" Wilson, Philip Nitschke, and Michael Irwin no longer confined their work to the bedside. Instead, they jumped into the public arena, regardless of the flak.

Dr. Jack Kevorkian I regard as a special case. Gutsy and flamboyant, he helped to die some 130 people who requested his assistance. The news media adored him. His one-man crusade aimed to shame the medical profession into being more merciful with dying patients. Unfortunately, it did not work. Too many doctors were upset at the speed at which he helped people, leaving no time for careful assessment of their needs.

Undoubtedly the most famous name in euthanasia, he pooh-poohed all legislative changes being worked on by others. It's the other people in this book who did—and are doing—the spade work on actual law reform.

Reading between the lines of the following portraits, one can perceive the makeup of these pioneers: compassionate, sensitive, strong-willed, and convinced that the world cannot be changed for the better without positive actions by themselves and as part of a team. They stepped forward. They are not without flaws and have sometimes made mistakes. They are the cream of the crop, well deserving of the recognition that this book at last brings to them.

The right-to-die movement has a long way to go before choice in dying is an option for all. From my position as a universal communicator on the subject, it is apparent that the movement was never stronger in membership, finances, and talent to continue the mission that those in this book started.

Derek Humphry
Eugene, Oregon
September 11, 2011

Preface

L ife has an expiration date. That we cannot change. Longevity, on the other hand, increases each year. Since the 1960s, medical science and technology have made astounding progress in curing diseases and extending the time we have to live. Unfortunately, the same technology has also prolonged the time it takes us to die—and agonizing pain and loss of autonomy often come with protracted, lingering death. The goal of the modern death-with-dignity movement is to create a peaceful path to the inevitable.

Establishing the right to die with dignity is the most recent battle in the long history of the struggle for civil rights and personal autonomy. Victories in the fight for colonial independence, the abolition of slavery and child labor, women's rights, racial desegregation, and anti-discrimination laws were all hard-fought against bitter, entrenched opposition. So it is for the fight for the right to die with dignity today.

The baby boom that followed World War II (1946-1964) produced a large and generally affluent generation of people. As demand for consumer goods rose, money flowed and jobs flourished. Boomers grew up accustomed to previously unknown levels of prosperity, individual choice, and self-direction. As they now start reaching retirement age, their choices may be more limited because of significant unemployment and the financial losses of the last decade. To make matters worse, their age makes them increasingly heavy users of healthcare services in an economy where healthcare costs continue to skyrocket and government funding dwindles. Yet they demand quality care despite the price tag.

As the cost of healthcare has risen, both public and private healthcare providers have been forced to decide what maladies would or would not be covered, for how long, and which treatments and drugs they would and would not pay for. The boomers' lack of planning for post-retirement medical care will place an undue economic burden on the children and grandchildren. The signs of that are already apparent.

In the generation before World War II, most people died at home in their own beds. Today, the majority die in expensive hospital rooms, where the out-of-pocket cost for a ten-day stay in an intensive care unit can easily exceed that of a new luxury car. Born in 1945, I am among the first in my boomer generation to face these issues. To me and the other members of my generation, they are very, very scary.

As one response to this fear, an international army of right-to-die activists has arisen to give people a direct choice of how, when, where, and under what circumstances they want to die. Their work has enabled the dying—and those with incurable, intolerable non-lethal suffering—to end their lives painlessly and peacefully when and where they choose, surrounded by loved ones. For many, this is a welcome contrast to enduring a lingering, painful, and expensive death in a hospital, connected to often-futile life-support machines after days, weeks, or months of being probed and prodded by strangers.

As with most members of my generation, I never thought of death as including any choices. It was something that just happened, whether you were ready for it or not. I first heard the term *euthanasia* (Greek for "good death") in 1996, when our vet told us that our beloved fourteen-year-old Siamese cat "Gato" had terminal feline leukemia. The veterinarian explained that "putting him to sleep" was the only humane thing to do when he could no longer prevail over the disease. Gradually, Gato lost his appetite and energy and began to rapidly fade away, losing strength and mobility by the day. Yet he always managed to purr at our every touch. I was in Dubai, United Arab Emirates, working on a book when my wife called me with the vet's confirmation that Gato's death was imminent. We agreed that the doctor should give him the recommended injection of Nembutal, a powerful barbiturate, to end his life. Within seconds, Gato died peacefully and painlessly in my wife's arms.

At the time, I knew as much about death and dying as the average American, which is to say, virtually nothing. My father died from leukemia, quickly and without great pain. My mother endured a slow, agonizing decline from amyotrophic lateral sclerosis (ALS), often called Lou Gehrig's disease in the United States and motor neurone disease abroad. But I had little first-hand knowledge of either death. My father slipped away so quickly and unexpectedly that I was not able to reach him until hours after he died.

As my mother's health deteriorated, she denied her diagnosis. It was "just a little stroke, that's all," she said. There was not a lot I could do to help because she was adamant about living in complete independence. Too soon, however, she could no longer manage unassisted, and my loving sister, Meredith, and an Indianapolis hospice saw her through her final year.

It took a chilling email on February 20, 2007, from The Reverend George Exoo, a Unitarian-Universalist minister, to introduce me to the world of planned, hastened death. A close personal friend (and my former pastor) with whom I had been out of touch for a decade, Exoo astounded me with the news that he might be arrested and extradited to Ireland for giving end-of-life information, directions, spiritual comfort, and a bedside presence to an Irishwoman as she gently ended her life in 2002.

During the phone call that followed his email, my perception of death began to change as Exoo explained his commitment to helping people die on their own terms and timetables. He introduced me to the concept of rational elective death. I learned that sometimes death was sought after, even welcomed, rather than being feared, avoided at any cost, or hidden.

Over the course of several months in 2007, I became intimately involved in Exoo's life, offering personal and professional support as he endured imprisonment in West Virginia, awaiting a verdict on his possible extradition. The day he was arrested, I volunteered to be his international media representative, fielding requests for information and refuting deliberately false and inflammatory statements about him, chiefly from the Irish and British media. The daily flood of phone calls and emails from Exoo's colleagues and supporters quickly connected me with a virtual *Who's Who* of the international death-with-dignity movement.

Until that point, I had been working for two decades as a writer, researching and writing well-received books in the fields of social history, biography, sexual abuse, terrorism, and espionage and creating an occasional novel. Just prior to Exoo's alarming email, I had been enthusiastically writing a long-planned historical novel set in a South Carolina cotton mill village during the Great Depression.

By November 2007, when the Irish extradition case was resolved in Exoo's favor, and having survived the personal media tornado created by his case, I was faced with a quandary. Should I finish the novel I had greatly enjoyed working on or temporarily shelve it to take on a new book?

Having been exposed by necessity to the right-to-die universe of euthanasia and assisted suicide, I inadvertently found myself in the perfect place at the perfect time. I had already met and interviewed many of the influential people who founded, led, and opposed the death-with-dignity movement.

Thanks to Exoo's detailed descriptions of his pioneering contributions to most of the currently used practices for achieving a peaceful death, I had gained unparalleled access to unique information and insights. Sharing this knowledge greatly appealed to the social historian in me, and writing about an underground subculture gave things a provocative twist. This was a story about an international group of individuals who were willing to sacrifice their careers and even face imprisonment in order to save their fellow men and women from needless and avoidable end-of-life torture. I could not let that story go untold.

I took the plunge, shelved the novel, and jumped into what would be a five-year, full-time research and writing odyssey, setting out to write a contemporary history of the international right-to-die movement, as seen chiefly through the eyes of its founders, pioneers, and leaders worldwide. This book presents their perspectives on death with dignity, with occasional insights and opinions of my own.

In countries where freedom of thought and choice are not forbidden by political or religious tyranny, the public demand for freedom of choice at the end of life has grown progressively stronger since the 1960s. It was in that era of fervent social change that people first started to ask, "Do we own our bodies or does the state or church?" If *we* do, we have the right to choose our own time and manner of death. But if the state or church does, then we are just pieces of government or religious property.

This book takes you deep into the lives of the leaders of the modern international death-with-dignity movement. It describes why they took up the cause and what they endured in the fight to allow this expression of free will. It also explores the convictions of those who oppose legalized euthanasia and self-deliverance for personal, professional, medical, political, or religious reasons.

It is my hope that this book will give you a new, more broadly informed, perspective on end-of-life care and the achievable option of a peaceful elective death.

Mt. Pleasant, South Carolina
April 15, 2012

– 1 –

The Parallel Universe

Mirrors are the doors through which death comes and goes.
— Heurtebise, in Jean Cocteau's *Orphée*

The email I received on February 20, 2007, left me speechless. "There is a good possibility that I will not be alive, c. Good Friday, via self-deliverance," it said. "Having lived a colorful life, which at times has reached the international news, I would like to tender you my personal and professional papers…. Are you interested?"

Shocked, I stared at the screen, uncomprehending, then reached for my phone. The message was from my close friend, George Exoo, a thoughtful man and an inspiring minister who cherished life more than anyone I knew. Self-deliverance? Suicide?

He answered on the second ring.

"George? What the hell—?" I heard a long sigh and then a once-hearty voice that was almost a whisper.

"It's time, Dick. All I want to know is if you'd like my papers." He sounded businesslike, his voice subdued, measured.

"Sure, but…." His papers would document the life of a vigorous social activist and advocate for the disenfranchised. He was Mother Teresa on steroids. His every brain cell was single-mindedly focused on helping others, with little regard for the often-damaging effects on his own life. Now he needed help.

"When can you come?"

After hopscotching around the eastern states, Exoo now lived in Beckley, West Virginia. I lived in South Carolina, more than four hundred miles away. Given the gravity of the request, I felt compelled to go.

A few weeks after the phone call, after rearranging a series of

1

book signings and speaking engagements, I started the long drive toward Exoo's home, hoping to find a tempest in a teapot. My Honda van, stripped of its back seats, was filled with dozens of document storage boxes, file folders, and a small arsenal of video and audio recording equipment. As I started climbing into the beautiful Blue Ridge Mountains, I recalled my long friendship with Exoo.

He had become an important part of my life when I met him in 1983 in Charleston, South Carolina. I had moved South to make a fresh start after a gut-wrenching divorce. He had arrived in 1977 to become the new minister of Charleston's Unitarian Church, the oldest of its denomination in the South.

At first, Exoo's education—magna cum laude diploma from Emerson College, bachelor's degree in sacred theology from Harvard Divinity School, and doctoral studies at the Graduate Theological Union at the University of California, Berkeley—was intimidating. My mother, for many years a secretary at Yale, hoped I would be accepted there, but the Yale admissions office diplomatically guided me elsewhere. Exoo's easygoing personality quickly put my intellectual inferiority complex to rest.

A man with boundless energy, he enjoyed letting his mind rove as much as I did. We were both transplanted Northerners. We both had unusual surnames. His was Dutch and mine French-Canadian. Few Americans pronounced or spelled either one correctly: his is EX-oh; mine ko-TAY. We quickly became close friends, sharing a bottle of pale-gold Bernkasteler Doktor *Spätlese* when we could, thinking great thoughts and concocting ways to save the world from itself.

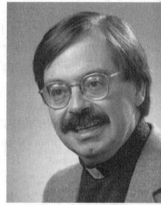

Rev. George Exoo

He was the first religious professional to show me that there was no inherent conflict between spirituality, free inquiry, and independent thinking. The spiritual and intellectual stew that he served up from the pulpit on Sunday mornings was the meal I had been craving for two decades. I soon joined his congregation.

In the ultraconservative, three-hundred-year-old Southern port city of Charleston, Exoo was a thoroughly radical figure. In addition to presiding over his diverse congregation of believers, agnostics, and atheists, he networked with neo-pagans, members of the Rev. Sun Myung Moon's Unification Church, spiritualists, and metaphysical New Agers. He championed the rights of the gay and lesbian community and stood up for people who were physically and mentally challenged. In the 1980s, his chief social mission was fighting the spread of AIDS.

When minority religious groups were discriminated against in the city, Exoo was usually the first (and often, the only one) to publicly defend them. He organized the first ongoing pulpit exchange between a black (Old Bethel United Methodist Church) and a white church (his) in South Carolina's history. He also established close ties with Kahal Kadosh Beth Elohim, America's oldest Reform Jewish synagogue. In addition, he served as a volunteer police chaplain and helped organize the Lowcountry Food Bank, which provides free food to the needy. A complex and both socially and theologically liberal man, his first seven years in conservative Charleston were often rocky.

Despite the liberal orientation of Unitarians, many of Exoo's views were unpopular in his congregation. As brilliant, progressive, and noble-minded as he was, Exoo proved to be far more effective as a social activist than as a parish minister. Sometimes he seemed aloof and oblivious to the needs of his church and its members. By the eighth year of his ministry in Charleston, his congregation had become polarized into pro- and anti-Exoo factions. In 1987, rather than see the congregation split, he resigned, delivering a gracious message of love and healing from the pulpit.

After he left South Carolina, he called me from time to time. For two years, he lived in the Hare Krishna community of New Vrindaban, near Moundsville, West Virginia. There, he had been promised a building to house his planned AIDS hospice. It was also there that he met the man who would become his life partner: Thomas McGurrin, a former Roman Catholic turned Krishna monk. Exoo and McGurrin were married in upstate New York in 2011, when that state passed its law legalizing same-sex marriage.

Quickly becoming disenchanted with New Vrindaban's self-aggrandizing and thoroughly unholy guru, Swami Bhaktipada (aka Keith Ham), Exoo and McGurrin denounced him and exposed his pervasive corruption and personal perversions. After their lives were threatened, he and McGurrin left the community for Pennsylvania.

In Pittsburgh, with the help of Tom Ammons, a producer for public radio, Exoo found a way to combine his extensive intellectual, theological, and musicological skills. In the early 1990s, he became a "church connoisseur," making unannounced visits to dozens of churches and synagogues in the greater Pittsburgh area, as well as in Milwaukee and Houston. Quickly dubbed "The Church Man," he rated congregations on the architecture of their buildings, the content of their ministers' sermons, the quality of their music, the extent of their social outreach, and their hospitality to strangers. His perceptive, often funny—and sometimes highly provocative—reviews aired on WQED-FM, one of National Public Radio's flagship stations, and were widely published.

The broadcasts brought Exoo national and international attention and an occasional scathing letter from ministers whose churches he had panned. He appeared on *Good Morning America* and on a BBC program and was profiled in *The Wall Street Journal* and *The New York Times*. In 1995, he earned a Gabriel Award from the National Association of Catholic Broadcasters and an alumni achievement award from Emerson College.

After several years of fulfilling but financially unrewarding work in Pittsburgh, Exoo and McGurrin moved to rural Beckley, West Virginia, where Exoo became the minister of the tiny New River Unitarian Universalist Fellowship. There he unsuccessfully attempted to supplement his meager salary with real estate sales.

Exoo's interest in euthanasia—literally, "good death"—surfaced shortly after he took the pulpit in Charleston. A life-long animal lover, he helped to found Spay Not Slay, an animal rights activist group.

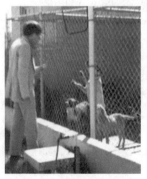

He successfully forced Charleston's animal shelter to abandon its barbaric method of killing unwanted pets: placing them inside a fifty-five gallon drum and gassing them with the hot exhaust fumes from a 1948 Dodge sedan. Painful death also haunted him because of his AIDS work. Although numerous terminally ill patients begged to die, many were too feeble to end their lives unaided. To help end their torment, they turned to fellow AIDS sufferers, pooling their supplies of prescription drugs and overdosing. However, at that time, primitive levels of knowledge about

Exoo at the Charleston animal shelter

how to die quickly and painlessly meant that many of those assisted suicides were botched, with horrible consequences.

Exoo had become a life member of the Hemlock Society USA in the early 1980s, shortly after the group's formation. Hemlock advocated the right to die when, where, and by whatever method a terminally or hopelessly ill person chose. *Final Exit*, written in 1991 by Hemlock's founder, Derek Humphry, taught Exoo that there were ways to ensure a painless, swift, and certain death for rational people who craved it. While living in Pittsburgh, Exoo decided to combine his passion for righting social wrongs with his humane attitude toward elective death. A decade before the Hemlock Society's Caring Friends Program was founded in 1998, Exoo became one of the nation's first "exit guides."

These guides counsel those who want to end their lives in a humane and dignified way and on their own schedules. Like Exoo, many of the early guides fell into their new calling before any established death-with-dignity organizations had developed training procedures. Therefore, guides had to train themselves and work independently. They had to decide, on a case-by-case basis, whether the suicidal person was acting impulsively and irrationally (for example, a depressed teenager who lost his girlfriend or a worker whose job was outsourced abroad) or rationally (or example, someone suffering from chronic or terminal pain or who had made a reasoned choice to die on his or her own terms and timetable).

Guides, who generally work *pro bono* or for out-of-pocket expenses only, deliberately keep a low profile and fly under the radar. As a result, they generally accept only clients whom they have questioned at length about their motives, who seem rational, have untreatable physical or existential pain, are close to death, or have other good reasons to end their lives. For these people, exit guides are generally willing, if requested, to provide specific information about how to achieve a dignified, painless death that does not result in a gruesome scene for those left behind.

Exoo's first experience with suicide came in 1987. While still in Charleston, he spent months trying to help a severely depressed member of his congregation whose financial assets had been wiped out. When his total net worth dropped to less than three hundred dollars, Exoo's congregant killed himself by sitting in his car with the engine running and the exhaust gases piped in through the car window. Exoo, who knew nothing about the man's plans, was indelibly marked by his inability to prevent the tragedy.

In Pittsburgh, seven years later, Exoo witnessed his first rational suicide. In 1994, sixty-eight-year-old George Koss, a fit, healthy, and vigorous man, began to feel weak. He fell while dancing with his wife, Josephine, and his voice, which rang out in the church choir every Sunday, turned into a squawk. His neurologist's diagnosis was unequivocal: Koss had amyotrophic lateral sclerosis (ALS), commonly known in the United States as Lou Gehrig's disease and abroad as motor neurone disease.

As the disease progressed, Koss would lose control of his muscles and would be unable to speak, swallow, breathe, or control any major bodily functions. Ultimately, he would become completely paralyzed and would likely die when his lungs could no longer deliver air. All of this would happen while he was still mentally alert and acutely conscious of his deteriorating condition. The disease, which destroys the body but not the mind, is one of the cruelest ways to die. I know this because my mother died of ALS.

When he began to fall often and had to ask his wife to help him perform his most basic bodily functions, George Koss could no longer bear to keep on living. He tried to asphyxiate himself with the exhaust gases from his car, but his wife intervened. After Koss convinced Josephine that his life had become too agonizing to continue, the question became when and how he should die. From Derek Humphry's 1991 book, *Final Exit*, the couple learned which medications could work, but, afraid of failure, Josephine Koss called the Pittsburgh chapter of the Hemlock Society. She was given the name of George Exoo, who served as chaplain of the group at the time.

At the Kosses' request, Exoo visited them. The couple's fears poured out. George Koss was terrified that the self-deliverance attempt would fail, leaving him even more debilitated. Exoo calmly agreed to be with him when he was ready to die.[1]

The call came several weeks later. On May 22, 1995, with Exoo present, George Koss mixed handfuls of crushed sleeping pills into a bowl of ice cream to mask their bitter taste and quickly downed the mixture. He knew that alcohol would speed up the action of the drugs, so Koss, his wife, and Exoo shared a pitcher of vodka and orange juice. Koss quickly became a very happy drunk. Soon all three people howled with laughter as he told tales of his life.[2] A short while later, Koss lay down on his bed. Unable to watch her husband die, Josephine Koss left the room. Then disaster struck.

Koss had miscalculated the amount of drugs it would take to kill him and did not quickly slip away. Aware of the dilemma, he did something completely unexpected. He pulled a plastic bag over his head. Exoo was aghast. He watched as Koss desperately fought for oxygen. Koss inhaled so hard that the plastic bag went up his nostrils. Three times the instinctive will to live took over with such force that Koss reached up to rip off the bag. And three times Koss forced his own shaking hands down. In the living room, his wife waited fearfully for the end.[3] When she heard Exoo's soothing voice reciting the Lord's Prayer, she knew that her husband had finally found peace.

George Koss' self-deliverance, and the drastic method he had to use when the pills failed him, was a turning point for Josephine Koss and George Exoo. In 1997, two years after her husband's death, they helped found Hemlock of Western Pennsylvania and West Virginia, an independent chapter of the Hemlock Society. On the same day, they founded The Compassionate Chaplaincy Foundation, Ltd., and registered it in the State of West Virginia.[4] Its stated purpose was "education, counseling, guidance and preparation (spiritual and non) for the hopelessly and terminally ill who wish to self-deliver."

Between 1997 and January 2000, Exoo and Koss served as exit guides, counseling people on how to achieve a dignified elective death and comforting them as they ended their lives. They discovered an enormous unmet need for accurate information and counseling services for suicidal people and decided to find ways to make people aware of their work. Ultimately, Koss moved on to other caregiving projects, leaving Exoo to forge ahead alone.

In 2001, he ran a small ad in four issues of *The New Yorker*, an expensive and risky choice for his foundation's underfunded euthanasia counseling service. It read, "Hopelessly or terminally ill? Want to stay in control as your life ends? If so, call the Compassionate Chaplaincy, The Reverend George Exoo at…." Between the advertisement and discreet referrals from the Hemlock Society, Exoo soon had all the requests he could handle.

By the time we talked in February 2007, Exoo had become one of the world's most experienced authorities on self-deliverance and had provided a pastoral presence or facilitated more than one hundred deathings in eight countries.[5] The term "deathing" was coined in 1984 by author Anya Foos-Graber, who used it to describe the ending-of-life process, the complement to birthing.[6]

The urgency in Exoo's voice on the phone had unnerved me. As I approached Beckley, I felt like Alice in Wonderland, falling down a magical rabbit hole leading to a parallel universe; one that revolved around peaceful elective death, not life. I found the former coal-mining town, home to about 17,000 souls, a drab, economically depressed place, doing the best it could with the little it had to work with. As my van pulled into the driveway of Exoo and McGurrin's weather-beaten wooden house, I was greeted by Winky, Exoo's excited cockapoo. Exoo quickly followed behind, and we exchanged hearty hugs.

Other than adding a few pounds (as had I), Exoo looked remarkably like the man I had known so well in Charleston. His five-foot-ten-inch frame was topped with straight, brown hair, which had thinned some and picked up a little gray. His dark-brown, Teddy Roosevelt mustache was also graying. At sixty-six, he still looked like the scholar he was. Behind his round, gold-rimmed, bifocal glasses, his blue eyes shone with welcome. His pace was brisk, and he wore his traditional fashion statement, a blue Harvard blazer with a striped tie and tan slacks.

Exoo then introduced me to his partner. Of medium height, with spectacles perched on the end of his nose; a jolly, ruddy face; a balding head; and an ample waistline, Thomas McGurrin looked like a combination of Friar Tuck, a laughing Buddha, and an introspective theologian, all of which mirrored his real life. All four walls of his small study were lined floor to ceiling with books on Eastern religions. Niches were reserved for intricate Buddhist mandalas, brass Vedic statues, and small, delicate prayer bells. It was not the room one might expect for an apostate Roman Catholic turned Hare Krishna monk turned Buddhist turned atheist. If Exoo's theology could be described as pluralistic and his personality effervescent, McGurrin's spiritual path was

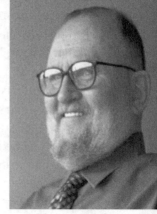

Thomas McGurrin

evolutional and his presence low-key and gently jovial.

With fond memories of the custom-designed, passive solar house in Charleston that Exoo had commissioned, built, and lost through foreclosure, I was shocked at his Beckley residence. A dilapidated 1930s Sears Roebuck kit house with peeling paint, it sat forlornly between a run-down auto body shop and the modest meeting hall of an apostolic Christian church. Like its neighbors, the house had settled into sedate decrepitude many years earlier. Its greatest asset was the free rent, thanks to an agreement Exoo had negotiated with his Beckley congregation. Because of his idealistic career choices and his inability to refuse anyone looking for a handout, Exoo was broke, and the house's appearance reflected it.

Sharing a bottle of New Zealand Chardonnay I had brought, we sat in his living room while the tape recorder rolled, and I listened to the story that had driven him to send his despondent email message and would ultimately make him the center of an international right-to-die controversy.

Exoo's euthanasia exit guide work came back to bite him hard in 2002 in the form of Irishwoman Rosemary Toole. Her attempts to end her life had started long before she met him. By 2001, she had decided with absolute certainty that she wanted to die. She had already attempted to kill herself once with an overdose of drugs but failed when someone found her. Instead of achieving the death she so desperately sought, she was locked up in a mental institution for six months.[7] The Dublin native did not want to try killing herself alone again for fear of failing, so she set out to learn how to take her life with the greatest efficiency and least pain. The latter was especially important because Toole had been in physical and emotional torment for as long as she could remember.

Early in her life, two tragedies lit a long-smoldering fuse that would eventually ignite deep-seated emotional problems, later complicated by medical ailments. When she was three years old, her father became mentally ill. He spent the remaining forty-eight years of his life in a psychiatric ward, and Toole's only contact with him was a single visit to the hospital. He did not recognize her. Shortly after her father was hospitalized, her mother also disappeared from her life, moving to England and later to Canada.

Fortunately, Rosemary was adopted by Owen Toole, a loving and generous stockbroker and former bank director, and his wife.

Despite the loss of both natural parents, Toole had what her adoptive father described as a carefree childhood and seemingly enjoyed life. She married in her twenties, but the relationship only survived for six months. Then she had a nervous breakdown in her mid-30s.[8] Toole was further disappointed when she made contact with her biological mother, who refused to meet her. Psychological problems went on to plague her second marriage, which also failed.

After working as bank teller for several years, Toole was forced to resign and was put on a disability pension because of prolonged acute depression. The depression was aggravated by Cushing's Syndrome, a rare, nonlethal brain malfunction caused by an overproduction of cortisol. The symptoms typically include fatigue, weakness, depression, mood swings, and panic attacks. Toole also suffered from severe heart problems and had a pacemaker.[9]

She became fixated on accelerating her death. To plan it, she contacted the Hemlock Society, then America's largest and best-known right-to-die organization.[10] However, Hemlock's Caring Friends Program offered self-deliverance information and counseling only for Hemlock Society members who were in extreme, untreatable pain or were terminally ill. Because they did not serve non-members or those suffering from depression, Hemlock declined to work with Toole.

After months of phone calls and internet searches, Toole found the basic answers to most of her questions in Humphry's book, *Final Exit*. Although she was confident that the helium gas inhalation method described in the book would work, she wanted an experienced exit counselor at her side for reassurance and support. Her research turned up the names of Evelyn Marie Martens, a thoughtful, patient Canadian grandmother who worked as a volunteer and exit guide for the Right to Die Society of Canada, and Dr. Libby Wilson, a retired general practitioner and founder of Friends at the End, a Scottish right-to-die activist group. She contacted both of them, seeking their active assistance in ending her life.

In November 2001, Wilson received an email from an Irishwoman who identified herself only as "Rosemary." She asked if Wilson could help her die. Believing that Toole was merely depressed, Wilson tried to dissuade her from killing herself. When it became clear that Wilson was not going to help her die, Toole turned to Martens. During an extended series of phone calls and emails, Martens also tried to discourage Toole from ending her life, telling her that she should seek further professional help for her depression. Toole remained convinced that her misery could only be ended by taking her own life. She asked Martens for a referral to an experienced exit guide.

Martens knew that George Exoo, who had a cordial professional relationship with the Right to Die Society of Canada, was willing to take risks that virtually everyone else would walk away from. Indeed, he was probably Rosemary Toole's only hope for a swift, painless, and certain death in the company of a sympathetic person. Martens put the Irishwoman in touch with his Compassionate Chaplaincy Foundation.[11]

Toole and Exoo began to communicate in late 2001. Through telephone calls and numerous Compassionate Chaplaincy Foundation emails, Exoo became convinced of the sincerity of Toole's wish to die, and Toole quickly came to believe that Exoo was the answer to her prayers.[12] For him, Toole's unending agony, extensive research on self-deliverance methods, and unwavering decision to take her own life were sufficient reasons to get on a plane and help her achieve the peace she sought.

Before Toole first talked to him, Exoo and McGurrin had already planned a trip to Europe. Exoo wanted to visit Holland, his ancestral homeland, and McGurrin wanted to see if he could find living Irish relatives. After agreeing that Toole's exit plan was rational, the men decided to combine both missions into a single trip.

Much to his later chagrin, Exoo did not investigate Irish law on assisting a suicide before he left. In the United States, providing information about self-deliverance is protected by the Constitution as an exercise of free speech. It is not a violation of any federal law as long as the provider takes no direct physical part in the death. However in Ireland, there is no such legal protection. Section 2 (2) of Ireland's Criminal Law (Suicide) Act, 1993, states that "a person who aids, abets, counsels, or procures the suicide of another . . . shall be guilty of an offense and be liable on indictment or conviction to imprisonment for a term not exceeding fourteen years."

On January 21, 2002, Exoo and McGurrin boarded a British Airways flight for the seven-hour trip to London and their subsequent flight to Dublin.[13] Rosemary Toole wanted to enjoy every minute of her final three days. She took Exoo and McGurrin sightseeing, and the three shared meals in local restaurants, toured Irish

craft centers, and enjoyed Irish music and
dancing. Toole carried on animated, nonstop
conversations and seemed to blossom before
the eyes of her two companions.

Exoo and McGurrin were amazed that
this woman, who had chosen to die just a
few days later, was so exhilarated. In light of
the suffering she had endured for years, her
euphoria was understandable. Knowing that
release from pain was now both certain and
imminent, Toole was jubilant. Whether or

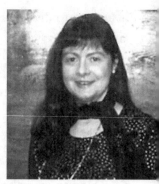

Rosemary Toole

not she was terminally ill later became a major controversy among
others, but it was irrelevant to her. She had exhausted all her medical and psychological counseling resources and was unwilling to live
through any more pain.

Friday, January 25, 2002, was Toole's planned exit day. That
morning, she and her two new friends met for breakfast at their
hotel. Then they packed their bags and drove to a townhouse Toole
had rented in a Dublin suburb for her final exit. She had left a suicide
note in her bedroom in the house in Dalkey that she shared with her
elderly adoptive father. He had approved of her plans, although he
would have preferred a more positive way to end her suffering.

It was late afternoon, and darkness was beginning to fall. Toole
changed into a gold lamé evening gown she had bought for the oc-
casion. The beauty she had not found in life would be hers in death.
When she was ready to proceed, Exoo carefully walked her through
a rehearsal of each step.

Only three things were needed for Toole's exit. The first was a
tank of helium, available from party supply stores as part of an inexpensive party balloon kit. Only one tank was necessary, but Toole
had purchased four, just to be certain. The odorless, inert gas would
pass through a plastic tube into a plastic "exit bag" specifically designed for the purpose by Canada's John Hofsess and manufactured
by his colleague, Evelyn Martens. The bag would fit loosely over
her head and be closed at the neck with a Velcro strap. Only one exit
bag was necessary, but Toole had purchased two. She did not want
a shortage of anything to jeopardize her plans. She also needed a
supply of powerful barbiturate sleeping pills.[14] She had a surplus of
these left over from earlier prescriptions.

About an hour before beginning her self-deliverance, Toole took an anti-emetic to prevent her from throwing up the overdose of barbiturates that would make her sleepy before she turned on the helium. Soon after washing down a large quantity of the ground-up pills with vodka to accelerate their effect, she began to get drowsy. Next, she picked up the exit bag, put it on her head, and pulled it down to her temples. Then she squeezed the air out of it and turned on the helium. As soon as the bag filled with the gas, she pulled it down and secured it around her neck with its Velcro strap. At that point, she was breathing pure helium.

McGurrin gently held her hand during the final minutes as Exoo read prayers. Deprived of oxygen by the helium, Toole quickly and painlessly fell unconscious from anoxia (oxygen deprivation, not suffocation). Her brain quickly died, having lost its oxygen supply. Within fifteen minutes, her tortured life had ended peacefully. The two counselors sat with her for about thirty minutes after her last breath to confirm that she was dead. Acting on Toole's prior request, they did not remove the plastic hood or the helium tanks because she wanted her death to be an obvious suicide. Then they drove to Dublin and checked into a hotel. The next morning, Exoo and McGurrin flew to Amsterdam to complete their European visit.

On the day after his daughter's death, Owen Toole dutifully opened the suicide note she had left for him and called the police. After breaking open the door and finding Toole's body, the authorities sealed off the townhouse as a possible crime scene. They dusted the apartment for fingerprints and quickly found those of Toole, Exoo, and McGurrin. Although there was no direct evidence linking Exoo and McGurrin to any active role in Toole's death, their fingerprints, which were soon verified by the FBI via Interpol, placed them at the scene and made them criminal suspects. In the eyes of the Irish police, the men were possible accessories to murder.[15]

When the authorities seized and searched the computer in Toole's bedroom at her father's house, they found numerous emails exchanged between herself and Exoo, and an extensive correspondence with right-to-die organizations worldwide. The messages she exchanged with Exoo left no doubt that he had been invited to be with her when she ended her life.

Irish law is clear about the prosecution of people who help someone commit suicide. Ireland's Director of Public Prosecutions (known as the DPP, the equivalent of the U.S. Attorney General) does not have any discretion over whether or not to investigate such cases. However, as a practical matter, prosecuting attorneys world-wide frequently consider a number of mitigating factors, including whether it is in the public interest to prosecute. Some aspects of the Toole case were problematic. Law or no law, if it was Toole's clearly expressed intention to commit suicide—which was not a violation of Irish law—should others be prosecuted for helping?

Had her self-deliverance been carried out in the company of close family members, the DPP might have let the case slip into obscurity. But those present were foreigners unrelated to the dece-dent. Furthermore, they were veteran professionals in their unique calling; men who had extensive experience with self-deliverance and whose expenses had been paid so that they could be present. As far as the DPP was concerned, there were no mitigating circumstances calling for leniency. Two foreign assisted-suicide activists had pub-licly thumbed their noses at the laws of the Irish Republic.

On the other hand, the circumstances of Toole's death would require an intense investigation because Exoo and McGurrin were not criminal hit men and might well be considered mercy killers by the Irish public, the majority of whom, by 2002, supported assisted suicide. As eager as the Irish police were to make an arrest and make an example of the two men, they were determined not to damage their case by being less than thorough.

More surprises surfaced when Toole's will was probated. When she directed the disposition of her personal property, valued at £627,113 GBP, she left 5 percent of it to Exoo's Compassionate Chaplaincy Foundation, 5 percent to Evelyn Martens and John Hof-sess of Last Rights Publications for the benefit of the Right to Die Society of Canada, and 1 percent to Derek Humphry's new group, the Euthanasia Research and Guidance Organization (ERGO). The rest was left to relatives.[16] Not only had Toole totally ignored the Irish assisted suicide law, she had rubbed salt in the prosecution's wounds by leaving unsolicited bequests of money to the very right-to-die organizations whose goals the law was designed to thwart.

The Irish High Court ultimately ruled that the bequests were not charitable donations under Irish law, and they were voided. But the DPP, incensed by Toole's postmortem defiance, declared war on the men who had helped her end her life.[17]

The "Rosemary Toole incident," as it came to be known, galvanized the Irish government into action and provided a nearly endless supply of lurid fodder for the tabloid press. Within days of the discovery of Toole's death, and based on information apparently leaked by the Irish police, the British and Irish news media unleashed a swarm of inflammatory reports, igniting for the first time a serious debate in Ireland over who had the right to die and whether anyone had the right to counsel or assist them in doing so.

Meanwhile, Exoo and McGurrin's return flight from Holland was long, and the men were tired when Exoo's old Mercedes rolled into the driveway of their home. Winky, Exoo's cockapoo, was thrilled to see them. As Exoo opened the gate on the chain-link fence, Winky leaped into his arms, licked his face, and peed on his jacket from sheer excitement. Then Exoo noticed a stranger standing nearby.

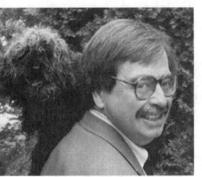

Exoo and Winky

"My name is Declan White," the man said. "I'm a reporter for *Ireland on Sunday*, a Dublin newspaper. May I ask you about your trip to Dublin and Rosemary Toole? You have changed the consciousness of Ireland."[18]

White showed Exoo and McGurrin a copy of the *Dublin Evening Herald* for January 31, 2002, which had run the story of Toole's self-deliverance as front-page news. Believing that he and his partner had nothing to hide, Exoo invited White into their home. McGurrin made them tea.

White recorded extensive interviews with the two exit guides during the next two days. He was soon joined by Dan Callister, a photographer working for the Splash News Agency of New York. My friend, the loquacious, naïve Unitarian minister, would quickly discover the difference between a well-researched feature story written to inform and educate by professionally trained, disciplined journalists and lurid tabloid pieces, written for their shock value by media hacks.

White's first story, emailed to his newspaper on the night of the first interview, filled the entire front page of *Ireland on Sunday*. Under the enormous headline, "The Angels of Death," it showed smiling head shots of the two exit counselors, standing in front of an oil portrait of Exoo in his Harvard Divinity School robes.

The first sentence set the tone of the article: "Pair who helped Irish woman kill herself assisted in 100 suicides." The photo's caption read, "These are the two self-confessed 'suicide assistants' who helped an Irish woman kill herself in a meticulously planned and clinically executed operation."[19] White and Callister would later give all their taped interviews, notes, and photos of Exoo and his house to the Irish police.

In the following days, Exoo, McGurrin, and even unsuspecting members of the New River Unitarian Universalist Fellowship where Exoo preached, were besieged by local, national, and foreign reporters looking for headlines. Within days, the story of Exoo and Toole had been broadcast and published throughout the world. Exoo's telephone rang unceasingly, until he let the answering machine take all the messages. In the interviews he did grant, Exoo remained implacable, not moving an inch from his position that helping Toole end her life was a humane and moral thing to do and that criminalization of the act was ludicrous.

When news of the alleged assisted suicide was first released by the Irish police, rumors spread in Ireland and England like a swarm of bats leaving a cave at night. Within days, Exoo was labeled "Reverend Death" and "another Jack Kevorkian" by a growing number of detractors. Wild tales emerged that Toole had paid the two men exorbitant sums to help her die, and they had spent the money on lavish jaunts around Europe. In fact, Exoo and McGurrin were paid $2,500, and that was simply reimbursement for the cost of their air travel, hotel rooms in Ireland, and the rental car they used for the days they spent with Toole. They were paid nothing for serving as her exit counselors or for their subsequent personal travel in Europe.

It soon became evident that the Irish media had already tried and convicted the two Americans, picked out the tree in Dublin from which they should be hanged, and were waiting for the opportunity to broadcast the execution on live television. Well before any official police information had been released, *Ireland on Sunday* was already portraying Exoo and McGurrin as imported murderers-for-hire.

After a period of fear that federal authorities, acting on behalf of the Irish government, might suddenly invade their home and arrest them, Exoo and McGurrin gradually started to relax when nothing happened. They did not know that the Irish police were still carrying out their investigation, building their case detail by detail, determined to pursue the apparent crime for as long as it took.

In October 2002, Ireland sent two veteran investigators, Detective Superintendent P. J. Brown and Detective Sergeant J. J. Kean, to West Virginia. On October 16, under a subpoena from the U.S. Department of State on behalf of the Republic of Ireland, Exoo and McGurrin appeared at the U.S. Attorney's office in Beckley's federal courthouse to make a deposition in response to questions from the Irish authorities.

Detectives Kean and Brown, accompanied by FBI Special Agent Michael A. Yansick, were present as an assistant U.S. Attorney, speaking on behalf of the Irish government, questioned Exoo and his partner. The Irish detectives could not interrogate the two directly because they had no legal jurisdiction in the United States. When asked about the events surrounding Toole's death, Exoo and McGurrin, on the advice of their attorney, invoked the Fifth Amendment of the Constitution, which gave them the right to remain silent. The interrogation was over in five minutes.[20] The detectives' trip from Ireland had produced nothing of value.

On December 18, 2002, the Dublin Coroner's Court found probable cause that the two Americans had violated Ireland's assisted-suicide law, and the DPP initiated extradition proceedings. He issued two warrants for Exoo's arrest: one for aiding and abetting the suicide of another and one for counseling the suicide of another. McGurrin, who had not given any incriminating interviews and did not have Exoo's high media profile, was not charged. Exoo was not notified about the formal charges filed against him, but his intuition left him fearful of what might lie ahead.

His close friend, Evelyn Martens, who produced the exit bag for helium for John Hofsess' Last Rights Publications in Canada, had been charged in 2002 with assisting the suicides of two women there. Believing that she was as fearful of the legal outcome of her trial in Canada as he would be if the Irish sought his extradition, Exoo invited Martens to join him in a double final exit in 2003. "He suggested that, if I wanted to, we could make the final leap together," she told me.[21] Although he did not know it at that time, his fears of extradition were well grounded.

In 2004, the Republic of Ireland forwarded a lengthy legal file to the U.S. Department of State, demanding Exoo's extradition to face trial in Dublin. In addition, Ireland requested "the seizure of all items by the police authorities of the United States of America which may be used as evidence for the purpose of prosecution of the aforementioned offences."

And then nothing happened.

The State Department was still dealing with the aftermath of the September 11, 2001, terrorist attack. Its staff was stretched paper-thin by the war on terrorism and the massive U.S. military involvement in Iraq. When compared with stopping attacks by Al Qaeda and Iraqi insurgents, the Irish plea to have a Harvard-trained U.S. clergyman extradited on an assisted-suicide charge was a very low priority. Nevertheless, the Irish government periodically queried the Americans about the status of their case.

Unaware that he was a wanted man, Exoo returned to work, counseling and assisting people who wanted to end their lives. He nearly forgot about the Toole case. But the Irish never did.

Few officials in the American justice system were aware of the case. When Exoo heard about rumblings from Ireland in early 2007, he had his attorney call the U.S. Attorney's office in West Virginia and the Department of Justice in Washington. Their spokespeople said they knew nothing about the matter.[22]

When Exoo sent me his grim email on February 20, 2007, he had a strong premonition that the Irish authorities were about to make their move. He feared that federal agents were going to burst through the door at any minute to arrest him. If the extradition warrant was approved by a federal judge, Exoo would be flown to Dublin in handcuffs to face a jury. It would have been the first time in history that someone had been extradited for assisting a suicide, an international legal precedent that Exoo had no wish to set.

It took me five days to finish my interviews with Exoo and McGurrin in Beckley and to pack up twenty-three document storage boxes stuffed with the personal and professional papers that I had promised to sort and transfer to the Harvard Divinity School archives. In a state of intellectual overload, I returned home to start transcribing the dozens of interview tapes and preparing the huge manuscript collection for Harvard.

Neither Exoo nor I knew at that time how well the Irish police had done their homework. After considering the hundreds of pages of legal paperwork prepared by the Irish authorities, Assistant U.S. Attorney Philip H. Wright directed that a warrant be issued to arrest Exoo and hold him until a judge could determine whether or not Ireland's extradition request was valid. On June 22, 2007, the warrant was approved, and Exoo was officially a wanted man.

Following a brash statement in 2002 that he would face an Irish court proudly and without shame for his role in Rosemary Toole's death, Exoo had begun to consider the realities of a possible fourteen-year prison term. A sensitive, altruistic man without a combative bone in his body, he knew that fourteen years in an Irish prison could be a death sentence. Being gay made him an obvious target for harassment, and being convicted of assisting in the death of an Irishwoman would make things even worse. He thought he would be dead within his first month behind bars.

When his tension level began to rise, Exoo planned to end his life in early April by drinking liquid pentobarbital, sold under the trade name Nembutal. It was a powerful, fast-acting barbiturate used by veterinarians to euthanize domestic and farm animals and was also the most sought-after self-deliverance drug in the world. The finalization of this plan led to his email to me. By the time I drove to see him in March, the exact date of his planned death had become less of an issue. Instead, Exoo explained the emergency exit plan he had ready in case the police arrived.

"They'll be here for me, not for both of us," Exoo told me, "so only Thomas is answering the door now. If it's police with a warrant, he'll call for me and say the police want to talk with me." He then opened his refrigerator to show me a plastic water bottle filled with liquid Nembutal from Mexico, mixed with Limeade powder and sugar to help mask the notoriously bitter taste.

"Thomas' signal will be my sign to chug-a-lug the Nembutal and go greet the authorities. I'll have about two minutes to say hello and chat with them before I drop dead in mid-sentence." Exoo saw this plan as a logical solution to his problems. But when put to the test, it failed. On the morning of June 25, 2007, McGurrin was sick, so Exoo went to answer a knock on the door.

Before he could attempt to get to the Nembutal, two FBI agents had him handcuffed and in the back seat of an ominous, gray, unmarked police car. For reasons unknown, the agents never attempted

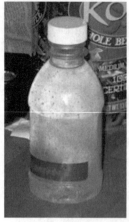

Exoo's emergency plan

to confiscate Exoo's computer or any of the documents the Irish had requested.

He was immediately driven to the U.S. Marshal's Service office in Bluefield, West Virginia. That afternoon, he appeared before U.S. Magistrate Judge R. Clarke VanDervort. Because he had no money to hire an attorney, Exoo was assigned to Edward H. Weis, a federal public defender. He was then turned back over to the federal marshals and driven to the West Virginia Southern Regional Jail.

It was Exoo's worst-case scenario come true. He was under arrest, pending the judge's ruling on his extradition, and no one could tell him how long he would be held. No bail was permitted under the terms of the extradition treaty, and there was no fixed date by which the judge had to make his decision. The legal case was mind-bendingly complicated.

Incarcerated, Exoo was miserable and frightened. His sexual orientation made him an especially vulnerable target, and he was tormented by prisoners and guards who viewed him as weak. He was threatened with murder, and nearly lost an eye after being pummeled with a barrage of paperback novels. Exoo's pleas to be placed in a protective custody cell were finally granted, and he was housed with two other at-risk inmates in a space barely big enough for two cots. He was allowed to leave his cell for one hour a day, during which he could shower, exercise, use the telephone, or visit the jail's law library. It was the closest thing to hell he had ever experienced.

Four days after his arrest, Exoo appeared at a detention hearing in Beckley. There, Judge VanDervort stated that he would remain in jail pending an August extradition hearing. Wearing torn orange jail clothes with shackles on his ankles, Exoo smiled gently and waved to his friends, including myself, who had turned out to show support.

At the hearing in August, the judge was expected to rule on whether or not Ireland had valid legal grounds to extradite him. Exoo, his hair neatly combed, wearing yet another ripped orange jumpsuit, was led into court in leg irons by two federal marshals. He seemed gratified by the presence of the friends and colleagues who filled the benches of the small courtroom. No representatives of the Irish government were present.

His dedicated and highly competent attorney, Edward Weis, turned out to be Exoo's greatest asset. Weis told the court that Exoo did not furnish any new information or any supplies to Ms. Toole, who had tried to commit suicide before and failed. She had contacted Exoo and paid his way to Dublin to have a compassionate person pray with her as she took her life. Since all actions taken by Toole were by her own hand, not his, Weis argued, Exoo had in no way assisted her self-deliverance.

Exoo had previously noted that hundreds of clergy have provided a compassionate spiritual presence and prayed with dying people who asked that their life support be discontinued. "If comforting and praying with a dying person is either a sin or a crime, then most of the ministers, priests, rabbis, and imams in America, Ireland, and the rest of the world must be sinners, criminals, or both," he said.[23]

The key issue facing the judge was whether there was a necessary "commonality of law" between Ireland's assisted suicide law and the assisted suicide laws of the United States. For extradition to take place, rigid legal criteria must be met. The alleged offense had to be a felony in both countries and had to carry a minimum prison sentence of at least one year.

Because there is no U.S. federal law against assisting a suicide, and no such law in West Virginia, Exoo's state of residence, Assistant U.S. Attorney Philip Wright, arguing for Ireland, maintained that the court had to determine whether a majority of states had such a law. If at least twenty-six states, a simple majority, had a law against assisting a suicide, Exoo could be extradited. If not, Ireland's petition would be denied, and he would be freed.

The case law evidence was so incredibly complicated that both the prosecuting and defense attorneys were ordered to prepare a detailed examination of each state's laws on assisted suicide to enable the judge to make his decision. Assembling this material and giving the judge enough time to complete his analysis proved to be a nerve-wracking, multi-month process. Because his decision would set an international precedent, Judge VanDervort paid extremely close attention to every detail of the case, while Exoo languished in jail, his fate unresolved.

For reasons he never understood, Exoo was shuttled back and forth between two different jails several times over a four-month period. Each time he was moved, he was stripped of his personal possessions and correspondence, even the legal correspondence with his attorney. Books ordered for him in compliance with West Virginia state prison rules were frequently returned to their senders. This left him with only the King James Bible and the right-wing, apocalyptic fundamentalist Christian books (chiefly the dismal *Left Behind* series of novels by Tim LaHaye and Jerry B. Jenkins) available in the jail library. Exoo's well-wishers frequently had their letters and books returned with a blunt "Not at this facility" stamp, as the West Virginia jail system made no attempt to forward inmate mail when they moved prisoners.

There were ten of us in Exoo's core support group. The most strident member was North Carolina resident Cassandra E. Mae, a controversial woman who had a house full of real and toy lizards. She had originally approached Exoo as a client. However, after his counseling, she decided that suicide was not the way to solve her problems. Instead, she became Exoo's volunteer understudy. When working as an exit guide, she sometimes used the alias "Susan Wilson." A dedicated idealist, Exoo had no idea what she would really do with her exit guide training, but he would soon find out.

Although she outwardly supported him and organized the first "Friends of George" mailing list after his arrest, Cassandra Mae quickly started to divert Exoo's clients to herself. As she proudly told Jon Ronson, a British film producer working on a documentary about Exoo, "He sees it as a calling. . . . With me it's a business. No cash, no help."[24] No other right-to-die group worldwide uses her cash-for-services model.

As the months went by, Exoo slipped deeper into depression. Convinced that his incarceration would never end, he began to plan his suicide inside the jail. He decided to starve himself to death but abandoned this idea when told that he would be force-fed through an intravenous drip. He then devised "Plan B": self-asphyxiation with a piece of plastic patched together from small bags and the adhesive tabs from Band-aids. It was a desperate, horrible way to take his own life, but one of the few available to prisoners.

Ultimately, Exoo's inherent drive to help others triumphed over his personal misery. Instead of dwelling morbidly on his own problems, Exoo worked to better the lives of his fellow inmates. He cared for their spiritual and emotional needs, taught peaceful conflict resolution techniques, and led prayer and meditation sessions.

Two months into his detention period, Exoo's hard-working public attorney discovered that a number of the case law citations presented to support the prosecution had been superseded by more recent laws decriminalizing assisted suicide. That seemed to tip the scales in Exoo's favor.

Both the prosecuting and defense attorneys worked on the case with great skill and dedication, spending hundreds of hours wrestling with the complex thicket of varying state laws. The judge was also meticulously fair. The Exoo case demonstrated American jurisprudence at its finest. In the media, however, the case was still being hyped like a circus freak show.

With the exception of two West Virginia newspapers and one in Charleston, South Carolina, the American media almost completely ignored Exoo's case. The U.S. papers that did print something usually repeated whatever was handed to them, questioned nothing, and did neither research nor fact-checking. The Irish newspapers and broadcast media were by far the worst of the lot. They went out of their way to point out that Exoo and McGurrin were gay (and, by implication, disreputable), a fact with no relevance to the story except to cast the two in a negative light. They were also labeled "Reverend Death" and "Angels of Death" by the same sources, for the same reason.

It was journalism at its rock-bottom sleaziest, from the gutter-raking British and Irish tabloids to Raidió Teilifís Éireann (RTÉ), Ireland's government-owned public broadcasting system. As late as December 11, 2007, more than five years after Toole's death, RTÉ was still reporting the falsehood that "Exoo and his partner admitted that they were paid $7,000 to support [Toole] to end her life," directly contradicting written statements from the Irish police.[25]

Judge VanDervort set Friday, October 6, 2007, as the date that his ruling would be announced. By that time, Exoo had been in jail for 121 days. Three reporters, including one from Ireland, and about two dozen of Exoo's supporters filled the visitors' section in the small Beckley courtroom.

After brief preliminary statements, the judge presented his ruling: "The Court finds that the conduct with which [Exoo] is charged in Ireland is not . . . felonious under the law of the preponderance of States and concludes that dual criminality therefore does not exist."[26]

In short, the prosecution had not demonstrated that a majority of states had laws equivalent to Ireland's law on assisting a suicide. The Irish extradition request was therefore denied, and the court ordered Exoo's immediate release.

Hoping fervently that his partner would be freed, Thomas McGurrin had brought a pair of shined shoes, Exoo's Harvard blazer, a burgundy dress shirt, a white clerical collar, and a pair of tan slacks to the courtroom. As soon as the judge finished his ruling, Exoo was released from his handcuffs and leg chains, and he traded his tattered jail jumpsuit for his minister's clothing.

For the first time in many months, Exoo smiled broadly as he walked out of the courthouse. With characteristic generosity, he offered his jail-issued brown-bag lunch—an unadorned bologna sandwich, an orange, and cookies—to the waiting reporters and was driven off to a celebratory luncheon by his friends.

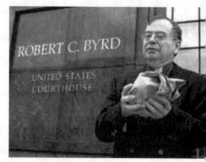

I emailed a report of his release to Derek Humphry, who sent it out worldwide to his international 1,800-member death-with-dignity email list. By the end of the follow-

Exoo's release from prison

ing day, people from fourteen countries had sent Exoo more than six hundred congratulatory emails. When we talked briefly on the phone on the afternoon of his release, a weary Exoo could not mask his joy at being freed, and he chuckled when I told him that I was officially resigning my nonpaying job as his international media representative, effective immediately.

After regaining his health, which had deteriorated while in jail, Exoo returned to his work of establishing a right-to-die hospice and resumed his parish ministry. As he looked back on the whole affair, Exoo was not bitter. But he is still bewildered as to why Ireland spent so much time and money seeking to punish him for something he viewed as an act of simple compassion. During his two decades of work in the death-with-dignity movement, Exoo has been struck by how few people care enough about the pain and suffering of others to risk violating the law to come to their aid. He wrote:

While there are those who stand only on the sidelines, often holding those who risk their freedom in disdain, some of us roll up our sleeves and jump right in when we learn of people suffering in body so much that they want out. . . .

We undertake our work of compassion always willing to risk our own creature comfort and our own safety. We do not care if there are enemies who revile us and our work. We do not care even if some of those who should be our supporters revile us. Being people who live for those strangers who contact us, we work as minorities of one. Our activism gives our lives meaning and often is our only reward.[27]

Exoo's departure from the limelight and return to relative obscurity happened as quickly as his arrest and incarceration. His grueling experience was only a link in a long chain of events. Thirty-two years before the Rosemary Toole case became a cause célèbre, one incident indelibly marked the beginning of the modern international right-to-die movement.

On March 29, 1975, British journalist Derek Humphry summoned the courage to do what his terminally ill, cancer-riddled wife, Jean, had requested. What evolved from that that single act of love and compassion changed the course of social history forever.

Good-bye, My Love

*Just as we need a midwife to bring a human being into the world,
we need helpers, wise women and men, to be there and to help him or
her leave it peacefully.* — Dr. Frederic Chaussoy

The man who has become an icon to millions—and the devil in-carnate to his opponents—does not spend all of his time as a fire-breathing social activist. On a recent, crisp fall morning, Derek Humphry faced an unusual problem. This time, at least, it was not a life-or-death situation.

Isabella, his Vietnamese pot-bellied pig, had found yet another way to get through the old wooden fence that separates Humphry's house in rural Eugene, Oregon, from the forests and fields that sur-round it. The godfather and guiding light of the international right-to-die movement found himself trying to coax the elderly neighborhood handyman into mending the fence quickly. The harried, overbooked man was not immediately available. Humphry was on his own.

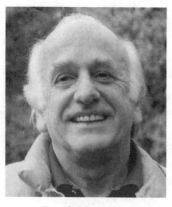
Derek Humphry

Undeterred, Humphry set out to search for Isabella, a once-cuddly piglet that had matured into a spoiled, fifty-pound mini-tank who could open drawers when she did not get what she wanted. Once the reluc-tant pig was coaxed back from a morning of gourmet dining on acorns, Humphry constructed a temporary patch for the fence and returned to his house.

There, in the small, overflowing office of the Euthanasia Re-search and Guidance Organization (ERGO), which he had founded in 1993, he dove into his work, dealing with a constantly ringing telephone and an overflowing email in-box. Both connected him to the world of the suffering, the dying, those contemplating suicide, and his fellow activists worldwide who were fighting to make death with dignity an inalienable civil right.

Two of his euthanasia books had become international best-sellers, and in 1980, he founded the Hemlock Society and built it into the largest right-to-die organization in the United States. His engaging, no-nonsense speeches and presentations drew thousands to the right-to-die movement.

The more his message of choice at the end of life took root, the more his opponents turned up the invective. A fundamentalist Christian news blog declared him the "February 2002 Anti-Christ of the Month" and described the videotape version of his self-deliverance book, *Final Exit*, as "sort of a cross between a low-key cooking class and that good-bye video from the Heaven's Gate Cult members."[1]

Humphry said, "Considering the source, the label was one of the most amusing ever applied to me."[2] The blogger who loathed him was probably influenced by Humphry's biographical sketch in *Who's Who in Hell*, a scholarly directory of high-achieving humanists, atheists, and freethinkers who were excoriated by organized religion. The list included Galileo, Voltaire, Darwin, Marie Curie, Salman Rushdie, fifty Nobel Prize winners—and Humphry.

When I first contacted him in 2007, after George Exoo's arrest, I was acutely aware of his reputation. My goal was simple. I needed his help in countering the gross and often deliberate media distortions of fact that arose during Exoo's incarceration. Humphry, who runs the world's largest internet-based euthanasia newsgroup, could regularly notify several thousand people about Exoo's predicament. After talking with me, he agreed to help, and I sent him regular updates on the case.

Four months later, the charges against Exoo were dropped, and that story was over. But my involvement with the subject of death with dignity had just begun. Because of Exoo's case and Humphry's extensive contacts, I had been introduced to leading right-to-die advocates all over the world. As a social historian and biographer with an amazing wealth of resources suddenly available, I could not pass up the unique opportunity to explore this controversial subject.

When I made the decision to write this book, one thing was clear. I would have to resume my dialogue with Humphry, for the simple reason that the story of the modern right-to-die movement began with him.

Derek Humphry is the death-with-dignity movement's uncontested patriarch. Born April 29, 1930, in the ancient Roman city of Bath, England, he is as influential today as ever, working to support the cause seven days a week. His understated British wit and his white hair, ruddy complexion, fluffy sideburns, firm handshake, and forthright manner create the aura of a character from a Dickens novel. But there is nothing fictional about his profound concern for the dying and for those who are willing to help them die peacefully.

Humphry was the younger of two sons of Bettine Duggan, a tall, slender Irishwoman reputed to have been a night club hostess and a fashion model, and her flamboyant husband, Royston (Roy) Humphry, a traveling salesman and the black sheep of his family. Both of Derek's parents embraced the high-spirited lifestyle of the Roaring Twenties and loved to drink and dance all night.

In the early 1930s, his parents began a bitter divorce and battled over custody of their two boys. Roy won. Bettine quickly remarried and moved to Australia in 1932, when Derek was two. Notoriously unreliable, Roy was never present in his sons' lives for long. Because of their feckless parents, the boys were often bounced around among the homes of begrudging relatives.[3]

Humphry's life played out as a classic Horatio Alger tale of pluck and perseverance. Virtually all of his education came from his love of reading and his passion for classical music. Throughout World War II, he listened intently to Alistair Cooke's *London Letter* and, after the war, *American Letter*, both on BBC Radio. Cooke recounted facts coolly, letting them speak for themselves. The broadcasts inspired Humphry to pursue a career in journalism, and his later writing reflected Cooke's style and tone.

Finding little satisfaction in his peripatetic schooling, Humphry longed to work as a newspaperman. By law, he was allowed to leave school after the age of fifteen, and a conflict with his family over religious beliefs made him eager to do so. His aunts and uncles were strict Anglicans who had decided that he would be confirmed in their church when he turned fifteen. However, the precocious young man had read the works of several iconoclastic thinkers, including H.

G. Wells. He concluded that if Wells' version of the beginning of the world was anywhere near correct, he could not accept the Biblical six-day version of creation. Then he read the works of Charles Darwin, which clinched his atheism.[4] The framework of his moral thinking was strongly shaped by the rationalism of George Bernard Shaw, who savagely attacked social hypocrisy, as Humphry himself would do later in life.

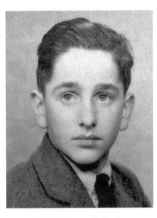

Humphry at fourteen

On his fifteenth birthday, Humphry ran away from home with the price of a one-way train ticket to London in his pocket. Good luck and audacity helped him find work as an editorial assistant with the London office of the *Yorkshire Post*. Despite his title, he quickly discovered that the job had little to do with writing or editing. He was the office flunky, and his primary duty consisted of running from pub to pub, trying to find tightly rationed cigarettes for the editors. His persistence ultimately paid off, and Humphry got to learn the journalist's trade.

In 1948, at the age of eighteen, he was drafted into the British army and stationed in Germany and Austria. He found the tour of duty extremely boring, except for one memorable evening when a willing Austrian girl relieved him of his virginity. After completing his military service, he returned to his career as a reporter, working for the *Bristol Evening World*. To broaden his perspectives before attempting the big leap to the prominent London newspapers, he moved to the north of England, where he pulled a hard-working stint at the *Manchester Evening News*.

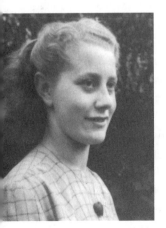

Jean Humphry

In 1953, he interviewed Jean Crane, a socially progressive, twenty-one-year-old woman. Born in the slums of Manchester, she had a childhood almost as bleak as his own. Humphry, then twenty-three, was immediately attracted to the shy, tall blonde and invited her to join him for a concert. Within six weeks, Humphry proposed. The couple married in a civil ceremony on May 4, 1953.[5] With a new wife, and two children born in quick succession, Humphry redoubled his efforts to support his aspirations and his family.

When he was thirty-seven, with over twenty years of journalistic experience under his belt, he landed a top-rank job writing feature stories for Britain's most prestigious newspaper, the *London Sunday Times*. He specialized in race relations, immigration, prison conditions, police brutality and corruption, and the war in Northern Ireland. As an outgrowth of his ongoing investigative reporting, Humphry co-wrote *Because They're Black* to explain the suffering of black immigrants to white Britons. The book earned him the Martin Luther King Memorial Prize for its contribution to racial harmony.[6] A number of other critically acclaimed books about social injustice followed. His family was completed when he and Jean adopted a mixed-race child in 1960.

In 1973, Jean, then forty-one, noticed a lump in her left breast, which proved to be malignant. She knew she was probably looking at a long, tortured path toward death because four aunts had died of the same disease, and her mother had died of lung cancer. Early diagnosis was uncommon at that time, as mammograms would not become routine until the mid-1970s.

The lump was significant, indicating an advanced cancer, and Jean was immediately taken into surgery. The disease had spread to her lymph nodes. After the operation, Jean burst into tears when she discovered that the doctor had removed her entire breast.

Knowing that life away from London would be easier on his wife, Humphry bought a large, three-hundred-year-old stone house in Langley Burrell, a postcard-pretty village in Wiltshire. Jean was in partial remission for the better part of a year and was able to run a small grocery store that came with the house.

Initially, radiation and chemotherapy seemed to help, but soon the cancer spread to Jean's bones. After two years of decline, she was almost completely bedridden. She asked Humphry to get an unambiguous prognosis from her doctors because she felt they were coddling her.

"She's going to die," one physician finally admitted.

When Jean asked her husband about the prognosis, he swallowed his emotions and repeated the doctor's bleak statement. The news was a terrible blow. For three days, Jean picked at her meals and said nothing. Humphry did not know how to react until a friend explained, "She is in mourning for herself."[7]

Soon after her worst fears were confirmed, Jean seemed more cheerful. She had accepted her imminent death and was determined to make the best of whatever time she had left. Her doctors were already using the most aggressive palliative care pain-management strategies available, but, having watched her mother's final ordeal, Jean knew how painful death was likely to be.

Soon she was in constant agony, and the powerful cocktail of painkillers she was taking rendered her unconscious most of the time. After a particularly bad episode, she was hospitalized, but she pulled through. However, her doctor understood that she was in final decline and did not want to live any longer.[8] A few days later, that is exactly what she told her husband.

"Derek," she said, taking a deep breath, "I simply don't want to go on living like this. I want you to do something for me so that if I decide I want to die I can do it on my own terms and exactly when I choose."[9] Stunned, Humphry said nothing.

Worried that the medicine she was taking would affect her decision-making ability, she continued, "I shall have a good idea when I've had enough of the pain. So I want you to promise me that when I ask you if this is the right time to kill myself, you will give me an honest answer one way or another. And we must both understand, both you and I, that I'll do it right at that very moment. You won't question my right and you will give me the means to do it."[10]

Jean had thought through the whole plan. "Find a doctor who will give us the lethal drugs," she said. "When I'm ready to go, you will hand them over without argument." Humphry agreed.

He sought out a physician in London whom he had interviewed for a story about problems in the British healthcare system. After a lengthy discussion, the doctor agreed that Jean had no quality of life left, and he gave Humphry the necessary pills, along with instructions on how to use them. Both men were acutely aware that they had just colluded to carry out a felony offense under Section Two of England's Suicide Act 1961, which is still in force. If discovered and found guilty of assisting a suicide, they could each be imprisoned for up to fourteen years.

Ironically, suicide or attempted suicide had been decriminalized in the United Kingdom in 1961 as a humanitarian measure so that suicidal people could seek help without fear of being thrown into a hospital psychiatric ward—a common fate for those whose suicide attempts failed. The logic of that time was simple: if you wanted to kill yourself, you must be crazy. Assisting a suicide, however, remained illegal. Humphry and the doctor were confronting a bizarre conundrum: they were committing a crime in order to enable Jean to carry out an act that was not a crime.

Soon Jean's cancer roared back, having spread to her vital organs. She was hospitalized, but the doctors could only treat her pain. With no hope of recovery, she chose to return home to die.

Her bones were as brittle as matchsticks, and one day, while bending to pick up a washbasin she had dropped, she broke three ribs. Now she was fragile, bedridden, and unable to reach the bathroom. Jean had always been an independent woman, and her loss of autonomy was the final straw.

Her condition put extremely heavy stress on her husband, who was now exhausted by the long ordeal. He raced from one assignment to another in London and then made the ninety-minute drive back home. "I realized that I was on my way to a nervous breakdown myself," he remembered. "Severe fatigue was my biggest problem, and I would fall asleep anywhere at any time as soon as I sat down. I dozed off in my car on the motorway to Oxford, awaking with a start to find myself overtaking another car at ninety miles an hour. Perhaps I only slept for seconds but I was frightened by this, pulled over, and fell asleep instantly."[11]

One morning Jean awoke in tremendous pain, unable to move. Humphry brought her painkillers, and after they took effect, she looked him in the eyes and asked, "Is this the day?"[12]

Taken aback, Humphry tried to come up with a reasonable answer. Then he repeated what the doctors had told him: her cancer was incurable, and there was nothing more to be done.

Jean responded immediately, "I shall die at one o'clock. You must give me the overdose and then go into the garden and not return for an hour. We'll say our last good-bye here but I don't want you actually to see me die. We can't alter what's going to happen and I'm quite happy. Of course I don't want to leave you but I can't take any more of this cancer. I'd rather die today in peace of mind, and in enjoying your presence and love in my own home than in some grim hospital ward after being knocked senseless with drugs for a couple of weeks."[13]

Jean's last hours were spent with her husband, reminiscing about the happy times in their long marriage. Jean then made Humphry promise that he would remarry. Tearfully, he managed to nod his assent.

"Stop crying," Jean told him gently. "Look at the time." At ten minutes to one, Humphry left the room and prepared the drugs that the physician had given him. Then he brewed a mug of strong coffee with milk and stirred in the lethal dose.[14] "Tears were streaming down my face," he recalled, "and I had to grit my teeth to do it. But, you know, there are some terrible things you have to do in this life. She'd been a good wife to me and a loving friend for twenty-two years. I owed her that action that she wanted, and she never backed off."[15]

As he set the tray down by Jean's bed, she asked, "Is that it?" Consumed with emotion, he could barely speak. She knew the answer. Humphry took her in his arms and kissed her. "Good-bye, my love," he said, tears streaming down his face.

"Good-bye, darling," Jean replied. She then picked up the mug, drank the contents, leaned back on her pillow, and closed her eyes. Within moments, she fell asleep, and her breathing became slow and heavy. Humphry chose not to leave her side, fearing that something might go wrong if the drugs did not work.

Then a frightening thing happened. About fifteen minutes after drinking the sedative-laced coffee, Jean vomited. Alarmed, Humphry thought she might not have kept enough of the drugs in her system. Two pillows lay on a chair beside the bed.

"I decided that with the first stirring of life I would smother her with them," Humphry wrote.[16] He would not break his promise to his wife, even if it meant doubly violating England's assisted suicide law.

As her husband kept his nervous, desperate vigil, Jean's breathing slowed. She needed no further assistance. With Humphry gently holding her hand, Jean died peacefully at 1:50 p.m. on March 29, 1975.[17]

After telling his sons that their mother had passed away, Humphry called the family doctor, who was familiar with Jean's condition. Without hesitation, the physician wrote out the death certificate, showing cancer as the cause of death.

Humphry threw himself into his work, hoping that it would help him overcome the pain of his loss. "Not once did the manner of Jean's death bother me," he confessed. "My conscience on that score was, and still is, clear."[18] Yet helping her choose a voluntary death had a profound effect on his perception of life, suffering, dying, and death.

His marriage to Jean had been warm and fulfilling, and he knew he would eventually remarry. Because his demanding schedule left him little time to meet eligible women, he turned to the personal advertisements. After several fruitless encounters, he was about to give up. Then he read an ad that began, "Attractive blonde, piquant, 33, about-to-be-divorced, Ph.D. student...."[19] Ann Wickett was indeed "piquant," highly intelligent, vivacious, and beautiful. She and Humphry had their first date five months after Jean's death.

As it was with Jean, Humphry's attraction to Ann was quick, strong, sensual, and mutual. The bright Boston divorcée and the accomplished British journalist rapidly fell in love. They were married in London's Marylebone Registry Office on February 16, 1976, less than a year after Jean's death. Photos taken that day show a radiant bride looking adoringly at a very happy groom.[20]

"I settled into my second marriage easily," Humphry said. Ann was ecstatic and responded to his charm and warmth with unbridled affection. However, both were on the rebound from different marital disasters and brought substantial emotional baggage to their union.

Humphry's British reserve and basic affability masked his turbulent emotional history. Ann had demons of her own. She suffered from deeply rooted abandonment issues stemming from several traumatic events. Her mother had treated her callously all her life. In addition, Ann had been forced to put her illegitimate, three-month-old son up for adoption because his father refused to marry her, and her affluent parents would not support her and the baby. Her failed marriage to Thomas Wickett, an aloof Toronto attorney, led to a suicide attempt that resulted in several months of treatment in a psychiatric ward.[21] For the rest of her life, this bright, educated, articulate woman felt like a complete failure, abandoned by her parents and unable to raise her own child.

Humphry, whose children were now adults and living on their

own when he remarried, looked at Ann and saw a beautiful, educated, outgoing, passionate woman, thirteen years his junior, un-
encumbered by children, and game for travel and adventure. Their
intellectual paths were quite different, but their achievements were
comparable. Humphry had dropped out of school at fifteen but had
worked hard to become a highly respected journalist and an award-
winning author. Ann had graduated *cum laude* from Boston University, had earned a master's degree from the University of Toronto,
and had completed everything but her dissertation for a Ph.D. in
English literature.

After learning every detail of the life and death of her husband's
first wife, Ann saw Jean's story as a romantic tragedy with the potential to be a powerful book. It would carry an important social
message—and it would provide a much-needed emotional catharsis
for her husband. She would help him create it.

Despite some initial hesitation, Humphry plunged into the work.
Writing the story was an emotionally wrenching and extremely
slow process for him and for Ann, who were both still living in Jean's
shadow. The resulting book, *Jean's Way*, portrayed her death as the
final act of mercy and compassion by a loving husband who fulfilled
the last request of his rational, life-loving wife. Eighteen years later,
Ann's biographer, anti-euthanasia activist Rita L. Marker, claimed
that Ann, under the influence of her strong-willed husband, had sof-
tened the details and sugarcoated the story to please him and make
the book more palatable to a wider audience, a charge Humphry
emphatically denied.[22]

After reading the manuscript, Humphry's literary agent and
most publishers were leery. "It's too depressing," they said. "It makes
people cry."[23]

Undaunted, Humphry took the book to Quartet, a small London
press. They offered him a paltry £500 GBP royalty advance, but
he took it. Fortunately, Quartet was interested only in the British
hardcover rights, leaving the paperback, foreign, and film rights to
Humphry, a decision the firm would soon regret.

Jean's Way was released in 1978 and became a runaway best-
seller. Its five-thousand-copy hardcover print run sold out in five
days. Another publisher quickly picked up the paperback rights, and
within a week, Columbia Pictures bought the film rights (although
the movie was never produced). The book also became a smash hit

in the United States and was ultimately translated into seven languages.

A television documentary featuring Humphry and the subject of assisted suicide aired shortly after the book's launch in Britain. It resulted in massive attention from the print media worldwide—and an official police inquiry into Humphry's part in his wife's death. When questioned, Humphry freely admitted that every detail of the book and the documentary was true. After months of investigation, the Director of Public Prosecutions (DPP) ruled that there was "insufficient evidence" to prosecute Humphry for assisting a suicide. The decision sent a clear message: prosecution in the case of an assisted voluntary death probably would not result in a trial. After all, a jury might reason, if suicide by a terminally ill person was legal, how could assisting such a suicide be illegal?

Immediately after the publication of *Jean's Way*, the battle lines formed. Humphry found himself defending assisted suicide daily, arguing against such formidable forces as the Catholic Church, the Church of England, fundamentalist Christians, medical organizations, and the British hospice movement.

The position of conservative Christian religious leaders was simple: only God can give the gift of life, and only God has the right to end it. Implicit in that viewpoint is the belief that people are commanded to live, and those who defy God by taking their own lives will face harsh judgment in the afterlife.[24] The Bible itself, however, is amazingly ambivalent on the subject.

Humphry found no merit in the "sanctity of life" argument. He believed that life was an experience, not a sentence, and that any true gift could be disposed of in whatever manner the recipient chose. To him, suffering for God's sake was ludicrous. He rejected any deity that would needlessly demand avoidable, excruciating pain and found no reason to believe in any form of afterlife.

British hospice representatives claimed that had Jean Humphry been in their care, her pain would have been better managed, and she would never have asked for a hastened death. In reply, Humphry pointed out that Jean had received every available palliative care pain-management therapy. She terminated her life only weeks before it would have ended naturally because her quality of life had diminished beyond her endurance.

When the first Australian printing of fifty thousand copies of

Jean's Way quickly sold out—an astounding quantity, considering the country's small population—Humphry was invited to Australia and New Zealand for a promotional tour paid for by the New Zealand Humanist Association and two Australian right-to-die groups.

"What impressed me most were the audiences, young and old, of varying educational backgrounds, who packed the meeting halls. *I must be saying something people wanted to hear*," Humphry mused.[25] He thrived on the response, becoming aware that he had a certain personal quality that made people want to listen.[26]

When *Jean's Way* was published in the United States in 1979, Humphry was invited to appear on major radio and television talk shows and received numerous invitations to speak to university groups, senior citizens' clubs, and Unitarian-Universalist congregations. At every event, he found people anxious—even desperate—to talk with him about their experiences with the loss of loved ones.

Humphry had developed a reputation for keen social insights, but he never thought of himself as a social activist. However, during his U.S. tour, the overwhelming support he experienced made him aware of the need for someone to fight for Americans' right to a chosen death. He asked the two main U.S. right-to-die organizations, Concern for Dying and The Society for the Right to Die, to begin advocating legal, medical, voluntary euthanasia and assisted suicide instead of merely publicizing the use of living wills.

"They declined, claiming America was not ready for this," he wrote. "I felt they were wrong because the evidence indicated a huge public interest."[27]

His experiences in America led to a one-year contract to write for the *Los Angeles Times* in 1978. He and Ann moved to California, but the *Times* turned out to be grossly overstaffed and let him go after the year was up. To support himself, he freelanced, mainly for the *London Sunday Times Colour Magazine.*

He parted with the magazine when the editor asked him to cover an aircraft disaster in the Antarctic. He refused the assignment only because it conflicted with the first public meeting of what would become the Hemlock Society. "At that moment I broke my ties with journalism and went with Hemlock," Humphry said.[28] He never looked back.

Derek and Ann Humphry had often discussed forming an American right-to-die organization. "She suggested that it be called

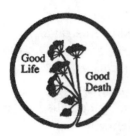

'Hemlock,' and I agreed, adding the word 'Society' as a clarification of what it was."[29] For its motto, they chose "Good life, good death."

She proposed the name as a symbol of the rational suicide chosen by the Athenian philosopher, Socrates. Convicted on a charge of corrupting his students through his social criticism, he was sentenced either to permanent exile or to death by drinking the sap of the hemlock tree, a natural poison. At the age of seventy, in the presence of weeping friends, Socrates drank the hemlock, choosing to die as a martyr to his beliefs. The wispy Hemlock flower became the society's insignia.

Humphry drafted a charter for the society and convened a group of like-minded people to review it. "I invited...everyone who had expressed sympathy for euthanasia whom I had met over the previous six months while writing a series of three articles titled 'The Quality of Dying in America' for the *Los Angeles Times*," he said.[30]

The initial gathering was held on the evening of July 16, 1980, in the large, comfortable home of Dr. Richard S. Scott. An intelligent, progressive physician-turned-lawyer, Scott had helped draft the world's first living will in the 1970s. About twenty people attended.

Humphry recalled, "Most were professional people: psychologists, doctors, nurses, and academics from the universities of southern California. I chaired the meeting and went around the room asking everybody for their opinion on whether we should start a right-to-die society which campaigned for voluntary euthanasia and assisted suicide for the terminal and hopelessly ill. Helping those with depression or mental illness was not even on the table. I took a vote on whether we should start up, and everybody said yes. Next I took a vote on who would join the group, and there was complete silence."[31]

One attorney summed up the feelings of many other attendees: "My God, they firebomb the houses of pro-abortion people! What do you think they'll do to us?"

Humphry was dumbfounded. Then, from the back of the room, a rich, resonant voice was heard. Dr. Gerald A. Larue, a professor of Biblical history and archaeology at the University of Southern California, asked, "How can we say we support euthanasia and not be willing to work for it? I will join."[32]

"Then I closed the meeting," Humphry said. "Enough had been said to encourage me to press on with idea of the radical movement."[33]

Larue recalled, "After the meeting, [Humphry] and I stood on the sidewalk and Hemlock was formed. I was voted in (two votes to my one) as the first president." The noted religious thinker went on to write *Euthanasia and Religion* and *Playing God* and served ably as Hemlock's president from 1980 until mid-1988.[34]

Journalists often asked how a professor of Biblical history could be president of a right-to-die group. "Of course what I didn't tell them was that Jerry was a respected expert on the world's religions but personally was a secular nonbeliever," Humphry said with a chuckle.[35]

Later that evening, Richard Scott agreed to be Hemlock's legal advisor and set up the group's charter and by-laws.[36] The core leadership of the society was now complete. Hemlock's articles of incorporation were filed several months later on March 10, 1981.[37]

The fledgling organization's headquarters was Humphry's tiny, one-bedroom, mass-produced, World-War-II-era house on 32nd Street in Santa Monica. The two-car garage became Hemlock's office.[38] Humphry was executive director and spokesman. His wife, who preferred research and writing, took on the roles of treasurer and newsletter editor.

The Hemlock Society was publicly launched on August 12, 1980, when Humphry and Larue walked into the Los Angeles Press Club for a press conference to announce the formation of the society. It was an unlikely time to begin such a venture. "Reagan was just taking over the presidency and the Rev. Jerry Falwell was in full song with his Moral Majority," Humphry recalled. "America had, it seemed, lurched to the far right, with liberals like us pushed aside."[39]

However, Humphry was optimistic about Hemlock's future. Toward the end of the news conference, a reporter asked how large the organization was. With considerable chutzpah, Humphry replied with a confident smile, "Small, but growing fast."[40]

His words were prophetic. By chance, Shirley Carroll O'Connor, a well-known California publicist, attended the event. Impressed with their mission, she handed Humphry a $20 bill and became Hemlock's first paying member on the spot. She remained an active volunteer in the movement for twenty-three years until her death in 2010 at the age of ninety-three.

Humphry's gut feeling was right. People had been waiting to hear his message for decades. The press conference generated numerous articles, which brought Hemlock hundreds of letters requesting information on membership—and hate-filled missives that consigned the group's founders "to some special region of Hell where they would meet an ugly end."[41]

As Humphry's reputation as an engaging speaker and a no-nonsense advocate for the right to die spread, sales of *Jean's Way* soared. Using royalties from the book, and the increasing financial fuel from membership dues, Derek and Ann Humphry gradually moved the Hemlock Society out of its home in their garage.

Ann immediately dove into her work. The first issue of *The Hemlock Quarterly* was published in October 1980. Its first editorial stated Hemlock's goals:

> First, Hemlock will seek to promote a climate of public opinion which is tolerant of the right of people who are terminally ill to end their own lives in a planned manner. Second, Hemlock does not encourage suicide for any primary emotional, traumatic, or financial reasons in the absence of terminal illness. It approves of the work of all those involved in suicide prevention. Third, the final decision to terminate life is ultimately one's own. Hemlock believes this action, and most of all its timing, to be an extremely personal decision, wherever possible taken in concert with family and friends. And fourth, Hemlock speaks only to those people who have mutual sympathy with its goals. Views contrary to its own which are held by other religions and philosophies are respected.[42]

As Hemlock's chief spokesman, Humphry was constantly on the road, lugging an overstuffed briefcase filled with books, brochures, and membership applications. He gave free lectures anywhere he could find an invitation. To get media bookings, he hired Irwin Zucker, a top-flight Hollywood publicist, and did as many as three hundred radio and twenty-five television programs a year.[43]

An articulate, polished, and unpretentious public speaker, he appealed to people of all backgrounds and education levels. Because of his personal experiences, his presentations, and his increasing collection of tragic end-of-life case histories, he rapidly became the leading spokesman for the right-to-die movement and its best-known writer. He would often be the single right-to-die proponent to face a panel of five or six antagonists.

People liked what they heard. Paying memberships started rolling in to Hemlock, and its numbers rose continuously during Humphry's eleven years as executive director. From a single dues payer in August 1980, the membership swelled to 144 by the end of the month and 700 by the end of the year. By 1992, when Humphry retired from Hemlock, the organization had more than 57,000 members and 90 local chapters.[44]

Hemlock got a huge boost with the 1980 publication of *Good Life/Good Death: A Doctor's Case for Euthanasia and Suicide* by Dr. Christiaan N. Barnard, the internationally known South African surgeon who performed the world's first successful human heart transplant in 1967. In his controversial book, Barnard spoke openly and compellingly of the patient's right to die, the family's right to turn off life-sustaining machines, and the doctor's right to participate in euthanasia as a humane and compassionate end to suffering. He also admitted that he had practiced passive euthanasia for years—on his own mother, in fact—and said that he would practice active euthanasia if it were legal.[45]

In response to a flood of requests from people begging for accurate information on how to achieve a painless, dignified, and legal death, Humphry wrote *Let Me Die Before I Wake: How Dying People End Their Suffering* in 1981. It included true stories of rational, sick, and dying men and women who decided to end their lives. By describing exactly what doses of which drugs these people used, it became the first book to provide accurate information on the effective use of lethal drugs for self-deliverance.

When released for general sale, the book's clear, detailed descriptions of self-deliverance infuriated religious conservatives and many physicians. The reviews, however, were generally positive. Time called it "a compassionate work." On *60 Minutes*, Diane Sawyer dubbed it "the Bible of euthanasia." *Let Me Die* ultimately sold more than 150,000 copies before being superseded by Humphry's landmark book, *Final Exit.*

For years, Humphry was Hemlock's only paid employee until Ann was finally put on the payroll for her substantial work. The royalties and direct sales of his books kept their rent paid and Hemlock afloat, as did numerous reprints of a 1988 *Hemlock Quarterly* article by British psychiatrist and right-to-die advocate Colin Brewer that included a table listing the lethal dosages of the drugs most suitable for self-deliverance.

By the late 1980s, Humphry's nearly bald head and wide, "ear-muff" sideburns were a familiar sight on television talk shows. However, his high media profile also made him the favorite whipping boy of everyone who opposed the death-with-dignity movement.

The controversy worked strongly in his favor. Media attention caused legions of people to ponder the subject of voluntary death for the first time. Humphry's core concept that it was an individual's right to choose when, where, and how to die—not a privilege rationed by doctors, church, or state—appealed to diverse groups who believed that personal autonomy trumped medical, religious, or governmental authority. The growing success of Hemlock's efforts in the United States was reflected in a scientific poll carried out in 1986 by the Roper Organization. Its face-to-face interviews with two thousand Americans showed that 76 percent believed a physician should be legally bound to obey a dying patient's living will, and 62 percent believed their physicians should be able to

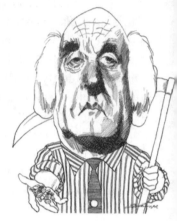

Humphry as the Grim Reaper

help them die when they were terminally ill. Opinions varied little from state to state, refuting the notion that places such as Florida and California, which have large elderly populations, were fueling the right-to-die movement.[46]

Hemlock's rapid growth put heavy pressure on the Humphrys' emotionally complicated marriage. Humphry said that problems began shortly after they were married. He alleged that Ann often flew into dish-throwing rages, especially when he spent time in the company of other women, which was frequent, given his heavy speaking schedule. He claimed that she scorned any relationship with his three sons, who returned her coldness in kind. He lamented that it was he who had proposed and welcomed the hasty match, then seriously considered a divorce within the first year of their marriage. He believed that insecurity, mental illness, and tranquilizer addiction were at the root of Ann's profound pain and explosive anger.

After a three-week argument over her demand that he fire two Hemlock directors who had criticized her, Humphry asked for a divorce. In retaliation, Ann threatened to create havoc for the organization. From 1984 on, Humphry fought to keep Hemlock from being dragged down by the domestic rancor. Marriage counseling failed. Ann's listless presentations on a 1986 book tour for the Humphrys' jointly authored book, *The Right to Die*, brought howls of protest from their publicist and from radio and television producers, who claimed that Ann was rude and uncooperative.

In 1986, Ann's elderly parents planned a double suicide and asked for her help. Arthur Kooman was ninety-two and suffered from congestive heart failure and a painful back. His wife, Ruth, was seventy-seven and had suffered several strokes, leaving her severely handicapped and almost unable to walk.

Despite their harsh treatment of her as she was growing up, Ann agreed to help her parents and asked for her husband's assistance. He obtained several hundred Vesperax pills (a combination of secobarbital and brallobarbital, no longer produced). Then he and Ann flew to Boston and carefully questioned the Koomans about their motives. Arthur was clearly dying, but Ruth was not. She had adequate funds for assisted living care, but she refused the option. "No, I want to go with Arthur," she repeatedly insisted.[47]

The Koomans died on July 21, 1986. After taking an anti-emetic to avoid throwing up the lethal drugs, they ate a light evening meal, had a few drinks, and went upstairs. Arthur kissed his wife good-bye and went to his bedroom, and she went to hers. Ann ground up about two hundred pills in a blender. Forty-five per person would have been a lethal dose. She mixed half of the pill powder into a bowl of applesauce, her father's favorite dessert, with the rest going into a large serving of coffee ice cream, which Ruth enjoyed.

Ann helped her mother die; Humphry helped her father. "I don't know how to thank you and Ann for what you are doing for us," Arthur said as he eagerly scooped up the applesauce. In a few minutes he was asleep. Within twenty minutes he was dead.[48]

Across the hall, Ann kept vigil with her mother as she slipped into her final sleep. Seven years later, Ann later told her biographer, Rita Marker, that the drugs had been insufficient. She is quoted as having said:

My mother started to die, and then something went wrong, and it was awful. Her breathing started to get sort of agitated, and I got really scared. And Derek had always said to me, you know, 'Just use a plastic bag or a pillow.' And I just did it because I was so terrified. There was a plastic laundry bag with her linens, her soiled linens in it, and I took the bag and I just very gently held it over her mouth. And I have never gotten over that. And she died very peacefully. But I walked away from that house thinking *we're both murderers and I can't live like this anymore.*[49]

Humphry disputed her damning statements. "Ruth had taken enough secobarbital to kill an ox," he wrote. "Ann did not mention it [the alleged smothering] at the time or in her fictionalized version of the event," referring to her 1989 Hemlock Society book, *Double Exit: When Aging Couples Commit Suicide Together.*[50]

In 1988, using part of the proceeds from her parents' estate, Ann purchased Windfall Farm, a beautiful forty-two-acre parcel of land in a small village north of Eugene, Oregon, and the Humphrys moved themselves and Hemlock's headquarters to the farm's cozy white-frame bungalow. For Ann, the move was a tonic, and she began to feel better about their chaotic marriage.

Over the next few months, however, the relationship spiraled further out of control. Then another tragedy struck. Ann was diagnosed with breast cancer. Fortunately, great medical advances had been made in the sixteen years since Jean Humphry's death. As had Jean, Ann underwent surgery, but she had a lumpectomy, thereby preserving most of the affected breast. Unlike Jean, Ann's tests showed no invasion of the lymph nodes, and her doctors were cautiously confident that, with proper treatment, the cancer was not likely to reappear. Despite the positive prognosis, Ann thought her husband should have shown more concern, raging, "You cried for Jean, why aren't you crying for me?"[51]

Three weeks after his wife's cancer surgery, Humphry announced that he was leaving on a business trip. He gave no phone number where he could be reached, and messages he left on Ann's answering machine were unequivocal. He was not coming back.

Ann was stunned. Abandoned in the middle of cancer therapy, with her job and medical insurance coverage threatened, she initiated divorce proceedings on November 22, 1989. Feeling callously neglected yet again by someone she loved, she briefly checked herself into a hospital for psychiatric help, her self-esteem in ruins. Anger became her driving emotion.

Her accusations and property demands, and her husband's denials and counter-accusations, soon played out in the media. Major feature stories about the fiasco appeared in the *New York Times* and in *People*. Then the tabloids joined the feeding frenzy. Every detail of the Humphrys' private demons, fights, charges, and counter-charges was reported.

About the time she filed for divorce, Ann poured out the intimate details of her tumultuous marriage to Rita L. Marker. A right-to-life attorney with an encyclopedic knowledge of the right-to-die movement, Marker befriended Ann. For many years, Marker had been a pro-life activist and vociferous opponent of euthanasia and assisted suicide. At the time Ann filed for divorce, Marker was the executive director of the International Task Force on Euthanasia and Assisted Suicide—renamed the Patients Rights Council in 2011—and one of Derek Humphry's most dedicated opponents. Marker was eager to hear anything Ann Humphry had to say.

Failing to get the story of her alleged mistreatment published by the *Los Angeles Times*, Ann asked a friend to approach the *New York Times*, adding the allegation that Humphry had stolen $40,000 from Hemlock.[52] Alarmed, Hemlock's board decided that both Humphrys, their only salaried employees, would no longer serve on the board, in line with the policies of most nonprofit groups.[53] The board commissioned a full audit, which found no money missing. In addition, the IRS audited Hemlock's books and found no irregularities. Ann's vindictive claims proved to be unfounded.

On January 6, 1990, Ann claimed that her husband had poisoned the minds of Hemlock's board members by saying she was mentally disturbed. The board ultimately granted Ann nine months' paid sick leave and replaced her as deputy director of Hemlock, thereby severing her last official connection with the society she had helped to found a decade earlier.

On October 19, 1990, after the divorce was final, Ann filed a $6-million personal injury lawsuit against her ex-husband, claiming that his actions had been intended "to impede and oppress [her] recovery from cancer itself and to induce [her] despair and suicide."[54] She further stated that he was guilty of "libel, slander, outrageous conduct, negligent infliction of emotional distress, and breach of fiduciary duty."[55] In 1991, Ann told her story in television interviews with television talk-show hosts Larry King and Sally Jessy Raphael.

Each of the feuding partners soon found a new companion. In 1991, Ann developed a caring relationship with an emergency room physician.[56] Derek found love with Gretchen Crocker, an Oregon farm girl, and they married in a civil ceremony on April 24, 1991.[57]

Ann's luck turned against her in early 1991. She elected to have both breasts removed to try to prevent the recurrence of cancer and opted for reconstructive surgery. Several days after the procedure, she came down with a massive infection that could not be treated with antibiotics. She was rushed into the operating room, and her new breast implants were removed. It was one more severe blow to her self-esteem.

In addition, her lawsuit against Humphry was failing. Her attorneys had not noted Oregon's $1-million cap on such suits. Then, in the discovery stage of the suit, where each side must reveal its proposed evidence, her lawyers found that Humphry's tax returns documented the frequency and amount of payments made to his wife's psychotherapists and psychologists over a fifteen-year period. Her attorneys would have to take time-consuming depositions from all of the mental health professionals.

Sensing a costly loss ahead, Ann's lawyers asked the court for permission to withdraw from the case because her resources would not permit the suit to go on. The judge agreed. Ann now believed she had only one recourse. She taped a video outlining the causes and extent of her emotional suffering and arranged for it to be distributed to the media. Then she typed an undated note to her ex-husband.

> There. You got what you wanted. Ever since I was diagnosed as having cancer, you have done everything conceivable to precipitate my death. I was not alone in recognizing what you were doing. What you did — desertion and abandonment — and subsequent harassment of a dying woman — is so unspeakable there are no words to describe the horror of it. Yet you know. And others know too. You have to live with this untiol [sic] you die. May you never forget. Ann.[58]

In October 1991, Ann, with her horse, Ibn, set out for her favorite place, the Three Creeks campground in Oregon's Three Sisters Wilderness Area. She parked her van, mounted Ibn, and rode several miles to a secluded spot. There she took off Ibn's bridle and saddle so that he could roam freely and sat down with her back against a tall pine tree. Next, she took a large overdose of the Vesperax left over from her parents' suicide and washed the pills down with Chivas Regal. Within a few hours, Ibn found his way back to the campground, triggering an intense search-and-rescue operation.

Four days later, on October 8, 1991, a search team found Ann dead, her head resting on a canvas saddlebag. The sheriff reported that she appeared to have simply fallen asleep. The news media immediately broadcast the story.

Humphry wrote, "Then followed perhaps the saddest television clip I had seen in my life…. Ann's body, slung over a pack horse, coming down the mountainside."[59]

In addition to bringing a mournful end to her turbulent life, Ann's suicide provoked a posthumous anti- versus pro-right-to-die furor. A few days after Ann's body was found, a copy of the suicide note arrived at Rita Marker's home.

In a handwritten postscript, Ann had written, "Rita: [These are] My final words to Derek. He is a killer. I know. Jean actually died of suffocation. I could never say it until now; who would believe me? Do the best you can. Ann."[60]

Marker interpreted the postscript to mean that she should tell Ann's story. She released a copy of the note to the media, along with a press release saying, "We hope that all this tragedy will cause people to wake up and to realize what Derek Humphry and the Hemlock Society now stand for."[61]

Humphry saw Ann's note and its postscript as a final hand grenade, thrown from the grave.[62] He assertively disputed all of her accusations, and Hemlock maintained a solid silence. Eventually, the uproar died down, but the controversy soon reignited.

A few months after the suicide, an ad appeared in the *Los Angeles Times*, offering Ann Humphry's personal journals and papers for sale. Ann had evidently stuffed these into a bag and thrown the bag into a dumpster. Someone had retrieved the papers and offered them to the highest bidder. Tabloid journalists viewed the material, but none made offers.

"The Hemlock Society eventually decided to offer $1,000 for the papers in order to destroy them," Humphry wrote.[63] He sent Cheryl

Smith, Hemlock's attorney, to read through them. What she found was shocking.

In her journals Ann revealed that she had "discussed with close friends paying a hit-man to have me assassinated, and then blaming the right-to-life movement for the murder," Humphry wrote. "Happily, there is no evidence that she went ahead with the plan, but it was yet another troubling revelation of her dark thoughts."[64]

After twelve years at its helm, Humphry resigned as executive director of Hemlock in 1992 to focus all his energy on writing. Given the tragic events in 1991, Humphry must have been relieved to have one spectacular success. The publication of his book, *Final Exit: The Practicalities of Self-Deliverance and Assisted Suicide for the Dying*, sent interest in the death-with-dignity movement skyrocketing.

"If *Let Me Die Before I Wake* was the 'guide' to self deliverance, *Final Exit* is the comprehensive shop manual," wrote reviewer David B. Clarke, director of Massachusetts Health Decisions.[65]

In unambiguous terms, Humphry described the most practical methods available for terminally ill people to end their suffering. The book also helped thousands of readers by providing specific instructions for doctors, nurses, and families on how to handle a patient's or loved one's request for assistance in dying.

Final Exit's most famous supporter was the science fiction writer, Isaac Asimov. He wrote, "No decent human being would allow an animal to suffer without being put out of its misery. It is only to human beings that human beings are so cruel as to allow them to live on in pain, in hopelessness, in living death, without moving a muscle to help them. It is against such attitudes that this book fights."[66]

The book ultimately succeeded because of immense public hunger for accurate information on its taboo subject, but it needed a boost. When the first run of 40,000 copies came off the press in January 1991, its arrival created a hollow thud. By mid-July, only 2,000 copies had been sold.[67] It did not grab the attention of the general public until a *Wall Street Journal* story appeared.[68] Three days later, Humphry's distributor ordered 100,000 more copies.[69] Within three months, 400,000 copies of *Final Exit* had been sold. The book stayed on *The New York Times* best-seller list for eighteen weeks.

Noted conservative William F. Buckley, Jr., a devout Catholic and the acerbic, erudite host of the PBS show *Firing Line*, invited

Humphry to be interviewed on September 17, 1991. Buckley questioned Humphry's authority to make moral judgments because, unlike Buckley himself, Humphry was not a college graduate and had never studied the works of the world's great intellectuals and philosophers.

Unintimidated, Humphry calmly replied, "I've derived my philosophy of life from what I've observed over the sixty years of my life and experience and observation, not philosophical study…. The law is wrong and I have set myself out with others to modify this law to be more intelligent. The law, I believe, must move with the times and must move with public opinion, and I think there is a welter of evidence that the public opinion seeks to modify the law on assisted suicide."[70]

Ironically, at the end of his life in 2008, Buckley, who suffered from emphysema and diabetes, actively pondered suicide and discussed it with his son, ultimately admitting that the religious aspect of the matter was prohibitive.[71]

Humphry's critics helped to guarantee book sales. Right-to-life organizations called for *Final Exit* to be banned, charging that it was a loaded gun, available to anyone who was mentally unstable, depressed, or impulsive. France, Australia, and New Zealand initially outlawed the book, but making anything forbidden only whets demand. By the end of 1991, *Final Exit* was number five on the list of best-selling nonfiction hardcover books in North America.[72]

Anti-euthanasia critics claimed that the book would be widely misused by allegedly "vulnerable classes of society" and that it would fuel the rate of suicide. But a November 1993 critical analysis in *The New England Journal of Medicine* found the predictions unfounded. A study led by Dr. Peter Marzuk of the Cornell University Medical College found that "In the year after publication of *Final Exit*, the number of suicides in New York City involving asphyxia by plastic bag [combined with helium or a barbiturate overdose] increased substantially, as compared with the numbers in previous years. [But] the overall suicide rate did not change…. It is therefore reassuring that despite the thousands of copies of the book in circulation in New York City, there was no increase in the overall rate of suicide." In other words, the availability of information on how to achieve a "good death" simply replaced the number of "bad deaths."

Research showed that in the United States as a whole, the number of suicides via plastic bags increased from 334 in 1990 to 437 in 1991, but overall suicide rates for 1991 actually dropped 0.9 percent from the previous year. In the decade after *Final Exit*'s publication, the overall national suicide rate also declined. In other words, *Final Exit* did not increase the suicide rate, but it allowed those who committed suicide to do so in a much more humane manner rather than using grisly methods previously available, such as guns, hanging, and household poisons.[73]

Because of its unique topic, *Final Exit* caused several unforeseen problems. It presented a particular challenge for Barnes & Noble, the world's largest bookseller, because they did not know how to categorize it. Ironically, they initially shelved it in the self-help section.[74] Today, it is found in the psychology section. Libraries had their own dilemmas. Many of their patrons checked out the book and then used it to "check out" themselves. As a result, many of the circulating copies were never returned.

Updated four times to keep it current, and available in print, video, DVD, and eBook versions, Humphry's magnum opus has sold more than 1.5 million copies in twelve languages, as well as Braille, and continues to sell steadily. In 2007, *USA Today* chose *Final Exit* as one of the most memorable books of the previous twenty-five years. Even in conservative South Carolina, where I live, the county library system owns and lends eight copies. The proceeds from Humphry's books have contributed more than $2 million USD to supporting citizen initiatives for state-specific death-with-dignity laws and furthering the worldwide goals of the right-to-die movement.[75]

Overall, his publications, his speaking tours, and the controversy and dialogue that his words provoked led to a major upsurge in the belief that choosing to end one's own life was a right, not a privilege. Despite ferocious opposition, Humphry, the Hemlock Society, and the people and groups they inspired created a fundamental paradigm shift in how the Western world viewed the right to die.

In 1992, a national Gallup Poll found that 75 percent of Americans approved of living wills; 66 percent believed that people have the right to end their lives when suffering great pain with no hope of improvement; and 58 percent—a clear majority—supported self-deliverance when someone has an incurable disease.[76] The approval ratings have steadily climbed ever since.

Derek Humphry had defined death with dignity as the ultimate civil right, but that was just part of the picture. Without laws that permitted assisted suicide and voluntary euthanasia, the movement could not succeed. Free of the duties of running Hemlock, Humphry publicly focused his energy on helping to create legal change.

Privately, he was also ready to tackle another project. Existing self-deliverance methods had major shortcomings. With Humphry's help, a small band of activists from Australia, Canada, and the United States, including two physicians, an anesthesiologist, a psychologist, a Unitarian minister, a former feature writer, and two scuba-diving technicians would soon make a quantum leap into the future of the death-with-dignity movement.

Euthanasia's Lightning Rod

He's a guy with great wisdom and no common sense.... If the
Nobel Prize committee is smart, they will give it to Kevorkian.
Provided I don't kill him first.
— Geoffrey Fieger, Jack Kevorkian's former attorney

Tick-tick-tick-tick-tick-tick-tick-tick. On the night of November 22, 1998, the familiar stopwatch announced the start of America's most popular television investigative news program, *60 Minutes*. More than twenty million people watched as correspondent Mike Wallace solemnly warned viewers about the visceral scene to come. They would see a videotape of Dr. Jack Kevorkian, a Michigan pathologist, euthanizing Thomas Youk, who suffered from end-stage ALS. It wasn't Kevorkian's first. Youk was, by estimate, Kevorkian's 130th deathing patient—but he would be his last. Kevorkian's dramatic appearance and Youk's on-camera death resulted in huge ratings and a heated discussion over broadcast ethics. The program galvanized the national controversy over the right to die and provoked yet another international frenzy over the man the media had branded "Dr. Death."

Dr. Arthur Caplan, director of the Center of Bioethics at the University of Pennsylvania, portrayed Kevorkian as "an explosion that came out of nowhere, a feisty doc basically saying, 'I'm going to take on the medical establishment. I'm going to take on the legal establishment and I'm going to do something unheard of. I'm going to assist people in dying publicly... then I'm going to dare somebody to come and prosecute me for it.'" [1]

Kevorkian considered physician-assisted suicide a civil right, protected by the Ninth Amendment to the Constitution. He unabashedly pushed the legal envelope to the limit, aiming at a single target: a Supreme Court decision that declared physician-assisted dying was legal nationwide.

Kevorkian was mystified as to why people found his logic and practices bizarre or threatening. He saw himself as a social welfare worker, dedicated to the betterment of humanity. Many heralded him as a genius, but his critics branded him a dangerous lunatic. Given his confrontational public persona and intensely held beliefs, intelligent people might have easily come to either—or both—of these conclusions.

Kevorkian was the son of Armenian immigrants who fled their homeland to escape their systematic extermination by the Turks between 1915 and 1918. Levon and Satenig Kevorkian raised three children in their new country. Their only son, Jack, was born on May 26, 1928, in Pontiac, Michigan.[2] With the smell of Middle Eastern oil in the air, the West didn't want to antagonize potential allies and refused to hold the Turks accountable for their genocide. As a result, Jack grew up in a household that perceived government as deceptive, blind to injustice, and unaccountable.

A precocious child, Jack was an avid reader, using what he learned to confront any statement that did not square with what he knew, taking on peers, teachers, and priests. People saw him as brainy but argumentative. His biographers noted that he could not connect well with other children or with most of his instructors because the subjects he was interested in were too complicated for them.[3]

His feeling of social isolation deepened when Kevorkian was promoted directly from the sixth to the eighth grade. Two years younger than his classmates, Kevorkian was at a complete loss when it came to social interaction. Instead, he poured his energy into his studies, further estranging himself from his peers. His formidable mind, implacable convictions, and uneasiness with human contact would define him.

His creativity found many outlets. With World War II underway, Kevorkian taught himself German and Japanese, becoming fluent in both languages. After graduating from high school with honors, Kevorkian was accepted at the University of Michigan, where he enrolled as a civil engineering major. He virtually lived in the library, studying philosophy, music, history, and any other subject that provoked his interest. Soon he questioned his choice of civil engineering, realizing that repetitive computations offered no "thrill of the hunt." He set his sights on medicine because great advancements were being made. Being part of a medical revolution suited him perfectly.

The University of Michigan's School of Medicine accepted him in record time. In his second year, Kevorkian became fascinated with pathology. As one biographer commented, "Without research or hands-on investigation of the human body [Kevorkian believed that] being a doctor would be no different than being an engineer." [4] Devoting almost all of his energy to pathology, and doing only what was necessary to pass his other classes, he graduated from medical school in the middle of his class in 1952 and was licensed to practice medicine in 1953. [5]

As an intern at Henry Ford Hospital in Detroit, he was exposed to human misery. The seminal moment when Kevorkian embraced euthanasia came soon after he started his internship. As he wrote in his autobiography:

> The patient was a helplessly immobile woman of middle age, her entire body jaundiced to an intense yellow-brown, skin stretched paper-thin over a fluid-filled abdomen swollen to four or five times normal size. The rest of her was an emaciated skeleton: sagging, discolored skin covered her bones like a cheap, wrinkled frock. The poor wretch stared up at me with yellow eyeballs sunken in their atrophic [withering] sockets. Her yellow teeth were ringed by chapping and parched lips to form an involuntary, almost sardonic 'smile' of death. It seemed as though she was pleading for help and death at the same time. Out of sheer empathy alone I could have helped her die with satisfaction. From that moment on, I was sure that doctor-assisted euthanasia and suicide are and always were ethical, no matter what anyone says or thinks. [6]

Upon completing his first year of internship, Kevorkian volunteered for medical service with the U.S. Army during the Korean War. In Korea, he saw men die because of a lack of blood for transfusions. The lives of others were prolonged for hours or days of needless pain before their inevitable deaths. He knew that there had to be ways to address such issues and vowed to find answers. [7]

Following his military discharge in 1955, he returned to the

University of Michigan as a first-year resident in pathology. He was eager to focus on research but was assigned the scut work that staff physicians did not want. Although the routine autopsies and examinations of surgical specimens were boring, they left him with hours to spend in the hospital library.

In 1955, there was no universally accepted medical definition of death. If a patient's heartbeat and breathing stopped, he or she was considered to be dead. Methods that would more accurately determine the point of death were needed to help decide whether or not to continue life-saving procedures.

Kevorkian took on the challenge of determining time of death. In dusty medical journals, nineteenth-century French doctors described the contraction of patients' retinas when they were near death.[8] Intrigued, Kevorkian decided that photographing the retina before, during, and after a person's death, could accurately determine the precise time of death—and define the difference between death and a coma.

With the consent of families and their physicians, he used an electrocardiograph to determine when dying patients' hearts stopped beating and then took pictures of their eyes with a sophisticated camera. His article on the results was published in December 1956.[9] Although his research was vital, advanced, and ethical, his innovative studies had nothing to do with saving lives and many of his colleagues found his work unnatural and creepy.[10]

Kevorkian's biographers wrote, "Soon the staff took to referring to the young resident's research as 'the doctor of death's rounds.' Within a few months, they simply began referring to him as 'Dr. Death.'"[11] Later, the moniker "Dr. Death" would come to taint virtually every story told about anything he did.

In a 2007 television interview, Kevorkian said that this nickname was affectionately given to him by his early medical colleagues. The nickname stuck—but the affectionate connotation did not. For the rest of his career, people would be repelled by the nature of his research. Its positive social value was largely lost in the distaste—the "yuck! factor"—it provoked.[12]

Judged a social misfit in his teenage years, Kevorkian was now viewed as a professional misfit as well. During his second year as a pathology resident, Kevorkian volunteered to trace the history of autopsy. His knowledge of German—the dominant language of science in the nineteenth century—enabled him to find references to the subject in obscure European medical journals. He learned that the kings of ancient Alexandria "decreed that condemned criminals were to be executed by submitting to dissection and experimentation in anatomical laboratories."[13]

The concept set Kevorkian's fertile mind abuzz. What if modern death-row inmates, after giving informed consent and being put under deep and irreversible anesthesia, could be used for experimentation and then donate their organs to science, after which the anesthesia would be increased until death occurred? Organ retrieval could not occur after the death because the methods of execution then in use made the organs useless.

The consent of the prisoners and the prison authorities would have to be obtained in advance. To see if this was feasible, Kevorkian drove to the Ohio State Penitentiary in October 1958. Soon the idealistic medical resident was sitting on a wooden stool, facing an inmate.

"I was quite apprehensive and suddenly unsure of myself," Kevorkian wrote. "What heretofore had been safe and comfortable philosophy had now become untested, down-to-earth reality.... There I was in the totally alien environment of death row, ready to start talking to a stranger about his excruciating extinction in the electric chair. What was I to say? How to start?"[14]

After listening as Kevorkian awkwardly explained his mission, the inmate said to a guard, "Maybe they could learn something from my body that might help my little daughter in the future." The prisoner agreed to anesthesia and experimentation, but the laws of Ohio forbade it.[15]

Kevorkian soon discovered that academic freedom often ended when taboos were challenged. When the University of Michigan gave him an ultimatum to drop his death studies or leave, he weighed the probable loss of his job against his right to conduct unfettered research and resigned, accepting a position as a third-year pathology resident at Michigan's Pontiac General Hospital.

There, Kevorkian's relentless research uncovered the fact that, since 1926, Russian medical personnel had successfully transfused blood from recently deceased patients into compatible living human recipients with virtually no ill effects. In addition, in the 1930s, Dr. Leonard L. Charpier, a surgeon in the Chicago area, had also successfully conducted such transfusions, but that information was never published in the United States.[16] Yet Kevorkian found it.

By 1937, the success of the Russian procedures had been presented to medical professionals in France and had been published in *The Lancet*, Britain's foremost medical journal. When Russia entered World War II, cadaver blood was used effectively in its battlefield hospitals, but the United States and its allies never accepted the idea.[17] Their rejection resulted in many preventable battlefield deaths, solely because Allied commanders were squeamish and unwilling to try the new procedure.

In 1961, Kevorkian published an article in the *American Journal of Clinical Pathology* describing four successful transfusions of cadaver blood that he and fellow researchers Neal Nicol and Edwin Rea had helped to perform.[18] Although his colleagues congratulated him, Kevorkian thought few laypeople would ever read the article.

To his surprise, *Time* magazine published an accurate and positive story on his work. Nevertheless, the writer stated, "U.S. doctors have shied away from [the use of cadaver blood] because of the prejudice against contact with anything taken from a corpse. The Pontiac pathologist hoped that this prejudice was weakening with wider acceptance of corneal grafting and the transplantation of bone and arteries from accident victims."[19]

Based on the success of his and the Russians' transfusions from cadavers, Kevorkian proposed that the procedure be used for soldiers during the Vietnam War. Under the right circumstances, dead soldiers could save their wounded comrades. The military, he thought, would finally leap on this concept. His research was published in *The Journal of Military Medicine* in 1964, but the Pentagon found the idea repugnant and turned it down.[20] Infuriated, Kevorkian vowed never again to waste his time seeking the approval of government agencies.[21]

Shortly after his plans for direct transfusion were rejected, Kevorkian learned that his mother had untreatable abdominal cancer. Her pain became so intense that he repeatedly asked the physicians to increase her morphine dosage. They refused, fearing that this might kill her or cause addiction. Delirious with pain, his mother lingered for several months before dying. Kevorkian became furious at the way people in terminal pain were treated.

With the agony of his mother's death echoing in the back of his mind, Kevorkian moved on. He served as the chief of pathology at Saratoga General Hospital in Detroit from 1970 to 1976. However, the medical genius in him finally burned out, and he moved to California to test another of his talents.

He used his savings and love of music to produce a feature film based on Handel's *Messiah*. An artistic flop, it never reached the theaters. Dejected and low on funds, he resumed his medical career. But he had learned a lesson that guided the rest of his life: "Don't do anything that takes a lot of money and people."[22]

As ascetic as ever, he abandoned hedonistic California and returned to a comfortable, minimalist lifestyle in his native Michigan. There his personal crusade focused upon changing end-of-life options. A no-talk, all-action man, Kevorkian believed that the legalization of physician-assisted suicide was the only reasonable way for suffering people to end their lives.

In 1986, he learned that euthanasia was being practiced by physicians in the Netherlands. Inspired, he traveled to Amsterdam, eager to learn from the Dutch and to share his ideas regarding medical experimentation on volunteer anesthetized prisoners immediately prior to their execution. The Dutch doctors, who had been practicing euthanasia (but decidedly not on prisoners) since the 1970s, were willing to share their expertise but had no interest in Kevorkian's prisoner-related research ideas.

Although widely used, euthanasia of the terminally ill was still illegal in the Netherlands, and physicians had no wish to call attention to their then-tacit *rapprochement* with the law. Dr. Pieter V. Admiraal, a pioneer of physician-assisted death in Holland, told Kevorkian what would happen if he took his proposals to Dutch authorities. "They'd hang you," he said.[23] Frustrated, Kevorkian returned to Michigan, vowing to put his theories into practice.

His reputation made it impossible to find work in any hospital. However, he still had valid medical licenses in Michigan and California. This left him with the privileges of a physician and an abundance of time to develop his plans, procedures, and equipment. In addition, his minimal need for creature comforts and lack of employment freed him to devote his considerable intellect to his causes. He was fifty-nine years old and in good health. His diet consisted largely of sandwiches. He slept on a mattress on the floor. For transportation, he rode a bicycle or drove a rusty, beige 1968 Volkswagen van. Unmarried and childless, he had no family responsibilities.

Although he bought his conservative wardrobe at thrift stores, he maintained it in such good condition that its humble origins were undetectable. While working at hospitals, he always wore a suit, conservative neckties, and a white shirt. On blustery days, he sported his signature porkpie hat.

In 1988, Kevorkian learned of David Rivlin, a thirty-eight-year-old Michigan man who had become a quadriplegic due to a surfing accident. Rivlin was unable to get enough funding from social services to pay for his home healthcare. After living in a nursing home for three years, unable to move, wash, or feed himself, Rivlin wanted to die, but his physician refused to disconnect his respirator for fear of legal liability. According to Kevorkian's close friend and colleague, Neal Nicol, Rivlin's plight inspired Kevorkian to create a solution: the suicide device that he named the Thanatron, Greek for "death machine." [24]

By the time Kevorkian visited him, Rivlin believed that he was out of options. Despite strong protests by right-to-life and disability rights activists, Rivlin asked for, and received, the state's permission to have his respirator turned off. Kevorkian thought that was a cruel way to die and raced to develop a machine that would provide Rivlin a gentle death.

After Rivlin ate his favorite meal—tortilla chips, guacamole, and salsa—Dr. John W. Finn, the medical director of the Hospice of Southeastern Michigan, administered a combination of Valium and morphine. Once Rivlin was unconscious, the respirator was turned off. Within half an hour, while three friends looked on, David Rivlin died on July 20, 1989. Had he been able to hang on just a little longer, Kevorkian might have spared him some of his ordeal. But although Kevorkian worked in a frenzy to create a functional deathing machine in time to help Rivlin die peacefully, he was unsuccessful. He completed his medical suicide device, which would soon become known as the Thanatron, on August 25, 1989. [25]

Because of his extensive knowledge of death by lethal injection, Kevorkian chose to build a machine that would deliver a fatal dose of chemicals through an intravenous (IV) line. When the patient was ready to die, Kevorkian would insert the line into a vein. Then he would start a harmless drip of saline solution.

Death would take place after the patient pushed a large red but-

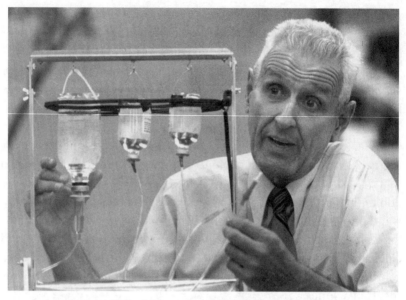

Kevorkian explains his Thanatron

ton, which stopped the flow of saline solution and started a flow of sodium thiopental, a fast-acting, sleep-inducing barbiturate. Unconsciousness would follow in twenty to thirty seconds. A timer would then release succinylcholine, a muscle paralyzer, mixed with potassium chloride, which would stop the heart.[26] Irreversible brain death from oxygen deprivation would usually occur within six minutes, and an electrocardiograph would quickly show the classic flat-line brain activity pattern seen in numerous television medical dramas.

Displaying both his thriftiness and inventiveness, Kevorkian built the first Thanatron using parts purchased at a Salvation Army store, flea markets, and garage sales and taken from his personal collection of medical supplies. Neither the prototype, which was completed in August 1989, nor the second attempt functioned properly. Kevorkian found better parts at a local flea market, and the third model worked perfectly. His total financial outlay had been about thirty dollars.[27]

Kevorkian opposed any form of euthanasia that could be easily used by depressed, irrational, or mentally incompetent people. His method had to satisfy three criteria. It must be able to produce a painless, certain death; be provided and supervised by a qualified physician; and be activated only by rational patients.

In 2009, when I asked him if terminally ill people should end their own lives using the latest gentle, painless do-it-yourself death-ing procedures that had been invented in the previous decade, Kevorkian replied, "Common sense shows the insanity of that statement! What medical service should the patient do on themselves? This [elective death] is a medical service." He went on to say that although the decision to elect death is the patient's choice, to carry it out without a doctor's assistance would be absurd.[28]

In order to distinguish the medical service he provided from rational self-deliverance or irrational suicide, he coined the term *patholysis* for it—and demanded that the American Medical Association adopt it.[29] They paid no attention.

In a 1988 Israeli medical journal article, "The Last Fearsome Taboo: Medical Aspects of Planned Death," he described a new branch of medicine that he called obitiatry.[30] It would provide planned deaths through a network of suicide clinics (*obitoria*) in each state. Patients would have the option of permitting medical experimentation and organ donation while under deep anesthesia prior to their deaths.

Kevorkian approached the Hemlock Society USA with a plan to open an obitorium in California, Hemlock's home state, where he would carry out physician-assisted suicides. Hemlock, he proposed, would refer dying clients to him. He met with Derek Humphry in Los Angeles and was astonished when Humphry was not at all enthusiastic.

"The place for voluntary euthanasia is in the home, accompanied by watchful friends and caring family as chosen by the patient, with the services of a willing doctor who possesses signed releases according to law," Humphry said.[31] He told Kevorkian that Hemlock was backing a voter initiative in California to allow voluntary euthanasia and physician aid-in-dying.

Kevorkian responded that if Hemlock supported his obitorium project, it would attract huge publicity for the initiative. When Humphry pointed out the conflicting goals of their two philosophies, Kevorkian petulantly stomped out of the meeting, muttering that Hemlock and Humphry were pathetically weak.[32] From that day on, Kevorkian scorned Hemlock and its founder.

To provide ethical standards for what he viewed as a universal civil right, Kevorkian drew up a list of mandatory protocols and procedures that he planned to follow and that other doctors assisting a suicide ought to use:

1. Foremost, the patient had to express a firm, voluntary, and unwavering wish to die.
2. A medical doctor was, and is, a necessity.
3. [An explicit] medical history must be obtained.
4. Consultation with family doctors and doctor specialists was a high priority.
5. Extensive and multiple consultations should be made.
6. The nearest relatives and/or best friends should be in attendance, when appropriate and feasible.
7. Psychiatric consultation was required to determine mental competency and lack of any psychiatric disorder.
8. Consultation regarding social interplay was necessary to detect personal or family disputes or irregularities, enabling a clarification of any financial problems among family members.
9. If requested by the patient, clergy would be involved.
10. The services provided would be pro bono (without fee), thereby eliminating any abuse for financial gain.
11. Legal consultations regarding testimonials were recommended.[33]

His protocols did not require the patient to be either incurably or terminally ill. After they were published in 1992 in the *American Journal of Forensic Psychiatry*, Kevorkian could rightfully lay claim to having developed the first formal set of ethical rules for conducting physician-assisted deaths.[34] Unfortunately, when he actually started helping patients die, he routinely ignored many of his own protocols.

Initially, Kevorkian had difficulty getting the word out about his euthanasia services. His classified ads in local newspapers read, "Death counseling. Is someone in your family terminally ill? Does he or she wish to die—and with dignity? Call physician consultant...." He got two responses: one from a man whose brother had been in a coma for six months and, therefore, could not give informed consent, and the other from a rambling young woman whom he judged to be mentally ill.[35]

To find suitable patients, he spoke with oncologists, offering them his professional card, which read, "Jack Kevorkian, M.D. Bioethics and obitiatry. Special death counseling, by appointment only."[36] Although some approved of his concept, they were predictably leery of supporting him publicly.

An initial meeting with three doctors and a small number of other medical personnel was held at a Detroit-area hospital, but a larger, official conference was quickly squelched by horrified hospital officials.[37] When Kevorkian submitted a professional ad to the *Oakland County Medical Society Bulletin* reading, "Doctor seeking patients for new practice of obitiatry," the society refused to run it.[38]

A story about the refusal to publish Kevorkian's ads caught the attention of two Detroit newspapers, and both ran feature stories about it. The resulting controversy produced a spate of interviews, one on *The Phil Donahue Show*, and the national press latched onto the unique news. Kevorkian was now on the fast track to fame, and his first patient was not long in arriving.

Oregon resident Janet Adkins was fatally ill with Alzheimer's disease. A woman of many talents, she had taught English and piano, taken up hang gliding, trekked the mountains of Nepal, and climbed Mount Hood. When the vibrant, fifty-four-year-old Hemlock Society member received her diagnosis, she was determined not to put herself or her family through the agony that lay ahead.

She first saw Kevorkian on *The Phil Donahue Show*. At her request, her husband contacted him on November 13, 1989.[39] Because he had yet to conduct his first deathing (he referred to them as "events"), Kevorkian wanted Adkins to explore all her other options. Over a period of several months, he discussed her case with three physicians in Portland, asking them to help her die. All three declined.[40]

Frustrated, Adkins decided to end her life quickly, before she lost the ability to care for herself. In June 1990, she and her husband flew to Michigan. They met Kevorkian at a restaurant, where he explained his procedure and decided that she was alert and able to understand the choice she wanted to make. Later, Kevorkian recorded discussions of her medical history, her medical records, and the data for his seven-page questionnaire. With two witnesses present, Adkins signed several detailed legal documents.[41] Then, she and Kevorkian made plans to meet the following Monday for her death, using his new lethal injection machine.

Only one problem remained—where she would die. "For two days Jack scouted locations to perform the medicide," his biographers wrote.[42] "He had little luck. Sympathetic people feared repercussions if they let him use their homes. Churches wanted no connection with him. He didn't want to use his own apartment or his sister Margo's for fear that they might be evicted or the landlords found liable. He was turned down by several motels, funeral homes, and landlords with vacant office space."[43]

Kevorkian had overlooked the obvious. If he was afraid to use his own residence for the deathing, how could he expect others to risk legal action and social ostracism and lend him theirs?

With no alternative in sight, Kevorkian was forced to use his Volkswagen van.[44] Though the exterior of the van was rusty, the interior was quite clean. He installed a cot and bought new sheets, pillowcases, and crisp yellow curtains. Supporters suggested that he drive the van to Groveland Oaks, a nearby public park and camping site that had an electrical hookup for his Thanatron and an electrocardiograph machine.

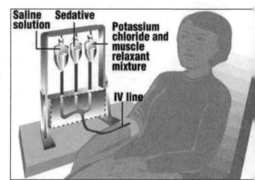

On June 4, 1990, just after 9 a.m., Kevorkian's sisters picked up Adkins at her motel. She was dressed in a white blouse, black suit, and a black-and-white scarf with a defiant dash of red. After exchanging tearful goodbyes with her loved ones, Adkins was driven to the campground. Almost two hours

How a Thanatron patient initiated death

later, after a nervous Kevorkian finished testing the Thanatron, she entered the van and lay down on the cot.

At Adkins' request, Kevorkian's sister read the 23rd Psalm.[45] Kevorkian then hooked Adkins up to an electrocardiograph. Next, he inserted the IV needle into her arm and started the saline drip. As he made the final preparations, she said, "Hurry."

He replied, "Have a safe journey." [46]

After he again verified that she was ready to end her life, he reminded her to push the red button to start the process, and she did. Just before she died, Adkins looked at him with grateful eyes and said, "Thank you, thank you, thank you." [47]

The saline drip stopped, the flow of thiopental began, and the courageous woman quickly became unconscious. Then the timer started the flow of drugs that would paralyze her muscles and stop her heart. Janet Adkins died six minutes after she pushed the red button.

After he confirmed her death with a stethoscope and the heart monitor, as well as the dilation of her pupils, Kevorkian disconnected the IV line, called the medical examiner's office, and told them what he and Adkins had done.

Kevorkian's precedent-setting use of the Thanatron exploded into the media the next day and quickly ignited a national debate over physician-assisted suicide. In an interview that appeared on the front page of the *New York Times*, Kevorkian said he had helped Adkins because he wanted to force the medical and legal professions to consider this idea.

Derek Humphry was attending the World Federation of Right to Die Societies' biennial congress in Holland when *Newsweek* phoned to ask his opinion on Adkins' death. Humphry replied, "It's not death with dignity to die in the back of a van. But what else could this woman do, because her doctors had deserted her."[48] *Newsweek* printed only the first sentence. Kevorkian was enraged. Even though Humphry called him to explain what had happened, Kevorkian was not placated, and his hatred for Humphry deepened.

On June 8, 1990, Kevorkian stood before Oakland County Circuit Court Judge Alice Gilbert. The prosecutor had asked for a temporary restraining order to prevent him from using his deathing machine again. Doing himself no favors, Kevorkian refused to use an attorney and defended his position from the witness box. There, he vented his anger against what he believed to be an archaic, patriarchal, and sanctimonious medical profession.

Showing his contempt for their "Dark Age mentality," he concluded, "If they could do it today they would burn me at the stake."[49] He promised that even if his medical license was revoked, he would build another device and use another system.[50] Unmoved, Judge Gilbert issued a temporary restraining order, which stated that until his case was resolved, neither Kevorkian nor anyone associated with him could use a suicide machine or in any way facilitate a suicide in Michigan. Kevorkian was later charged with first-degree murder in the Adkins case, but the charges were dismissed on December 12, 1990, when District Judge Gerald McNally ruled that Michigan had no law against assisted suicide.

This was the first of a swarm of trials that Kevorkian would endure in the following eight years, never wavering in his position on personal autonomy. "Personal choice is what it is all about. Quality of life, as opposed to maintaining existence," he told *Vanity Fair.*[51]

In 1991, Washington State's Initiative 119 (I-119) regarding death with dignity was headed for the polls. If it passed, the bill would make Washington the first state to legalize physician-assisted suicide for terminally ill patients. The initiative had heavy statewide support, and Humphry's Hemlock Society had provided considerable funding for the cause. Knowing of Kevorkian's high media profile, supporters of the bill repeatedly urged him not to rock the boat by assisting any more suicides before the November 5 vote.

Kevorkian thought otherwise. Much of his anger at Hemlock was fueled by professional jealousy. Humphry, a mere journalist, not a credentialed physician, was a center of world attention when it came to euthanasia and assisted dying. Humphry was also the respected leader of the nation's largest right-to-die activist group.

Then there was the matter of book sales. In 1991, both men had published euthanasia books. Humphry's *Final Exit* had taken off as a wildfire best-seller, gaining international attention, and heading the *New York Times* best-seller list. Kevorkian's book, *Prescription Medicide: The Goodness of Planned Death*, languished on the shelves, with *Publisher's Weekly* describing it as a "self-dramatizing, often strident manifesto."[52]

Kevorkian told Washington's Ralph Mero, who wrote the first draft of the initiative, "I believe Proposition #119 deserves to lose and I have no interest in supporting its aims."[53] On October 23, less than two weeks before the vote, Kevorkian helped two women die within minutes of each other. Marjorie Lee Wantz, fifty-eight, married, and a former elementary school teacher, complained of intense, untreatable pain following what she described as ten surgeries to remove vaginal tumors and her uterus and ovaries.

She had already attempted to kill herself three times using the exhaust gases from her car, not knowing that the addition of automobile catalytic converters in 1975 eliminated virtually all the toxic carbon monoxide that had formerly enabled many car suicides. She desperately feared another botched suicide attempt. With her husband by her side, she told Kevorkian that by using his services, "I feel it's going to be done right. It's going to be fast, no mistakes."[54]

Sherry Ann Miller, forty-four, a divorcée whose two young children lived with their father, suffered from multiple sclerosis and felt she had no reason to live. A former clerical worker living on disability, she had moved in with her parents because she could not care for herself. By the time she chose to die, she weighed only eighty-nine pounds.

This time, because of the difficulty he had in finding a place to help Janet Adkins die, Kevorkian chose a very private setting—a rustic cabin in Bald Mountain State Park near Lake Orion, Michigan. The women would lie on cots, close together. Kevorkian would sit between them and would use the Thanatron.

The next day, Wantz died by lethal injection as planned. But Miller's emaciation made it impossible to find a usable vein for the IV line. So Kevorkian helped her die using a carbon monoxide inhalation backup system he had invented. This device became known as the Mercitron ("mercy machine"), and Miller was the first of many patients to use it.

Kevorkian was reluctant to publicize the Mercitron carbon monoxide method because it could easily be made and used without physician assistance. The simple system consisted of a face mask connected by a plastic tube to a tank of carbon monoxide gas.

Kevorkian's colleague and biographer, Neal Nicol, who accompanied him on

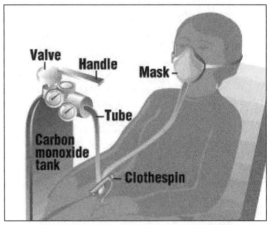

How a Mercitron patient initiated death

many of his missions, owned a medical supply business. This gave him ready access to suppliers of inert gases. Nicol asked a welding supply company to custom-mix cylinders of gas containing 9.5 percent carbon monoxide and 90.5 percent nitrogen, as concentrations above 10 percent incur more restrictive shipping requirements.[55] "When the carbon monoxide concentration rises to 10 percent or more," Nicol said, "it becomes explosive.... We bought it in lots of ten tanks. We never had to use more than half a tank per patient."[56]

The Wantz-Miller deathings shocked the nation and contributed to the narrow defeat of I-119. By helping to derail the initiative, a defiant Kevorkian had gotten his revenge against Humphry and Hemlock. But in doing so, he helped scuttle a law that would have furthered the very cause he championed: elective death.

On July 21, 1992, a circuit court judge dismissed the charges against Kevorkian in the deaths of Miller and Wantz because Michigan still had no law against assisting a suicide. Kevorkian soon stepped up the frequency of his highly publicized deathings. One problem dogged him. He was forever short of available places to carry out the deathings of his patients. Several months after the deaths of Wantz and Miller, he asked his friend Neal Nicol if he could use his house for the death of Lois Hawes. Nicol agreed. "Eaten up" by cancer, Hawes arrived with two of her closest friends and died there on September 26, 1992.

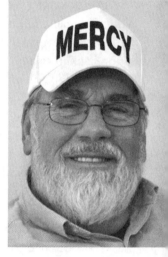

"The feeling of satisfaction that I got from that was so great," Nicol told me, "that I knew I could never do anything wrong by helping a person that much in need."[57]

In a bizarre turnaround, scarcely two years after thumbing his nose at Hemlock and trying to derail the Washington death-with-dignity voters' initiative, Kevorkian kicked off an unsuccessful ballot initiative to legalize physician-assisted suicide in Michigan. "This is really a right that already exists, and we already have, but which we

Neal Nicol

have to put into writing because of human irrationality," he told an audience of seven hundred in suburban Detroit. "Every reasonable adult is going to have to realize that if he votes 'no' on this, he is throwing his right away."[58] It was a speech that could have been cribbed directly from the media releases for Washington's I-119, which he had successfully helped to torpedo.

In 1991, just before the Adkins case was thrown out, the Michigan State Board of Medicine revoked Kevorkian's medical license, although there had been no complaints or disciplinary action against him in the forty-seven years he had held it. The revocation was irrelevant to Kevorkian. He still had a valid California medical license, which enabled him to order legally controlled drugs.

Even the 1993 revocation of his California license—the state's

attorney general declared him "fundamentally unfit to practice medicine"—had no effect on his activities.[59] He had already developed
the Mercitron, which did not require controlled substances. In addition, Kevorkian still had a supply of lethal drugs, and both patients
and right-to-die advocates gladly donated additional drugs to him.

On December 3, 1992, the Michigan legislature passed a hastily
written bill making assisted suicide a felony, carrying a jail sentence
of up to four years. The statute and its successors were expressly
written to stop Kevorkian, but the law had so many loopholes that
his lawyers easily found ways to work around them, and the law
barely even slowed Kevorkian down.

On August 4, 1993, Thomas Hyde, thirty, a landscaper and carpenter dying from ALS, chose death on his own terms in Kevorkian's van in Belle Isle, a Detroit park. Kevorkian promptly reported
the death and was charged with violating the new law. Unfazed, he
attended the deathing of cancer patient Donald O'Keefe, seventy-
three, in Redford Township, Michigan, and was later acquitted of
Hyde's death.

Anti-euthanasia groups were livid over Kevorkian's ability to
escape conviction on any of the charges filed against him. Nicol recalled a private attempt to trap him. "The group run by Rita Marker
[then known as the International Task Force on Euthanasia and
Assisted Suicide, and now as the Patients Rights Council] attempted a sting operation on Dr. Kevorkian back in the early 1990s by
submitting a fictitious medical history in the hopes of entrapping
him," Nicol wrote.[60] The ruse was detected and failed.

Continuing in his quest for the ideal setting for assisted suicides,
and finding no support for his suicide clinics, Kevorkian rented a
vacant building on a rural highway in Springfield Township, Michigan. He named it The Margo Janus Mercy Clinic after his late sister,
who was one of his staunchest supporters. On his business cards for
the clinic, he listed his name, his late sister's name, Neal Nicol, and
a phone number. On the back was a handwritten explanation of the
clinic's name and purpose: the "<u>M</u>ovement <u>E</u>nsuring the <u>R</u>ight to
<u>C</u>hoose for <u>Y</u>ourself."[61]

His first and only Mercy obitorium client was Erika Garcellano,
sixty, a nursing home aide who had been suffering from ALS for
three years. She was brought to Kevorkian's obitorium by her two
sons and a friend, all of whom were with her when she died.[62] Upon

learning of Garcellano's death, the owner of the building demanded that Kevorkian vacate the property.[63]

Kevorkian did have some supporters among the medical community. In 1995, he announced the formation of Physicians for Mercy, a small group of doctors who were sympathetic to physician-assisted suicide. Among the first members was bluff, good-natured Dr. Georges René Reding, a Belgian psychiatrist who had practiced in Belgium and New York prior to moving to Michigan. He and Kevorkian were two of the five physicians present at the deathing of Austin Bastable, a prominent, terminally ill Canadian. Reding, a practicing Catholic, is the only doctor who admitted to having helped Kevorkian with deathings outside Michigan. He had previously helped patients die in Belgium. Later, in the United States, he assisted with five of Kevorkian's deathings, starting with Bastable's on May 6, 1996.[64] Reding fled to Europe after being indicted for murder in the 1997 assisted suicide case of Donna Brennan in New Mexico. A district attorney there sought his extradition to the United States for prosecution, but the case remains unresolved.

Even with the loss of his suicide clinic, Kevorkian seemed unstoppable. By 1998, he had helped an estimated 130 people die, all in Michigan. After three different juries refused to convict him of any crime associated with the deaths, Kevorkian began to think of himself as legally invincible. His lawyer, however, knew better.

Kevorkian's courtroom personality was totally unpredictable, and he was often his own worst enemy. One memorable spectacle took place in May 1995. The Michigan Supreme Court had ruled that the state had no law explicitly banning assisting a suicide, but it decided that this was a felony under common law and reinstated four previously dismissed cases. At his arraignment hearing, Kevorkian arrived in homemade stocks, from which hung the sign, "Common Law of the Middle Ages! What's next—the Inquisition?" The rest of his mock-colonial costume consisted of tights, a powdered wig, and shoes with huge buckles.[65]

During another case, he withdrew entirely from the fray and let his lawyer, Geoffrey Nels Fieger, do all the talking. "To him it was all a farce and a game.... While Fieger thundered, trying to set the stage for a decision as momentous as *Roe v. Wade*, his client intently studied vocabulary lists of Japanese verbs."[66]

Kevorkian had successfully avoided prison because he had the good fortune to be represented by a highly skilled attorney who could work around his client's eccentricities. Like Kevorkian, Fieger was outspoken, audacious, and tenacious—and shared P.T. Barnum's passion for showmanship.

Unlike Kevorkian, who thought the field of law was asinine unless it coincided with his personal vision, Fieger maintained a laser-like focus on his goal: keeping his client out of jail. Kevorkian and his lawyer were known for their catfights, but the feisty pathologist knew the value of his hard-hitting attorney and, sometimes against his better judgment, stuck with Fieger—until the most important case in his life came to trial: Michigan v. Jack Kevorkian, 1998.

Thomas Youk's heavily publicized death ended Kevorkian's career as an obitiatrist. This time, Kevorkian did play God. Instead of helping Youk take his own life, he deliberately crossed the line by directly injecting him with fatal drugs and videotaped the entire process. Despite Youk's fully informed consent, that act made the procedure a straightforward case of active euthanasia, a first for Kevorkian. It brought about not only the death that Youk so fervently wanted but also a verdict from which Kevorkian thought he was immune.

Believing that he owned the moral high ground on the subject of physician-assisted suicide, Kevorkian was ready to celebrate one final victory and shock the medical and legislative world into changing the law. By filming himself injecting Thomas Youk with lethal drugs and handing the evidence to the world via *60 Minutes*, he dared the courts to try him. They obliged.

Three days after *60 Minutes* aired, Michigan charged him with committing first-degree murder, violating the assisted suicide law, and delivering a controlled substance without a medical license. Then the overconfident Kevorkian made the worst decision of his life. Over the impassioned protests of his supporters, he dismissed Fieger and insisted on defending himself, despite having the "legal knowledge equivalent to that of your average space alien," according to one observer.[67]

Without Fieger, Kevorkian failed to spot the prosecution's forthcoming tactical move. He planned to call Youk's widow and brother to testify how greatly Youk had suffered, how rational his decision was to seek Kevorkian's help, and how strongly they supported Youk's choice. That was the strategy that previously led jury after jury to effectively nullify Michigan's assisted suicide law.

But this time, the charges were different. The prosecutors chose to try Kevorkian only for murder and illegal distribution of controlled substances. Kevorkian was stunned when the judge ruled that the testimony of his two witnesses was inadmissible. Kevorkian mistakenly agreed to allow charges of assisting a suicide to be dropped. This doomed his case because, in a murder case, the condition of the patient was not relevant.

"In assisted suicide cases, the defense can call evidence of suffering and choice, whereas in murder cases this cannot be done," wrote Derek Humphry, who had studied hundreds of similar cases worldwide. "In a murder case, only evidence of the action and who did it can be admitted."[68]

Kevorkian had no other witnesses to call. The jury had the video showing Kevorkian directly injecting Youk with the lethal chemicals that caused his death. The judge charged the jury solely to decide if Kevorkian had willfully given Youk the chemicals that killed him—and of that, there was no doubt. The "case of the century" lasted only a day and a half. The jury had nothing to deliberate. They found Kevorkian guilty of murder in the second degree and of delivering a controlled substance.

On April 14, 1990, Circuit Court Judge Jessica Cooper read the riot act to Kevorkian before sentencing him to ten to twenty-five years in prison:

> Based upon the fact that you publicly and repeatedly announced your intentions to disregard the laws of this state, I question whether you will ever cease and desist. The fact that your attorney in a pre-sentence investigation says you're out of business from this point forward doesn't negate your past statements. . . .
>
> Perhaps even a stronger factor in sentencing is deterrence. This trial was not about the political or moral correctness of euthanasia. It was all about you, sir. It was about lawlessness. It was about disrespect for a society that exists and flourishes because of the strength of the legal system. No one, sir, is above the law. No one.
>
> So let's talk just a little bit more about you specifically. You were on bond to another judge when you committed this of-

fense; you were not licensed to practice medicine when you committed this offense; and you hadn't been licensed for eight years. And you had the audacity to go on national television, show the world what you did and dare the legal system to stop you. Well, sir, consider yourself stopped.[69]

Kevorkian wanted to be prosecuted and convicted so that he could argue his case before the Supreme Court and win once and for all. The tactic failed. Because there were no procedural errors in the murder trial and no constitutional issues, appeals to higher courts were pointless. As a result, seventy-year-old Jack Kevorkian became a convicted murderer and prisoner #284797 of the State of Michigan.

In 2005, prison doctors told Kevorkian that he was suffering from hepatitis C, which he had contracted while researching cadaver blood transfusions forty years earlier.[70] He was up for parole at that time, and an MSNBC poll revealed that 88 percent of the respondents thought he should be freed. Despite his medical condition, and numerous pleas from his legions of supporters, the parole board denied his request for an early release.

Two years later, Kevorkian prevailed. The parole board announced that he would be released because of ill health. In addition to hepatitis C, he had diabetes and was painfully thin. His attorneys alleged that he had less than a year to live. His skeptical opponents decried the board's decision. Stephen Drake, spokesman for Not Dead Yet, a disability rights group that vigorously opposed assisted suicide in general and Kevorkian in particular, predicted, "We expect that Kevorkian will show 'near miraculous' recovery from his alleged grave medical problems." He also prophesied that "Mike Wallace or Barbara Walters can be expected to do a very sympathetic and biased interview with Kevorkian . . . and portray him as some kind of martyr."[71] Drake's predictions proved to be totally accurate.

On Friday, June 1, 2007, Kevorkian, seventy-nine, walked out the front door of Coldwater State Prison. Slightly stooped, dressed in his signature blue cardigan sweater, a white shirt, and a striped tie, he was upbeat in his brief statements. The first to greet him was *60 Minutes* reporter Mike Wallace, who embraced the former pathologist and playfully asked, "What do you say, young man?"

After the CBS crew quickly ushered Kevorkian into a large white van, Wallace conducted the first interview with him as they drove him home. Refuting a *New York Times* description of Kevorkian as "deluded and unrepentant," Wallace declared, "The Jack Kevorkian I know is a warm, engaged, thoughtful and compassionate individual who speaks Japanese, plays the flute, reads voraciously and is of academic bent."[72]

For the duration of his parole, Kevorkian was forbidden to directly advise anyone about assisted suicide or assist a suicide him-

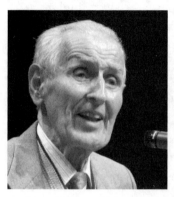

self. However, he was free to discuss and campaign for the right to die. Reflecting in the first minutes after his release, he said, "I'm going to work with activist groups trying to get [euthanasia] legalized. . . . Either through legislatures or through courts if possible."[73]

However, his apparently new willingness to work with others for law reform quickly evaporated. In a press conference at Kutztown University on September 20, 2009, his last national appearance, Kevorkian lashed out at existing death-with-dignity laws be-

Kevorkian at Kutztown University

cause of their restrictive procedures. When I asked him, "Will you work to extend those laws to other states?" he had a feisty reply.

> That would be like a law extending torture. It's crazy. [Euthanasia] has nothing to do with law. Those three states— Washington, Oregon, and Montana—are doing it wrong. A doctor can't even participate [except to evaluate the patient and prescribe the lethal drugs]. He can't help the patient [take the lethal drugs] if the patient is crippled or paralyzed or can't put the pill in his mouth…. That's a medical service? Why do we perpetuate suffering like that unnecessarily?[74]

Kevorkian's parole restrictions expired in 2009, two years after his release from prison. The media, and those who knew him well, waited expectantly to see if he would resume his euthanasia activities. In a 2010 interview with Neal Nicol, Kevorkian's long-time colleague and friend, I asked, "Am I correct in assuming that Jack Kevorkian's direct involvement with helping people die on a hands-on basis is over?" I did not expect Nicol's response.

"He still gets requests for help, but no, he is not participating. At first it was a condition of parole, so he had no choice. But I think he would, still. If the right case came along, he would do it," Nicol told me.[75]

On July 1, 2010, Rev. George Exoo, head of the Compassionate Chaplaincy who was still trying to establish an AIDS and right-to-die hospice, received an unexpected email from Nicol, who wrote, "Surprise, surprise. Had a meeting with Jack this morning along with his attorney and proposed that Jack align himself with you in your efforts. This is in an effort to keep Jack in the forefront of a movement to allow patients to self-determine their fate. He suggested a meeting with you and I to discuss details of your plan.... If this is agreeable with you, get together any supporters and select a couple dates and we will try to set it up."[76] Ultimately, Kevorkian changed his mind about the proposed alliance, never met with Exoo, and nothing came of the proposal.

Jack Kevorkian remains an iconic figure and hero to legions of people. On the morning of June 3, 2011, I received an unexpected email from Neal Nicol. He wrote that Jack had died at 2:30 that morning from a pulmonary embolism. It happened while Kevorkian was being treated at William Beaumont Hospital in Royal Oak, Michigan.[77] He had been hospitalized for pneumonia and kidney cancer in May 2011 and returned to the hospital about a week later. He developed pulmonary pneumonia thrombosis, and a blood clot that had formed in his leg made its way to his heart and killed him. Kevorkian was eighty-three. His death, by an odd quirk of fate, occurred on my birthday. At the exact time of his death that morning, I had, quite by chance, been finishing the final edit of this chapter.

Kevorkian had long considered the outcome of his own mortality. "You don't know what will happen when you get old," he said in a 1998 interview with *60 Minutes*. "I may end up terribly suffering. I want some colleague to be free to come and help me when I say the time has come. That's what I'm fighting for, me. And if it helps everybody else, so be it."[78]

He never chose to ask for a hastened death. "Ultimately, it came peacefully and pain-free in the hospital. During his last two hours, the nurses in the ICU piped in music by Johann Sebastian Bach, one of his favorite composers. "We did it because we knew it would make him happy," said his friend and attorney Mayer Morgenroth.

Anti-euthanasia activist Wesley J. Smith implied that Kevorkian should have ended his own life in the same way that he assisted others to end theirs: via an assisted suicide. "His death had a certain irony," Smith wrote. "Despite being in declining health, he never took the out that he offered to other people."[79]

Smith's position was specious. The reason Kevorkian did not choose a hastened death for himself was obvious. He did not *need* any extreme measures to achieve a peaceful death, and hence, did not ask for any. The right-to-die community—part of which supports Kevorkian's method of operations and part of which does not—has made it clear for decades that it seeks to legally *empower* any rational adult to *choose* a hastened death should life become unbearable, not to *force* it upon someone. Kevorkian's unaccelerated natural death was a testament to personal autonomy and the fundamental concept that an assisted, hastened death should be a civil *right* for any rational adult, not a *requirement*.

The world holds widely divergent views of Kevorkian and his astonishing beliefs and deeds. Many who chronicled his headline-making career had reduced their ambivalent conclusions about him and his work to a four-word mantra: "Right message, wrong messenger." On the day after Kevorkian's death, Brian Dickerson, a *Detroit Free Press* journalist who had often interviewed him, wrote, "Today that strikes me as too pat. History is seldom made by those who are reluctant to break rules or to challenge popular conventions."[80]

Kevorkian remains an iconic figure and hero to legions of people. Until his health took him off the streets of Detroit, people regularly stopped him and asked for his autograph—and he always gracefully obliged. Yet, while many of those who fervently believe in the right to die with dignity applauded his courage, they winced at his refusal to work with others to achieve their common goal and decried his arrogance and his failure to employ his own list of safeguards. And the question of whether Kevorkian ethically served the best interests of his patients will likely remain a relevant topic of debate for a long time. One thing is certain: the family members of those whom Kevorkian helped end their lives were and remain his staunchest public supporters, and none of them ever came forward to rebuke or sue him for what he did.

Kevorkian's outrageous antics and extreme statements forced the mainstream right-to-die movement to distance itself from him and fine-tune its message in the 1990s. In comparison to state-based death-with-dignity legislative proposals, his in-your-face, renegade tactics made the more conservative legislative proposals look moderate in comparison. To that extent, he did the movement a favor. Portland attorney Eli Stutsman, who was deeply involved in drafting the death-with-dignity laws in Oregon and Washington, noted, "In the end he was helpful because we used his approach as an example of a problem," he said.[81]

Under Derek Humphry's leadership, the Hemlock Society USA disavowed him, but several succeeding Hemlock leaders embraced him. Some Hemlock members revered him as a savior; others saw him as a public menace.

Marilynne Seguin, founder of Dying With Dignity, Canada, and an early Kevorkian supporter, wrote in 1994, "I am repelled by his publicity seeking, which flies in the face of the need to respect each person's right to privacy and compassion. Such behavior simply makes a spectacle—a circus—out of the desperation and despair of vulnerable people in our otherwise civilized society."[82]

Despite the fact that he had drawn the public's attention to the issue of physician aid-in-dying, Kevorkian's contempt for the law and brief acquaintance with most of his patients scarcely qualified him to be the poster child for the death-with-dignity movement. Yet, as John Hofsess said, "Jack conveyed a message . . . about people exercising a fundamental right. In that, he lit a flame, a tribute to freedom of choice, and that will be his legacy."[83]

But there is another significant vantage point for the perception of Kevorkian's work: the harm principle. As described in *On Liberty*, the work of the eminent English thinker, John Stuart Mill, "the harm principle states that individuals are free to act in any way —so long as that behavior does not harm others. The only purpose for which power can rightfully be exercised over any member of a civilized community against his will, is to prevent harm to others," Mill wrote. "In the part which merely concerns himself, his independence is, of right, absolute. Over himself, over his own body and mind, the individual is sovereign."[84]

Kevorkian did not ask for any commemoration of his passing. Nevertheless, a public memorial service, followed by a small private burial service, was held for him on June 10, 2011, at the White Chapel Memorial Cemetery in Troy, Michigan, near his former home.

"We weren't going to do anything," said Mayer Morganroth, "but we started getting calls from all across the country and from foreign countries, too."[85]

The chapel, which has a capacity of about two hundred mourners, filled to overflowing. Kevorkian's casket was draped with a U.S. flag, a right he had earned by his service in the Korean War. A large photograph of him smiling stood nearby. His surviving sister, Flora Kevorkian Holzheimer, and his niece, Ava Janus, attended the ceremonies. Later that day, he was buried beside his parents and his other sister, Margaret "Margo" Kevorkian Janus.

"After all the years of fighting the medical and legal establishments, and falling way short of his goals, Kevorkian is finally at peace," a friend said.[86] Kevorkian had asked that any memorials be donated to The Salvation Army, in whose thrift stores he bought his clothing and what little furniture he owned.

So what is Jack Kevorkian's legacy? John Hofsess, founder of the Right to Die Society of Canada, said, "He served a unique purpose at a time when most other people in the so-called 'right-to-die movement' were just talking and doing nothing."[87]

Without question, Kevorkian made a huge and indelible imprint on the world's consciousness. The title of the 2011 television movie made about him, *You Don't Know Jack*, will be accurate for a long time. It will be decades before any consensus will be reached about the degree to which he was a compassionate, visionary medical pioneer or a menace to society.

The description that Kevorkian himself might have enjoyed most came from *Detroit News* journalist, Jack Lessenberry, who had covered Kevorkian for over two decades. In a blog posting written shortly after Kevorkian's passing, he summed up Kevorkian's impact succinctly. "He was the crank who made us rethink how lives should end."[88]

– 4 –

The Twilight Zone

The story of Terri Schiavo should be disturbing to all of us.
How can it be that medicine, ethics, law, and family could work so
poorly together in meeting the needs of this woman who was left in a
persistent vegetative state after having cardiac arrest?
— Dr. Timothy E. Quill

Hundreds of thousands of people worldwide are trapped between life and death, locked into unstoppable medical decline, progressive dementia, or persistent or permanent vegetative states. These people are powerless in the hands of others, often confined without a voice in institutions controlled by inflexible rules or impersonal regulations.

They become shackled by these invisible chains because they live in places where culture, laws, or religions prohibit them, while still competent and able, to make legally enforceable decisions on their behalf or to designate proxies to do it for them when they can no longer do it themselves. The campaign to enact laws that empower people to designate in advance what kind of medical procedures they do and do not want if catastrophic disease, injury, or incapacitation strikes, and who may speak for them if they are no longer physically or mentally able to do so for themselves, has been at the top of the death-with-dignity movement's agenda since the 1970s.

Even where advance healthcare directives are legal, most people do not make plans for future incapacitation while they are mentally competent. If they do not, and the need arises for someone they trust to have the legal authority to make end-of-life decisions for them, it is too late.

With the advent of dramatic medical measures such as cardiopulmonary resuscitation (CPR), respirators, extraordinary new drugs, and tube feeding of food and fluids, people once doomed to certain death can be kept alive, although not necessarily restored to health. Today, many patients fall into a medical "twilight zone": technically alive, but not capable of sustaining life without constant and intense artificial assistance.

A vegetative state occurs in comatose patients with severe brain damage. After being in a vegetative state for four weeks, unable to react to external stimuli, a patient is usually classified as being in a persistent vegetative state. If his or her condition does not improve within one year, and is not likely to improve, the diagnosis is usually reclassified as permanent vegetative state. In the United States, it is estimated that 15,000 patients are in a permanent vegetative state, and more than 100,000 others are in a minimally conscious state.[1]

Twenty-first-century medicine has thoroughly blurred the line between life and death. The need to define that line becomes progressively more important. Explains American physician James Murtagh, "Doctors [feel] a 'technological imperative' to do 'everything possible' [to preserve a life], regardless of whether an intervention could work, and regardless of whether a patient wanted a futile intervention."[2] Hospitals increasingly apply high-technology, high-cost heroic measures to delay death, knowing that the measures will not bring about any healing. In some cases, this amounts to "futile care": extreme treatments that have little chance, if any, to cure the patient or extend a meaningful life. In some cases, decisions about using extreme medical technology have moved from "Because we can, we should consider it" to "Because we can, we must."

In response to these medical and ethical dilemmas, new legal tools have been developed to enable people to have direct control over end-of-life events in case they are not able to do so personally due to severe medical problems. They are known as "advance medical care directives," and educating the public about their value and use has for decades been the highest priority of right-to-die groups worldwide. There are three main types of these documents.

The first is a *living will*, which states an individual's preferences regarding cardiopulmonary resuscitation, life-sustaining treatments, and options for palliative care and/or physician aid-in-dying, where legal. It takes effect if the patient is unable to make competent medical treatment decisions. The creation of the first living will in 1967 is generally credited to Luis Kutner, a Chicago human rights attorney and cofounder of Amnesty International.[3] The California Natural Death Act of 1976 was the first legislation to specifically validate the legality of living wills.[4] Now, all states and most progressive countries have enacted an equivalent legally enforceable document, and the forms for all states can be downloaded via computer for free. James L. Park, an existential philosopher who maintains an extensive website exploring the ethical, philosophical, and practical realities of self-deliverance, said:

> At the end of each of our lives, most of us will eventually become so debilitated by our disease or by simple old age that others will have to make our medical decisions for us. If we do not care what will happen to us medically speaking, then we do not need any Advance Directive for Medical Care. We will simply be treated according to the standard operating procedures of whatever hospital we happen to go to and of whatever members of the medical profession are called upon to treat us. But if we have developed any sense of our own medical preferences, then we should put our ideas about medical care into a written document.[5]

The second tool is a *durable healthcare power of attorney*, a document through which a patient authorizes a legal proxy and trusted representative to make healthcare decisions should the patient temporarily or permanently lose decision-making capacity. Dr. E. James Lieberman, of the George Washington University of Medicine, recommends that because it is impossible to specify all possibilities that might arise in an emergency, a living will should be specific about major choices, such as "do not resuscitate" (DNR) orders, but should not be overly detailed. This allows the proxy, who has the latest information, to make real-time decisions on the spot.[6]

The third is the *Physician's (or Medical) Order for Life-Sustaining Treatment* (POLST or MOLST orders). These are written instructions from a physician, printed on brightly colored paper for quick recognition. They notify other health professionals about life-sustaining treatment the patient wants or does not want to receive at the end of life. Cardiopulmonary resuscitation is one example. Having such written orders immediately available to medical personnel is critical, as healthcare professionals are required to attempt CPR when a patient's heart or breathing stops unless they have medical orders to the contrary. In addition, patients who fall into a persistent vegetative state may find that their caregivers automatically intubate them (insert breathing or feeding tubes) unless written advance medical directives and/or POLST/MOLST orders are in place to prevent it.

As valuable as these documents are, they are sometimes disregarded through ignorance or neglect. Some institutions go so far as to categorically refuse to honor them, despite being legally obliged to do so. If your healthcare institution is governed by Catholic medical and religious directives, for example, your end-of-life wishes may not be honored.

On November 17, 2009, the U.S. Council of Catholic Bishops (USCCB), through a change in its Directive #58, "Ethical and Religious Directives for Catholic Healthcare Services," ordered Catholic institutions to initiate and maintain artificial feeding and hydration in permanently unconscious patients, regardless of their advance directive instructions or family wishes. According to Compassion & Choices, the largest U.S. death-with-dignity group:

> The USCCB order runs counter to written instructions in hundreds of thousands of Advance Directives and the clear wishes of many individuals with no written document. The primary consideration in healthcare decisions should always be the individual's values, beliefs, and desires, not fixed doctrine of any one religion. We respect the beliefs of all Catholics, but we do not respect an attempt by Catholic Bishops to override the health care decisions of a majority of Americans.[7]

In the United States, Compassion & Choices drafted a legally enforceable document to ensure that if treatment within the bounds of a patient's advance directives was refused, the patient would be transferred to another healthcare institution that would honor it.[8] Their *Directive Regarding Health Care Institutions Refusing to Honor My Health Care Choices* is available without charge from www.compassionandchoices.org.

In addition to intolerance from those who wish to impose their religious views on persons not of their faith, same-sex couples face other challenges. Their marriages or civil unions may not be respected under the laws of many states or countries. In a recent New Jersey case, two gay men who had lived together for twenty years had each named the other as their proxies in their durable healthcare powers of attorney. Both men's blood relatives had shunned them decades earlier. By mutual consent, the sick partner and his proxy agreed that a DNR order should be posted at the foot of his bed. The doctor and the hospital complied, as death seemed imminent. Without warning, the dying man's parents—who had not spoken to him in twenty years—arrived and demanded that the DNR notice be removed and wanted "that pervert" banned from the son's room. New Jersey's laws do not yet recognize same-gender marriage partners, so despite all the legal documents being at hand, the son suffered alone for weeks although there was no hope for recovery.[9]

Many extraordinary cases worldwide have brought wide media attention to the heart-wrenching dilemmas caused by the absence of advance medical directives. In 1973, Aruna Ramachandra Shanbaug, twenty-five, was thrown into existential limbo, trapped in a permanent minimally conscious state. The pretty, bubbly, and spunky young woman, a highly regarded nurse at the sprawling King Edward Memorial Hospital in Mumbai, India, was professionally on the rise. She was engaged to be married to Dr. Sundeep Sardesai, a local physician. But the day before starting a vacation to prepare for her wedding, she was assaulted by Sohanlal Bhartha Walmiki, a hospital ward assistant who was angry because she had reprimanded him.

In revenge, he attacked her, choking her with a dog chain and brutally sodo-

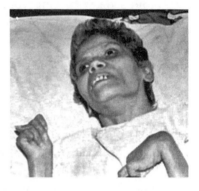

Aruna Ramachandra Shanbaug

mizing her. The choking cut off the oxygen supply to her brain, resulting in brain stem and cervical cord injuries, as well as leaving her blind.[10] Because of the social stigma—the "blame-the-victim" syndrome—frequently attached to rape victims in India, Shanbaug was totally abandoned by her family, fiancé, and friends.

Since the attack, Shanbaug has lived for decades as a blind, comatose, minimally conscious ghost in an obscure corner of the hospital where she was once a rising star, alone except for a group of dedicated nurses who care for her, force-feeding her twice a day by spooning liquid nourishment down a throat that cannot swallow. Author Pinki Virani took up her case, tracked down the details, and wrote *Aruna's Story*, a powerful book about medical negligence and hospital cover-ups that rendered her a living non-person. Only in

2009 did the Supreme Court of India accept a petition by Virani to permit Shanbaug to die by withdrawal of food and fluids, as Shanbaug was "devoid of any human dignity."[11] Dr. Surendra Dhelia, a member of India's Society for the Right to Die, said that "even a miracle would not possibly save her. She definitely needs a peaceful exit." Dhelia was no stranger to anguished deaths. His own father spent two years in a permanent vegetative state, ultimately dying from a combination of diabetes, prostate cancer, and dementia.[12]

"A barrel-thumping brigade comprising doctors, religious figures, lawyers, and assorted commentators has piously and passionately upheld life," wrote Bachi Karkaria in the *Times of India*. "Yes, only God (or biology) is entitled to take away what he (it) has given. Yes, the medical profession is committed to prolonging life and to terminate it willfully is to betray the Hippocratic oath to which doctors are sworn. But ivory tower grandstanding faces the awkward problem of coming undone when confronted by brute reality. What sounds noble in abstraction acquires ghoulish dimensions in fact."[13]

On March 7, 2011, the court denied Virani's petition to end the thirty-seven years of artificial nutrition and hydration for Shanbaug. In its ruling, however, the Supreme Court set out rules where passive euthanasia cases might be allowed in the future.

"Aruna was ours, and will always remain so," said Agnes Thomas, a nurse who has been working in the hospital for the last thirty-five years. "Her family stopped visiting her some years ago. She belongs to our family. We are not under any obligation to care for her but we do it because we feel a kinship towards her."[14] At the hospital, Shanbaug's fellow nurses, who had cared for her so long, rejoiced by sharing sweetmeats, a traditional Indian expression of joy and goodwill. On April 25, 2011, Auxiliary Bishop Agnelo Gracias of the Diocese of Bombay presented its annual pro-life award to Shanbaug's nurses. Rejecting the growing demand for the right to die with dignity, the bishop stated that "We have no right to die—neither with dignity nor indignity. After God has brought us to life, we have a right to live with dignity and we die with serenity, surrendering our life to God at the proper moment."[15]

The tragic case did, however, push Indian legal reform a small increment forward. On March 7, 2011, a two-judge bench in India's Supreme Court ruled that removing life support for long-term comatose patients under exceptional circumstances was allowable, provided that the request was from family and supervised by doctors and the courts.[16] There is no way to determine whether Aruna Shanbaug felt that the church's position and the court's decision to consign her to an indeterminate fate for the rest of her life was a blessing or a curse.

The 1975 case of Karen Ann Quinlan, then twenty-five, took a different course. The court in this case affirmed that in the United States, life-sustaining extraordinary measures could be discontinued if a comatose patient diagnosed as being in a permanent vegetative state had virtually no likelihood of reassuming the capability of self-awareness and interaction with the outside world.

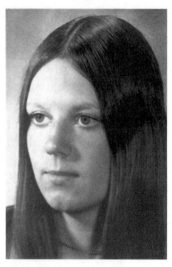

On April 15, 1975, Quinlan, who had been on a drastic weight-loss diet, felt faint at a party after consuming several alcoholic drinks and one or more drugs. Her friends took her home and put her to bed. When they checked her about fifteen minutes later, she was no longer breathing. They attempted mouth-to-mouth resuscitation and called an ambulance. During transport to Newton Memorial Hospital, CPR was administered

Karen Ann Quinlan

by the emergency responders. In all, she had ceased breathing for at least two fifteen-minute periods.[17]

Upon admission to the hospital, Quinlan's pupils were unreactive, and she was unresponsive even to deep pain. She was put on a respirator and remained there in a coma for nine days before being transferred to St. Clair's Hospital, a larger New Jersey healthcare facility. There a nasal feeding tube was inserted, and she was diagnosed as being in a persistent vegetative state resulting from severe brain damage due to oxygen deprivation. Her EEG was not flat, but it showed only abnormal slow-wave activity. Over the next five months, her weight dropped from 115 to 80 pounds, and she was declared to have entered a permanent vegetative state.

After several months, Quinlan's Catholic family concluded that she was beyond hope of recovery and decided to remove the ventilator, an option within the ethical bounds of Pope Pius II's 1975 declaration that "if it appears that the attempt at resuscitation constitutes in reality such a burden for the family that one cannot in all conscience impose it upon them, they can lawfully insist that the doctor should discontinue these attempts, and the doctor can lawfully comply."[18]

However, St. Clair's Hospital refused to remove the ventilator. The Quinlan family took the case to the New Jersey Supreme Court, which ruled in their favor in 1976.[19] The court identified a right to decline life-saving medical treatment and held that life support could be removed if the physicians and a hospital ethics committee agreed that a patient had no reasonable possibility of returning to a cognitive, responsive state.

Karen Quinlan surprised many by continuing to breathe unaided as her brain stem, which controlled primary body functions such as heartbeat and respiration, continued to function. She never regained consciousness, remained in a permanent vegetative state, was fed via artificial nutrition for nine more years, and ultimately died of multiple infections and pneumonia on June 11, 1985.

The court ruling affected the practice of medicine and law around the world. The Quinlan case "was hugely significant in part because it was the first state high court decision to permit a refusal of life-sustaining treatment based upon the Fourteenth Amendment right of privacy. It was also unique because the facts of the case made clear to the courts what had long been known in the medical profession—that medical technology increasingly enabled physicians to keep patients alive without any restoration of health."[20]

On January 11, 1983, twenty-five-year-old Nancy Cruzan lost control of her car, was thrown out, and landed face-down in a water-filled ditch in southern Missouri. Paramedics found her with no vital signs and restored her breathing, but after several weeks in a hospital, she was still in an eyes-open coma and was diagnosed as being in a persistent vegetative state. Doctors inserted a feeding tube, and her husband and parents hoped for a recovery, but after four years, her family accepted the grim reality that there was no hope left. However, Bill Colby, the lawyer who represented Cruzan's family, said, "The idea of letting nature take its course had fallen by the medical-technology wayside."[21]

Her family petitioned the Missouri courts for permission to have her feeding tube removed to let her die. Lower courts denied the request, citing a lack of definitive evidence that she would not have wanted futile care. However, in 1989, the U.S. Supreme Court was persuaded to hear Cruzan's case—the first right-to-die case ever considered by that august body. In a 5 to 4 decision, the court chose not to rule on the request to have the feeding tube removed. Instead, it focused on the lack of evidence that Cruzan would not want life-sustaining treatment, upholding the Missouri courts' right to pre-serve life in the absence of verifiable proof that the person would choose to die.[22]

Because the Supreme Court's verdict left the door open for the family to pursue further appeals, Cruzan's case was finally resolved in 1990, when three of Cruzan's friends went before a Missouri circuit court to present clear and convincing evidence that Nancy would not have wanted to exist in a persistent vegetative state. Cruzan's feeding tube was removed on December 15, 1990. In front of her hospital, protestors waved signs proclaiming "murderers," and satellite TV trucks captured the emotional scene. Cruzan died eleven days later.

In 2005, inside the Woodside Hospice in Pinellas Park, Florida, forty-one-year-old Theresa "Terri" Schindler Schiavo finally died after a fifteen-year coma. The events leading up to her death fractured America along multiple lines: her parents vs. her husband, conservative religious activists vs. medical science, Congress vs. the judiciary, and the right-to-life movement vs. the death-with-dignity movement.

On February 25, 1990, Schiavo, an insurance clerk, collapsed in her Florida apartment. Emergency medical technicians responding to her husband Michael's 911 call found her unconscious and not breathing, with no pulse. After attempting resuscitation and defibrillation, they transported her to a nearby hospital, where a feeding tube was inserted, and she was put on a ventilator. Her time without oxygen led to profound brain injury, and Schiavo was comatose for several months, after which she was diagnosed as being in a permanent vegetative state. Her husband was appointed as her legal guardian.

At first, Michael Schiavo, with the blessing of her parents, Bob and Mary Schindler, tried numerous types of therapy in hopes that his wife could recover at least some of her normal functions. However, over the next few years, multiple neurologists examined her, confirmed her diagnosis, and concurred that she had no chance for

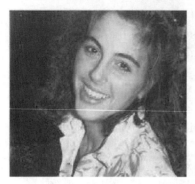

Terri Schiavo

improvement. In 1998, Michael filed a petition to have his wife's feeding tube removed because she would not have wanted to live in a permanent vegetative state. The Schindlers strongly objected.

A complex series of court battles ensued during which Terri Schiavo's lack of a living will played a key part. A court inquiry was held in January 2000 to determine whether Schiavo would have wanted life-sustaining procedures. Eighteen witnesses testified regarding her medical condition and her end-of-life wishes. Her husband claimed that she would not want to be kept alive by machines, with virtually no hope of recovery. Her parents maintained that she was a devout Catholic who would not wish to violate the church's teachings on euthanasia. In February 2000, Judge George Greer issued an order granting Michael's petition for authorization to discontinue artificial life support for his wife.

The Schindlers appealed, and the court battles escalated. Schiavo's feeding tube was removed, then reinserted, and the court ordered her reexamined by five neurologists. In 2002, a court-ordered hearing was held to determine whether new therapy treatments could help her regain any cognitive function. A CAT scan showed severe cerebral atrophy. An EEG showed no measurable brain activity. The court concluded that her permanent vegetative condition was "factual and not subject to legal dispute."[23] Her parents nevertheless continued their fight.

In the interim, Schiavo contracted a urinary tract infection. Michael halted most of her therapy and requested a DNR order, believing that there was no hope for her recovery. The disability rights group Not Dead Yet protested his actions, stating that she was a disabled person, and to let her die without any proof that she would have wanted it would negatively impact other people with disabilities.[24]

In 2003, the court again ordered the disconnection of the feeding tube. With the case now nationally notorious, Florida's legislature hastily passed Terri's Law, giving Governor Jeb Bush the authority to have the tube reinserted—thereby overruling multiple court decisions. Terri's Law was quickly ruled unconstitutional by the Florida Supreme Court because it violated the separation of powers of the judiciary, the legislature, and the governor.

By early 2005, the hospice that Terri Schiavo had been moved to became Ground Zero for a malignant circus. Angry pro-life crowds swarmed the perimeter, chanting and waving signs. A child was used to try to gain access to the hospice with a cup of water for Schiavo, who, had it been administered, would likely have choked to death. Two attempts were made to smuggle cameras into Schiavo's room. After the hospice manager, Annie Santa-Maria, received death threats, a police perimeter was established to prevent attacks on the staff and the building.[25]

Right-to-life supporters offered massive amounts of cash to bribe Michael Schiavo to relinquish custody of his wife to her parents. Michael prepared a secret exit from his home in case it was stormed by zealots.[26] Television reporters flocked to the site, providing hourly rumor-by-rumor commentary.

Then, in a bizarre and highly controversial move, both houses of the U.S. Congress attempted to take the matter out of Florida's hands by passing a bill transferring jurisdiction of the case to the federal courts at 12:41 a.m. on March 21, 2005. President George W. Bush, the brother of Florida's governor, flew back from his vacation in Texas and signed the bill into law that same morning.

His signature changed nothing. The presiding judge in Florida ordered a stay in moving Schiavo out of the hospice.[27] The feeding tube was duly disconnected, and Terri Schiavo died on March 31, 2005, fifteen years after her initial collapse.

Dr. Timothy E. Quill wrote in the *New England Journal of Medicine* that he believed, "both [Schiavo's] husband and her family, while seeing the situation in radically different ways, were trying to do what was right for her."[28] Death-with-dignity advocates were primarily concerned with "the willingness of the executive and legislative branches at both the state and federal levels to usurp the judiciary role . . . in an effort to promote a 'culture of life.'"[29]

While controversy swirled around Terri Schaivo, Piergiorgio Welby, an Italian right-to-die activist, was alert and actively seeking the right to have his own life support equipment turned off. Welby was diagnosed with muscular dystrophy at the age of seventeen. For many years he supported himself as a poet, painter, and painting instructor. In 1997, at the age of fifty-two, he fell victim to a respiratory condition that worsened to the extent that he depended on mechanical ventilation to breathe, received artificial nutrition through an implanted tube, and communicated through a keyboard-actuated voice synthesizer.[30]

He rapidly became a vigorous euthanasia activist, posting messages on various internet forums and on his own blog. On May 1, 2002, he posted the message, *Eutanasia*, which read in part, "Worse than the desert of the Tartars.... While staring at the horizon.... Terminal patients like me.... Envy the Dutch people.... WAKE UP!"[31]

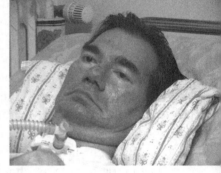

Piergiorgio Welby

In April 2006, he lost the ability to interact with his computer, severely limiting his communication. At that juncture, he decided to publicize his request to die, hoping to start a nationwide debate on euthanasia. In September 2006, he sent an open videoletter to Italian President Giorgio Napolitano that was broadcast on television and could be downloaded from the internet.

> I love life, Mr. President. Life is the woman who loves you, the wind through your hair, the sun on your face, an evening stroll with a friend. Life is also a woman who leaves you, a rainy day, a friend who deceives you. I am neither melancholic nor manic-depressive. I find the idea of dying horrible. But what is left to me is no longer a life.[32]

A number of prominent Italian disability rights activists strenuously opposed Welby's request and urged him to go on living. An equal number of death-with-dignity proponents supported his wish to die. His court request to be permitted to refuse medical treatment was denied, although several prominent physicians said that his right to do so was granted by the Italian constitution.

Anesthetist Dr. Mario Riccio, after assuring himself that Welby's request was genuine, volunteered to disconnect the respirator.[33] On December 20, 2006, with his wife and Riccio at his side, Welby asked to listen to Vivaldi's *The Four Seasons*. Because that selection was not available, he chose Bob Dylan. After Welby was sedated, the respirator was removed at 11 p.m. and he died forty minutes later.

Liberal politicians expressed relief for the end to his suffering. Conservatives criticized Riccio and the use of Welby's death for political ends. One demanded the immediate arrest of the doctor and "Welby's murderers."[34] However, both the committee of the local medical association and the criminal court judged Dr. Riccio's conduct to be legitimate, establishing a legal precedent in Italian law.[35] Welby was denied a religious funeral by the Catholic Church, which noted that he had "repeatedly and publicly affirmed his desire to end his own life, which is against Catholic doctrine."[36] His heavily attended civil funeral was celebrated in a public square in Rome.

Of all the major European right-to-die cases that captured the world's attention, none gained more notoriety than that of Ramón Sampedro, a commercial fisherman from Galicia, Spain. As a result of a diving accident, Sampedro was left a quadriplegic at the age of twenty-five. Unwilling to accept the limitations this catastrophe imposed on him, he spent the rest of his life—twenty-nine years—fighting for his right to a legal assisted suicide.

He fought unrelentingly in the Spanish courts, claiming that he was the victim of disability-based discrimination because he did

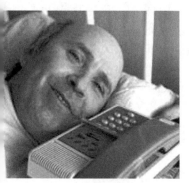

Ramón Sampedro

not have access to the suicide options available to the able-bodied. They could physically and legally end their own lives, but without assistance, he could not.

After exhausting all legal avenues, he concluded that he would have to borrow the hands and legs of others to accomplish his goal. Had it been unassisted, his self-inflicted death would not have violated Spanish law, but the complicity of others would turn it into a criminal act for the helpers.

Sampedro chose to die by drinking liquid potassium cyanide through a straw. To ensure the freedom of his friends, Sampedro devised an ingenious and intricate division of labor, whereby all the actions were separated into individual acts, with each participant knowing only his or her part. Since no individual knew who carried out any other part of the plan, they would be unable, even if required by law, to reveal the roles of their coconspirators. María José Guerra explained:

> He entrusted a very specific task to each one: to buy the cyanide, to analyze it, to calculate the dose, to transport it, to pick it up, to prepare the beverage, to pour it in a glass, to place the straw in the glass, to bring the glass to him, and to receive the final letter, which he had written with his mouth. The eleventh task, the most dangerous one because Spanish law requires a person to come to the aid of someone in danger of death, was to prepare the videotape of the last moment, in which Sampedro was the only protagonist. At the end, he remained firm in his decision to die, but he did not do so sadly. He did not seem a desperate man, on the contrary, he seemed calm and serene. In the end he became an activist defending the dignity of people and their right to die.[37]

Sampedro died on January 12, 1998, in Boiro, Spain. Ramona Maniero, one of his coconspirators, was arrested and charged with assisting his suicide but was released due to lack of evidence. No one else was ever detained. Seven years later, after the statute of limitations on the "crime" had run out, Maniero admitted to being the person who handed the cyanide-laced drink and a straw to him. She had also been the one behind the camera that recorded his last words.[38] In 2004, his story was eloquently told in *The Sea Inside*, an Academy-Award-winning film. Sampedro's legacy is simple: even in the face of the most complex obstacles, where there is a will, there is a way to overcome them.

– 5 –

Who Owns My Life?

I want to ask you, gentlemen, if I cannot give consent to my own death, then whose body is this? Who owns my life?
— Sue Rodriguez to a Canadian parliamentary committee, 1992

In 1991, Sue Rodriguez, then forty-one, was at her physical peak. Five feet eight inches tall and weighing 135 pounds, she embraced the outdoor life. Hiking, rock climbing, and skiing gave her great joy. Having served in several responsible business positions, she was accustomed to taking charge and making her own decisions. She was then separated from her second husband, biochemist Henry Rodriguez, and living in Victoria, British Columbia, Canada, with her son, Cole. She had no idea that in one year she would be confined to a wheelchair and that in three, she would be dead.

In April 1991, she noticed a strange tingling and twitching in her hands, but her overall good health led her to dismiss this as a temporary condition, probably brought on by the stress of her impending divorce and her new status as a single mother. As the twitches lingered on, and other puzzling physical oddities started to appear, she consulted two physicians, but neither detected any significant underlying cause other than stress. When she also started to feel tightness in her arms and pain in her neck and lower back, she decided to see a specialist.

On August 22, 1991, Dr. Andrew Eisen delivered the chilling news: she was suffering from ALS. The incurable condition was an automatic death sentence with no provision for appeal. In horror, Rodriguez learned that as her brain and spinal cord degenerated, she would progressively lose control of her muscles. Then, trapped in a physically nonfunctioning body, but with her mind still acutely aware of what was happening, she would die.

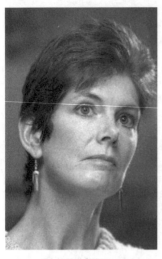

Sue Rodriguez

On the day of her grim diagnosis, her physician told her that the average time between diagnosis and death was three to five years. But none of the brochures he gave her offered a realistic picture of what was in store for her as the disease progressed, and the only mention of death was in a section referring to hospices.

Discarding the pamphlets, Rodriguez attended a meeting of a local ALS society to find support. The youngest and least afflicted person there, she was further dismayed to see the drooling, physically atrophied people. Appalled by this portrait of her future, she fled. In April 1992, after attending a number of meetings of the ALS Society in Victoria, she decided to end her life and bought Derek Humphry's how-to manual, *Final Exit.* [1]

For Rodriguez, the ability to control her body was integral to her identity. In *Uncommon Will,* which she and Lisa Hobbs Birnie cowrote, she stated, "If I cannot move my own body, I have no life." [2] Birnie explained, "Slowly, Sue was moving toward the position that she would steadfastly and publicly maintain for the next two years— that the quality of life is the essence of life, and that a life deprived of quality was not worth living." [3]

As long as she was physically able to do so, Rodriguez could have legally committed suicide without involving anyone else. But the rapid decline in her muscle control soon made that impossible. Less than a year after her initial diagnosis, she was confined to a wheelchair, her fingers curled up and immobile. Unable to carry out the steps necessary to end her life, she needed a physician to hasten her death. In May 1992, she asked her doctor about his attitude toward euthanasia. Hemming and hawing, he gave her no clear answer.

Three weeks later, she got a call from a Vancouver anti-suicide quick response team. Her physician had tipped them off that she might be suicidal. Feeling betrayed (and noting the irony that a "quick response team" took three weeks to respond), she asked to have her medical records transferred to a new doctor. The second physician told her that he was not prepared to risk everything he had achieved to help her die.

At that point, Rodriguez realized the medical establishment would be of no use to her. Instead, she sought information and assistance from Dying With Dignity (DWD), Canada's oldest end-of-life educational organization, formed in 1980 by a small group of people who held deep concerns about the quality of care given to the dying. The founders, including Marilynne Seguin, a registered nurse, came chiefly from the fields of academia, law, and health care. They had experience with end-of-life issues because of their affiliations with similar groups from other countries, notably the United States and the United Kingdom.

One of their most prominent supporters was Derek Humphry, who attended DWD's first organizational meeting in Toronto in 1980. "At the end of the meeting," Humphry said, "the audience voted to support voluntary euthanasia and assisted suicide but then voted not to say so publicly."[+] Humphry, whose views had been widely reported in the media since 1975, was shocked by DWD's reticence to publicly declare its position, although the initial supporters of the Hemlock Society had reacted the same way. Seguin, on the other hand, sensed that a low public profile would enable the organization to grow and carry out its work without making any more enemies than necessary.

In 1982, DWD incorporated as a registered charity, with the objective of raising awareness of end-of-life options throughout Canada. Seguin became its first paid executive director three years later and served until 1997. In her fifteen years of service, she worked tirelessly with the medical community to make death with dignity possible for numerous people. Restrained by DWD's conservative board and membership, however, she could not speak out as strongly as she wished on euthanasia issues.

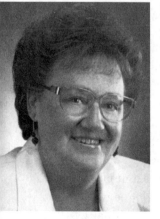

Although DWD's approach left some Canadian euthanasia activists and members frustrated, Seguin employed an astute strategy. To counteract the limitations under which she worked, she frequently brought in Derek Humphry, who spoke out fearlessly on issues that she could not discuss.

"No one else in the Canadian right-to-die movement came near to emulating Mari-

Marilynne Seguin

lynne's work for DWD," Humphry wrote. "Throughout the 1980s, Marilynne invited me to Toronto and Vancouver to say the sort of things she dared not say out loud. But the truth was that, quietly and secretly, she was constantly at the bedside of many terminal people."[5]

In 1982, DWD's first major project was promoting the use of living wills in Canada. An innovative feature was a wallet card that would alert emergency medical care workers to the critical directives in the living will. Next the group introduced a durable power of attorney for health care and a voluntary euthanasia declaration for DWD members. During the 1980s, it carried out numerous studies of end-of-life hospital care and held several public forums. But at that time, most groups involved in end-of-life counseling knew little about reliable, humane methods of self-deliverance. They could talk about preparing for death but had virtually no technical knowledge of how to bring about a peaceful death on demand.

DWD's first decade was a constant struggle for survival. Branches in London, Vancouver, and Ottawa all evolved and dwindled by 1991, at which time all operations were consolidated in Toronto. Despite these setbacks, DWD's membership grew steadily, due largely to Seguin's vigorous work, warmth, concern, and nonthreatening public rhetoric.

It was to DWD and Marilynne Seguin that Sue Rodriguez first turned as her ability to manage life slipped away. Accompanied by her mother, she attended a DWD meeting at a Unitarian church in Victoria in April 1992. Seguin was a speaker, and Rodriguez was deeply disappointed when the talk focused only on advance health-care directives and living wills. Intimidated by her surroundings, she had her mother ask Seguin a question on her behalf. "What do you think of someone's assisting a terminally ill relative to commit suicide?"[6] The room instantly turned silent as all heads turned to look at Seguin.

She was trapped. It was the kind of question she would answer candidly in private but dared not address in public. "Many of us may regard it as unfortunate," Rodriguez recalled Seguin as saying, "but assisted suicide is punishable by up to fourteen years' imprisonment." She added, "We believe that through ongoing dialogue with governments at different levels, we can change the laws eventually."[7]

Rodriguez felt the response as a blow to her solar plexus. *What good to me is 'ongoing dialogue with governments at different levels?"* she thought.[8] A short time later, she called DWD, hoping for clarification on where it stood on assisted suicide and euthanasia. Their representative, Clem Finney, replied that if she was interested in those issues, she should talk to the Right to Die Society of Canada (RTDS-C).[9]

It took Sue Rodriguez six weeks to work up the courage to call the RTDS-C in August 1992. In response, one of its members, Anita Bundy, quickly came to her home to help her review her options. She was soon introduced to the society's founder and director, John Hofsess, who had also attended the meeting where Seguin had been cornered by Rodriguez' question. Hofsess helped chart an end-of-life strategy for Rodriguez. The six months that they worked together ignited a boiling debate in Canada over death-with-dignity issues and the fundamental question: Who had the authority to control her choice to live or die?

By the time he met Sue Rodriguez, confronting authority head-on to achieve social justice was already a way of life for John Leonard Hofsess. Born in Hamilton, Ontario, on May 27, 1938, the only child of Jack and Gladys May Hofsess, he was two when his father abandoned the family.[10] Although his mother had to support herself and her son on her $23 CAD weekly salary as a waitress, Hofsess never felt poor. On his tenth birthday, at great financial sacrifice, his mother gave him a handsome, leather-bound set of *The Book of Knowledge,* and he reveled in the stories of Huckleberry Finn and Robin Hood.

In 1965, at McMaster University in Ontario, Hofsess served as the student editor of the magazine *Muse Quarterly* and arts editor for *Silhouette,* a student newspaper.[11] In the next two years, he wrote and directed two counterculture films. The first was a ten-minute anti-war short, *Redpath 25.*[12] It was later incorporated into *Palace of Pleasure,* a dual-projector 16-mm film, which won the Best Experimental Film prize at the Vancouver International Film Festival in 1967.[13]

One of his first experiences with inciting controversy came in 1969, when Hofsess and other members of the McMaster Film Board shot a film called *The Columbus of Sex,* based loosely on *My Secret Life,* a risqué Victorian novel. When it was first screened at the university on August 8, 1969, it got a dramatic reception—from the police. The Ontario Board of Censors promptly outlawed it, giving it the distinction of being the first Canadian film ever banned.

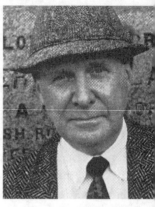

Because of his demonstrated talent, the notoriety did not hurt Hofsess' career. In the 1970s, he found fame as a writer, assistant editor, and film critic for *Maclean's* magazine, a highly respected periodical. While working as a critic in Toronto, Hofsess befriended Canadian film director Claude Jutra. When Jutra developed Alzheimer's disease in 1985,

John L. Hofsess

he asked Hofsess, who had written about euthanasia, to help him die. Hofsess knew nothing about assisting a suicide, and could not bring himself to do so. Jutra disappeared on November 5, 1986. Five months later, his decomposed body was found on the bank of the St. Lawrence River, after he had apparently jumped to his death from a bridge. Hofsess never forgot his friend's desperate plight.

The final event that launched Hofsess into full-blown euthanasia activism was the 1990 death of an elderly couple who committed suicide by tying themselves together and jumping off the fourteenth-story balcony of a building in Victoria. Although the event made little lasting impact on the public consciousness, it made a profound impression on Hofsess.[14]

In 1990, Hofsess was a highly paid advertising copywriter who was tired of wasting his talent writing commercials for chocolate-chip cookies. Despite the substantial salary, he left his Toronto-based career to care for his eighty-year-old mother, Gladys, who lived in British Columbia. Her physical decline provoked him to think about the needless suffering of so many dying people. For inspiration, he needed only to look south to California, Oregon, and Washington, where social transformation was rapidly accelerating.

In Oregon, Derek Humphry's voluminous writing, tireless campaigning, and never-ending public speaking and media engagements had built the Hemlock Society into the largest death-with-dignity organization in North America. Humphry and Hofsess were very much alike in significant ways. Both were veteran professional writers and communicators, committed right-to-die activists, and risk-takers. Hofsess admired Humphry's active, take-charge attitude and soon became his protégé. He approached Humphry about establishing a branch of the Hemlock Society in Canada, but Humphry thought it better to keep the groups separate, due to the differences in culture and politics in the two countries. "I wanted Hemlock to be a solely American thing, but encouraged John to start a separate organization, which I would back," Humphry said, and made good on his offer with both funds and numerous speaking engagements in Canada.[15]

On September 29, 1991, Hofsess launched The Right to Die Society of Canada to meet the need for an aggressively activist choice-in-dying group. He founded it as a private organization to avoid the restrictions imposed on tax-free, charitable groups. The society's high-profile inaugural event was a program at the University of Victoria, featuring Derek Humphry; Svend Robinson, M.P., who gave the first public address on euthanasia by a major Canadian politician; and a number of other prominent Canadians. To spread the word, Hofsess published *Last Rights Magazine* as the society's voice. The group grew quickly, but predictably, Hofsess' high media profile attracted vehement opposition from anti-euthanasia activists, who viewed him as a menace to society.

Until 1972, even attempting to commit suicide in Canada was a criminal act, punishable by an unspecified jail sentence. But both suicide and attempted suicide were decriminalized in that year, when the government realized that a successful suicide leaves no one to prosecute, and attempting to punish someone whose suicide attempt has failed increases the risk of another attempt. However, assisting a suicide was another matter. That remained a criminal offense. This left Canada, along with many other western countries and many states, with the paradox that it was illegal to help someone do something that was perfectly legal.[16]

One of Hofsess' first agenda items for his new organization was to directly challenge Section 241 of Canada's Criminal Code, which banned euthanasia or assisted suicide and made either a felony offense. The law stated, "Every one who (a) counsels a person to commit suicide, or (b) aids or abets a person to commit suicide, whether suicide ensues or not, is guilty of an indictable offence and liable to imprisonment for a term not exceeding fourteen years." Canada, Australia, New Zealand, Scotland, Northern Ireland, and Ireland all originally adopted their laws on euthanasia and assisted suicide

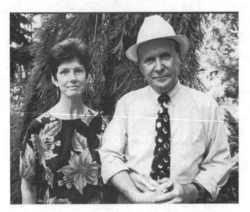

Sue Rodriguez and John Hofsess

from British common law, and all use nearly identical wording and levy the same penalties in their present-day laws.

In order to provoke changes in the law quickly, Hofsess needed a dramatic legal challenge, centered on a dying person willing to spend his or her last months fighting for the right to die amid the flashbulbs and unblinking eyes of television cameras. He would first take his case to court in British Columbia, and then, if he lost the case there, move on and appeal the verdict to the national parliament in Ottawa, which wrote the criminal code. If those steps failed, he would ultimately appeal the case to the Canadian Supreme Court.

Hofsess was certain that he had public support for his cause. Although vehemently denied by anti-euthanasia factions, objective professional polls repeatedly found that a majority of Canadians supported physician-assisted suicide for terminally ill people. By 1992, the figure was 78 percent in favor.[17] However, without obtaining the necessary majority of votes in the national parliament, Hofsess could not strike down the anti-euthanasia law.

In Rodriguez, Hofsess found his perfect test case. She was willing to be the public face of the Canadian assisted suicide law reform movement, and he was willing to put his money where his instincts told him he should. "John was impressed by Sue's practicality, dignity, and determination. Sue was impressed by John's kindness, straight talk, and experience with questions of death and dying. Both had a strong sense of a meeting of the minds," said Lisa Birnie.[18]

"Sue and I made a contract that she would get help in dying if she would let me publicize her case," Hofsess said. "We wanted her story to be like a two-act play. In the first act, she'd become very well known. In the second [if the law couldn't be changed], she'd be actively helped to die—either by myself or someone within the society—in a completely open manner, so either charges would be brought and I'd be convicted or jailed, or I wouldn't be charged, but because I had been so open about it, the law would have been sorely tested in the process."[19] Her case was the first major assault on Canada's ban on assisted suicide, and it became both a national and international media event. But for Hofsess, it would also lead to a professional disaster.

He and his supporters put up approximately $25,000 CAD to pay for Rodriguez' legal expenses. In the October-November 1992 issue of *Last Rights*, he declared, "I, John Hofsess, do agree to assist Sue Rodriguez in terminating her life at a time of her choosing, preferably by permission of Canadian law but if failing that, by moral authority of personal conscience."[20] The gauntlet had been thrown at the feet of Canada's legal system. With or without the blessing of the law, Sue Rodriguez was going to end her life at the time, place, and by the method of her own choosing.

In addition to being willing to be tried for assisting a suicide, Hofsess publicly promised to find Rodriguez a physician who would help her take her life if the law could not be changed. Dr. Scott Wallace of Victoria, a medical consultant to RTDS-C, announced his willingness to fulfill this role, even if he would be breaking the law to do so.[21] "[Hofsess'] plan," wrote ethicist Ian Dowbiggin, "was to dare the government into bringing charges against the physician, and later win a dramatic court victory for the right to assisted suicide."[22]

Hofsess began by taking the fight to the Supreme Court of British Columbia. There, Rodriguez' attorney, Christopher M. Considine, would argue that Section 241(b) of Canada's Criminal Code violated her civil rights as guaranteed under the Canadian Charter of Rights and Freedoms because it discriminated against disabled people who were not physically able to end their own lives, whereas able-bodied people could.

In November 1992, as the case was going to court, a national parliamentary committee in Ottawa was revising the Canadian Criminal Code, including the laws relating to euthanasia and assisted suicide. It was the perfect time for Sue Rodriguez to testify. Too weak to travel, she videotaped her address, asking the committee for the legal right to end her own life with the assistance of a physician. Staring directly at the camera, she posed the question around which her entire case revolved: "I want to ask you, gentlemen, if I cannot give consent to my own death, then whose body is this? Who owns my life?"[23] That question resonated with the Canadian people and reverberates worldwide to this day.

On December 30, 1992, Justice Allen Melvin of the Supreme Court of British Columbia dismissed Rodriguez' challenge without a ruling, stating that the case was a public-policy issue that should be decided by elected officials, not the courts.

Considine immediately filed suit to have Melvin's opinion overturned. In February 1993, the case was heard by the British Columbia Court of Appeals, but the original ruling was upheld by a 2 to 1 vote, with Chief Justice Allan McEachern the dissenting judge. Undaunted, Considine and Rodriguez planned to make their final appeal to the Canadian Supreme Court.

Two groups immediately opposed the issue. One was Cheryl Eckstein's Compassionate Healthcare Network (CHN), founded in 1992. It opposed "all programs, policies and perspectives which may threaten or weaken the physical existence of any person who is sick, disabled, infirm, dying or otherwise medically at risk."[24] Eckstein, a college-educated, deeply religious Pentecostal Christian and mother of seven children, had quietly infiltrated Hofsess' inner circle. "I was a mole in Hofsess' organization for a few years," she wrote to me. "He didn't have a clue, until that story was released."[25]

"That story" concerned a decision Hofsess had made to get his cause rolling quickly. He naively revealed in the April-May 1991 issue of the RTDS-C newsletter, *Last Rights*, that he had invested nearly $19,500 of his own funds in the society and that much of this money came from an $18,000 grant provided by the Canadian government to enable him to write *Requiem: Death and Dying in Canada.* Instead, he used the grant to support the launch of the RTDS-C and help pay for Rodriguez' defense. The book was never completed. Eckstein saw an opportunity to discredit her enemy and notified the media in September 1992.[26] Hofsess was angered by the exposé —while Eckstein was delighted—but Hofsess had not yet identified Eckstein as a mole, and she was not finished with her work.

Hofsess' other opposition came from the Campaign for Life Coalition (CLC), then led by Sabina McLuhan and the political wing of the Canadian pro-life movement. Its position was clear: "We defend the sanctity of human life against threats posed by abortion, euthanasia, doctor-assisted suicide, reproductive and genetic technologies, cloning, infanticide, eugenics, population control, and threats to the family."[27] Because Eckstein's CHN was small and lacked significant recognition, she pitched in to work with the better-known CLC.

As part of its testimony to the parliamentary subcommittee for the recodification of Canadian criminal law, CLC played a portion of a well-known 1941 Nazi propaganda film, *Ich klage an* (*I accuse*), which justified involuntary killing of "undesirables," such as chronically or mentally ill and disabled persons. The attempt to link the proposed change of Canada's anti-assisted suicide law to Nazi mass-murdering of Jews, Gypsies, and the mentally disabled who might contaminate the gene pool of Hitler's planned "master race" was a seedy and discredited propaganda trick that seriously undermined the CLC's credibility.[28] "Playing the Nazi card" had by then become a stock-in-trade tactic used by anti-euthanasia groups in an attempt to link Nazi state-directed mass murder with the elective right to die.[29] The ruse had no discernable effect on the committee.

In early 1993, Hofsess made a decision that would haunt him for the rest of his tenure as head of the RTDS-C. Infuriated by the lack of support from the ALS Society and similar disability groups, and hampered by Rodriguez' waning ability to maintain a high media profile, he wrote a letter in her name. Published in January 1993 in the *Vancouver Sun*, it lashed out at some members of the ALS Society for their lack of support.[30]

Hofsess' misguided act caused immediate problems. Cheryl Eckstein, who held no personal ill will toward Rodriguez, sensed that the letter's combative tone and Rodriguez' dignified, resolute character did not match. She pressured the *Vancouver Sun* to verify the letter's authenticity.

When she learned the truth, Rodriguez was outraged and broke all ties with Hofsess and his organization. When the *Sun* contacted Rodriguez about the letter, she denied writing or authorizing it.[31] "I did not make those statements, nor would I, and I am sorry that they were said," she told the newspaper.[32] Hofsess wrote her a letter of apology, but the damage was done. He had lost the leadership of the battle for legislative change and would never play out the heroic role he had envisioned for himself.

With Rodriguez' health in daily decline, Chris Considine appealed her case to the Canadian Supreme Court in the fall of 1993. By this time, it was the hottest news story in Canada, and almost every pro- or anti-euthanasia group in the country wanted to be a part of it. *Amicus curiae* (friend-of-the-court or intervener) status was granted to two pro- and seven anti-euthanasia groups. That status allowed each party to submit formal briefs to the justices stating their positions, hoping to influence the outcome of the lawsuit. The two pro-euthanasia groups were the RTDS-C and DWD. Allied against them were the Pro-Life Society of British Columbia; Pacific Physicians for Life Society; the Canadian Conference of Catholic Bishops; the Evangelical Fellowship of Canada; the British Columbia Coalition of People With Disabilities; People in Equal Participation, Inc.; and the Coalition of Provincial Organizations of the Handicapped.[33]

As the fierce court battle continued, Rodriguez stayed above the fighting and was accorded tremendous admiration for her courage. When she emerged from a press conference one day, traffic and pedestrians stopped, and a spontaneous burst of applause reverberated among the buildings, reflecting the enormous affection people had for the fragile invalid.

Earlier that year, Rodriguez had attended a fundraiser for her legal costs, the local premiere of the play *Whose Life Is It Anyway?* about a paralyzed man's fight for the right to die. As she was wheeled onstage, the audience burst into applause. She was presented with the Canadian Humanist of the Year Award for her "courageous fight to gain legal recognition for the inalienable right of the individual to determine the time and nature of their own death, including the right to seek qualified assistance in the termination of life where such termination reduces human suffering."[34]

The outpouring of public support was not enough to sway the legal system. On September 30, 1993, in a landmark decision, *Rodriguez v. British Columbia* was defeated in the Canadian Supreme Court by a 5 to 4 vote. When he wrote the majority decision, Justice John Sopinka expressed sympathy for Rodriguez, but he ultimately ruled that she could not be exempted from the law. "No consensus can be found in favour of the decriminalization of assisted suicide. To the extent that there is a consensus, it is that human life must be respected."[35] That human life must be respected is, of course, of paramount importance. But according to the great majority of all Canadians, it is equally important that no law should force a citizen to bear unendurable or unwanted terminal suffering and that a physician should be empowered to end such suffering if requested by the patient.

The legal loss was a catastrophe for the Canadian right-to-die movement because it seemed to rule out future appeals to request physician-assisted suicide. Any change in the law would, it seemed, have to be made directly by Canada's national parliament. Eighteen years would pass until the fuse was lit for the next frontal attack on Canada's assisted suicide law.

Undeterred, Rodriguez had planned her final exit strategy. "I'm not afraid of death at all," she said, "But I fear gasping for breath, panicking, being in a situation where I am hooked up to a respirator, unable to swallow, unable to move, unable to do anything for myself."[36]

The morning of Saturday, February 12, 1994, was cold and overcast. Sue Rodriguez' ex-husband, Henry, came to her house to pick up their son, Cole, then almost nine years old, so that he would not be a witness to what was to come. Later that day, Rodriguez drank a fatal barbiturate cocktail through a straw, defying the law by ending her life at the time, place, and by the method of her choosing.

Her companions for her last act were Svend Robinson and (allegedly) a doctor—never identified—who supplied her with the lethal drugs: a massive overdose of morphine taken with seconal capsules.[37] It was a dramatic ending for the woman who had galvanized Canada and elicited widespread support for the right to legally die with dignity. Although Robinson, Hofsess, and senior members of the RTDS-C were investigated by the police, no charges were ever brought against them.

The loss of the Rodriguez case was a profound disappointment for Hofsess. Defeated on the legal battlefield, he lost all interest in legislative reform. Instead, he decided to put the best possible information on euthanasia and assisted suicide directly into the hands of those who wanted it. He published the North American edition of Chris Docker and Cheryl K. Smith's *Departing Drugs* in 1993, followed by *Beyond Final Exit* in 1995.[38] In his next attempt to educate the public, Hofsess completely leapfrogged the authority and control of the government censors by making himself an information mogul in cyberspace. He set out to master the unregulated, rapidly growing international free market of online information, and succeeded to an extent never before imagined possible.

Even though, at that time, only a tiny fraction of Canadians had modems capable of connecting to the internet, Hofsess sensed that the information genie was already out of the bottle. His advanced grasp of the power of this new technology was soon evident.

In April 1994, Hofsess established a special interest group about the right to die on the Victoria FreeNet. By September 1994, Hofsess' Last Rights Information Center offered information and links to numerous euthanasia newsgroups. His first fully functional website, DeathNET, went online on January 10, 1995. It offered unrestricted access to euthanasia information. Canadian content was provided by Hofsess, and U.S. information was supplied by Derek Humphry. Hofsess wrote, "We embrace the internet as virtually the only place where people can learn the deeper and fuller truth about the 'right to die' issues."[39]

Within weeks of its launch, DeathNET produced alarm, outrage, and outright terror in anti-euthanasia groups. In October 1995, *HLI Reports*, a Catholic news agency, wrote, "The Culture of Death has arrived on the internet.... Four different avenues try to convince visitors to adopt a pro-death position [including a homepage with] bright colors and a basic platform which looks far more like something you would see in a video arcade than in a funeral home."

"Whole sections of the site," the agency continued, "are dedicated to testimony gathered at pro-euthanasia hearings and court decisions involving right-to-die cases [and the site] proposes several means for making death more emotionally palatable for those considering suicide and their families."[40] Not everyone was appalled at DeathNET's frank discussion of end-of-life issues. In 1995 and 1996, it was named "Best Health/Medical Site" by the Canadian Internet Awards.[41]

Adding more fuel to the fire, Hofsess created a page on the DeathNET site for Windsor, Ontario, resident Austin Bastable, who suffered from progressive multiple sclerosis and whose motto was, "carrying on where Sue Rodriguez left off." Using Elvis Presley's rendition of "My Way" as the theme song for his web page, Bastable succeeded in bringing assisted suicide back onto the front burner. Unable to find final exit help in his own country, Bastable made his way to Michigan, where he became Dr. Jack Kevorkian's twenty-eighth client in 1996.[42]

By 1998, Hofsess had turned over most of the management, counseling, and speaking operations of the RTDS-C to Ruth von Fuchs in Toronto. She assumed the leadership of the society in 2001 and still serves as its unpaid president. She had been active in the society since it was founded in 1991. Membership duties were handled by Evelyn Martens, Hofsess' colleague and neighbor in Vancouver, where Martens also manufactured Hofsess' exit bags and shipped them and his literature worldwide.

Other than believing that death with dignity ought to be recognized by law as a civil right, the Canadian right-to-die groups had no common philosophy, goals, methods, agendas, or spokespeople. In order to communicate with each other, they launched a joint newsletter, *Free to Go*, in 1999. It was edited by Ruth von Fuchs and provided space for the four groups then active: Choice in Dying chapters in Ottawa and White Rock/Surrey; DWD; The Goodbye Society; and the RTDS-C. Despite high public approval levels for the right to die, membership in the Canadian activist groups waned after the loss of the Rodriguez case. By the mid-1990s, there were fewer than two thousand members in all of the groups combined.

Dying With Dignity lost its hardworking and dynamic leader, Marilynne Seguin, in the winter of 1998. Seguin's own battle with diabetes, rheumatic fever, bacterial endocarditis, and uterine cancer made her a candidate for the humane self-deliverance she promoted for others. In 1994, she wrote, "No matter how much support and love surround a person, the experience of serious illness is painfully lonely. Another revelation I was unprepared for was that at a certain point I would find myself con-

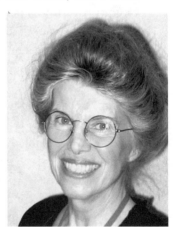

Ruth von Fuchs

sidering that most difficult of all choices: whether to continue the struggle for life or pursue the alternative—to choose to die."[43] That January she had written, "I have very strong feelings about my right to autonomy and self-control and I find no fear in the concept of death. . . .What I do fear is the concept of being alive but not living. . . . Either I will manage my own death or I will have an assisted death."[44] Over the course of twenty years she had reached out and educated thousands of people at public lectures and in private, had counseled over two thousand dying people and had been at the bedside to comfort more than three hundred and fifty of them.[45]

Seguin practiced what she preached and meticulously planned

her self-directed death. Two weeks before her exit, after suffering through several diabetes-related comas and severely impaired vision, she celebrated her planned departure with a warm-hearted, upbeat "living wake" with champagne for about twenty friends.

On September 9, 1999, surrounded by several of her closest friends, including Dr. Richard MacDonald, the Hemlock Society's medical director, she made her final exit with a sleeping pill overdose. "Her death was one of the most memorable for me in the planning, the carrying out of her explicit wishes, and the absolutely peaceful final hours when she had close friends whom she trusted. . . .Without hesitation, when the time appointed by her arrived, she took the medication."[46]

Her death was front-page news in Toronto, and her legacy lives on. Her work is commemorated every two years by the World Federation of Right to Die Societies, which presents the Marilynne Seguin Award to a person who has excelled in advancing the death-with-dignity cause worldwide.

The loss of Seguin was a major blow to Canada's struggling right-to-die movement. To overcome the leadership vacuum, John Hofsess took on the role of pathfinder. Although sidelined by his mistakes as a leader, he reinvented his mission and became a cutting-edge, right-to-die technology activist. An innovative, imaginative thinker, he assembled a brilliant, state-of-the-art technical staff and created a radical self-deliverance research and development team. Its mission: invent and develop deathing technologies that would enable people to control their own destinies without any interference from the government or the medical establishment.

This approach would turn the entire international death-with-dignity movement on its ear and give immediate hope to thousands of people frustrated by the legal and medical status quo.

The revolution began quietly in Hofsess' Victoria apartment. There he met with Dr. Rob Neils, an American clinical psychologist and inventor from Spokane, Washington. These two right-to-die radicals would be joined by eight more to found an astonishing team that would reshape self-deliverance worldwide. They named it NuTech.

Ω

Robbing Death of Its Sting

What's driving groups like this is our opponents, who have worked
so hard to overturn good law.   — Dr. Philip Nitschke

The most radical transformation of self-deliverance since the 1991 publication of Derek Humphry's *Final Exit* began on August 21, 1997, at an informal, private meeting of two dedicated, little-known right-to-die activists in Canada. Its ambitious goal was to harness the minds of the world's widely separated euthanasia researchers to develop methods and technologies that anyone seeking a gentle death could use. The result of the meeting was the formation of the New Technology Self-Deliverance Group, whose name was quickly (and mercifully) shortened to NuTech.

Its goals were both audacious and daunting: to develop legal, peaceful self-deliverance methods that would be inexpensive and easy to obtain and use, would not physically or legally endanger any second party, and would reliably produce a rapid, painless death that did not leave a gruesome scene behind. NuTech was totally consumer driven. It would serve those people facing unacceptable futures who wanted a certain and effective way to end their lives.

NuTech's founder, John L. Hofsess, sought to grant people the right and ability to die with dignity without breaking the law. He recalled:

> I began investigating inhalants, injectables and ingestibles, toxic venoms—anything that looked possible as a way of eliminating the need for a doctor or pharmacist, and always with the idea of staying one step ahead of the law. New technology doesn't need the law to be changed, as suicide is legal already. What we need are means of empowerment for people that are difficult for politicians to control, but that remain within the law.[1]

A colleague wrote of Hofsess, "He believes that with so many suffering members, right-to-die advocates have nothing less than a 'moral obligation' to investigate 'new and realistic means' of death."[2]

Before effective self-deliverance technologies could be developed, one huge practical obstacle had to be overcome—an almost total lack of communication between widely separated researchers. The search for a simple, humane suicide method was still the province of individuals working alone. This inevitably led to duplication of effort, lack of access to recently developed concepts, and wasted time. An international think tank was needed where ideas and information could be freely shared and nurtured.

The NuTech Group answered that need. It was born at the apartment of John Hofsess, in Victoria, B.C.[3] His first collaborator was Rob Neils, Ph.D., a clinical psychologist who specialized in grief, dying, and catastrophic events. He was also founder and president of the Dying Well Network, an all-volunteer, nonprofit, right-to-die organization based in Spokane, Washington. Neils was a pioneering advocate for strong safeguards against the misuse of deathing technology. He and a colleague, Valerie Snipes, had developed a psychological screening test to help medical professionals differentiate between people with rational suicide desires and those with irrational motives.[4] His insistence on safeguards would play a major role in his later dealings with NuTech.

Hofsess freely admitted that he was no medical or engineering mastermind. "I have absolutely no technical skills whatsoever. I don't even drive a car," he said.[5] He was, however, a tireless advocate for change and a cutting-edge computer user. He became NuTech's sparkplug and intellectual catalyst: a research visionary who could inspire and communicate good ideas and bring talented people together to develop them.

By the late 1990s, two mutually exclusive schools of thought had evolved within the international death-with-dignity movement. The conservative majority believed that educating the public about living wills, advance directives, and changing laws to permit physician aid-in-dying were the best ways to bring about reform. To achieve their goals, they used the traditional tools of social change: public speaking, publications, protests, educational outreach programs, and ballot initiatives. Euthanasia radicals, however, most of whom were libertarian and/or anti-authoritarian by nature, wanted immediate results. They embraced a direct-action, do-it-yourself, personal autonomy approach, and their basic philosophy was simple: "Keep the authorities out of our lives—and deaths." They knew that every day that politicians dragged their feet over enacting responsible self-deliverance laws their constituents wanted, hundreds of thousands of dying people worldwide would suffer in untreatable and unnecessary agony.

Suicide methods developed before 1997 had significant limitations. In the early 1980s, British psychiatrist Colin Brewer suggested taking a large overdose of barbiturates, typically sleeping pills. Just before falling asleep, the person would pull a large plastic "turkey roasting bag" over his or her head and close it with a rubber band or a necktie, shutting down the available supply of fresh oxygen. As the oxygen inside the bag was consumed and the percentage of exhaled carbon dioxide inside the bag rose, the patient would automatically react by breathing faster and harder to get more oxygen, and soon the brain would trigger a panic response. But if the patient was in a barbiturate-induced sleep, this alarm response would not register with the brain, and the person would die painlessly from anoxia: oxygen deprivation to the brain.[6] However, overdoses of pills could cause vomiting, which sometimes led to botched suicides, and insufficient doses would not put the patient to sleep quickly enough to make the bag effective.

In the late 1980s, the plastic bag method was improved when experts found that taking an anti-emetic drug half an hour before taking the barbiturates could reduce the chance of vomiting up the drug overdose. Derek Humphry and others published accurate information on what doses of barbiturates would be most lethal and stated that alcohol would speed up the effect of the pills. However, the method still relied on prescription drugs and sometimes, despite the best precautions, death was not always quick or certain. During the process of learning how to bring about a peaceful, certain end of life, about one in seven guided attempts was unsuccessful. "Failures were horrible situations, most dreadful, requiring great courage and willingness to sacrifice freedom in pursuit of 'changing the face of death,'" said one NuTech researcher.[7]

Other technology pioneers were also at work. On August 29, 1989, Jack Kevorkian finished building the first of three prototypes of his Thanatron lethal injection machine, and soon thereafter, he developed the Mercitron, which delivered carbon monoxide gas through a partial face mask.[8] But both were designed for use only by a physician, and the carbon monoxide method left the body with a flushed red skin color likely to arouse the suspicion of coroners.

Dr. Philip Nitschke's computer-controlled Deliverance Machine, developed in 1995, had the same drawbacks as the Thanatron, from which it had evolved. Using the sophisticated medical device required prescription drugs and a doctor's direct involvement. The result was physician aid-in-dying, not unaided self-deliverance.

John Hofsess created an "exit bag" in 1995 that was specifically designed to be used with a deliberate overdose of prescription drugs. Its elasticized collar, fleece-lined neckband, and adjustable Velcro strap to hold the neckband closed made self-deliverance more comfortable. In response to horrified reactions from right-to-life groups, he replied, "The 'Exit Bag' is no more controversial a device for its intended purpose than the use of condoms to prevent sexually transmitted diseases."[9]

Derek Humphry's continuous flow of how-to books, especially *Final Exit* and its periodic updates, set the high-water mark for do-it-yourself self-deliverance manuals. *Final Exit* was followed by other works, each further exploring different aspects of the self-deliverance puzzle. The wide-ranging writings of Cheryl K. Smith, Christopher G. Docker, Dr. Bruce Dunn, and John Hofsess were collected in *Beyond Final Exit: New Research in Self-Deliverance for the Terminally Ill* in 1995.

All this information was well-known by the second NuTech meeting, which was held from November 8-9, 1997, also in Victoria. A fly on the wall would have seen four creative and dedicated middle-aged people with their mental shirtsleeves rolled up, trying to solve a huge, somber, and knotty problem: every day, people were dying in avoidable agony while legal reform moved at a glacial pace.

The expanded working group was made up of Canadians Hofsess and Martens, American Rob Neils, and Australia's Dr. Philip Nitschke.[10] "Nitschke was visiting the U.K., where he had been invited for a speaking engagement," Hofsess said. "I asked him to consider flying home to Australia by way of a stopover in Canada. I wanted to get his views on what was at the time an idea in gestation: the debreather."[11] Neils brought for demonstration the critical core component of his debreather concept: a water-based carbon dioxide scrubber.[12]

In two days, the team conducted a free-wheeling review of every existing self-deliverance option, including World War II cyanide pills used for suicide by the Nazi elite, most famously Hermann Göring, Eva Braun, and Heinrich Himmler. All U.S. B-29 atomic bomb flight crew members carried cyanide suicide "L-Pills" in case they were shot down over Japan, captured, and tortured for information.

Next was saxitoxin (mollusk poison) pressed into the tiny grooves of suicide needles that were given to pilots of U-2 spy planes to use if they were shot down and captured during the Cold War. Hofsess also identified tetrodotoxin, a natural poison found in Japanese blowfish and the venom of Australian Taipan snakes.

Readily available poisonous plants included the oleander, the azalea, and the Carolina jessamine, all signature decorative plants of the American South. The three are among the most poisonous and deadly of the commonly grown garden plants in the world. When it came to using the toxins from naturally occurring plants and animals, the challenge to NuTech was great because many of the most toxic natural substances would cause horribly painful, prolonged deaths.

NuTech also considered the use of exit bags and inert gases, which were much less problematic.[13] They also discussed reevaluating barbiturates that had been rejected during research trials because of possible lethal side effects. To doctors, "lethal" was a bad thing. To those who wanted a quick, peaceful death, lethal side effects might instead be the answer to a prayer. Many of the methods NuTech considered were quickly ruled out because they were impractical, unavailable, would take a long time to develop, or would bring about a very painful death, but the master list of all possible avenues of research was NuTech's jumping-off point.

Led by Hofsess, the group soon defined its goal. In his *Victoria Manifesto*, dated April 17, 1998, Hofsess threw down the gauntlet before opponents of elective death. He decried church-led opposition and spineless politicians who refused to support the will of the majority of the population, who wanted legal euthanasia and assisted suicide. He also scolded the conservative elements of the right-to-die movement itself.

Addressing the latter, he said, "The current 'politically-correct' method of self-deliverance by a massive overdose of hard-to-obtain medication . . . is about as advanced a method of suicide as a Model T Ford is as a means of transportation."[14] After lambasting those who blocked progress, Hofsess laid out NuTech's agenda for change. "When it comes to developing new and better methods of voluntary dying, we are dealing with a problem that clearly CAN be solved with a modest financial investment—and imagination."[15]

Dr. Pieter Admiraal, a distinguished anesthesiologist and euthanasia pioneer from the Netherlands, agreed to serve as an official consultant and advisor to NuTech.[16] The group quickly embarked on its ambitious plan to create life-ending procedures that would not only work but would also meet twelve critical goals derived from Rob Neils' Dying Well Network's definition of a good death:

1. Death would be swift, gentle, and painless.
2. The method would enable the decedent to say good-bye and die in the company of friends and family.
3. The method would be simple enough for the average person to understand and use alone.
4. The method would guarantee a failure-proof death.
5. The method would be inexpensive.
6. The method would be nonviolent and would not cause seizures, disfigure the corpse, or leave behind a revolting or traumatizing scene for others to find.
7. The method could be used by terminally or incurably ill people who could not swallow pills.
8. The required supplies could be obtained legally, without a prescription.
9. The use of the method would not physically or legally endanger anyone present at the deathing.
10. The method would not require the permission or the involvement of any government authority, medical practitioner, or pharmacist.
11. The method would result in intentionally self-inflicted death, which is not a crime, rather than an assisted suicide or mercy killing, which are illegal in most places.
12. The method would leave little or no evidence that the death was not from natural causes.

These criteria created a truly daunting challenge. However, if NuTech could accomplish its goal without government funding or foundation research grants, it would establish self-deliverance as a *de facto* personal right, whether or not anyone else agreed with it.

Of all the methods evaluated at the early NuTech meetings, Hofsess' preferred choice was his own invention, the Hofsess De-Breather. It was a reverse-engineered derivative of the rebreather, a well-known underwater breathing device used by scuba divers. Normal air consists of about 78 percent nitrogen, 21 percent oxygen, and 1 percent argon and other trace gases. A debreather would allow a person to breathe a fixed amount of normal air and consume the oxygen. Then it would scrub (remove) the carbon dioxide in the exhaled air. This was crucial because the presence of abnormally high amounts of carbon dioxide in the air supply triggers automatic panic attacks. Without carbon dioxide buildup, the body is unaware that it is no longer receiving sufficient oxygen. Soon, the person would be breathing almost pure nitrogen, which does not sustain life. With the carbon dioxide removed, there would be no panic, no feeling of suffocation, and no gasping for air. In just a few minutes, the oxygen level would drop to about 10 percent, and the person would peacefully become unconscious. When the oxygen level dropped below 5 percent, the person would die painlessly, typically within twenty minutes.

Hofsess had previously discussed the development of debreather technology with Rob Neils, and the two stayed in touch, working along parallel tracks to develop prototypes.[17] Hofsess' version quickly evolved as a closed-system breathing device consisting of a face mask connected by soft plastic "accordion" tubing to a carbon dioxide scrubber and an air bag. His team, comprised of Canadian professional rebreather diving technicians, decided to scrub out the carbon dioxide by passing exhaled air through a coffee-can-sized plastic container filled with Sofnolime, a professional grade of soda lime designed for scuba-diving rebreather use. The scrubbed air was then stored in a plastic or rubber bag. When the user inhaled, the stored air was sucked out of the bag and back again through the Sofnolime, removing virtually all remaining carbon dioxide, and was then rebreathed. With each breath, the user consumed a portion of the oxygen, exhaling carbon dioxide, nitrogen, trace gases, and what was left of the oxygen. As a result, the oxygen content of the air dropped rapidly.

Neils' Dying Well Network researchers were testing a some-

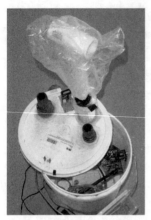

The Kick-the-Bucket Machine CO_2 scrubber

what different system, which sought to scrub out the carbon dioxide through a solution of calcium chloride dissolved in water. The prototype of their device was housed inside a five-gallon plastic bucket. The network's engineers wryly nicknamed their creation the "Kick-the-Bucket machine."[18] Both Hofsess' and Neils' systems successfully scrubbed carbon dioxide out of exhaled air, but the development of Neils' device was significantly slowed by the impracticality of his water-based system and his lack of trained technical manufacturing staff.

Adam Smith,* Hofsess' lead design and construction engineer, and his technical colleagues, Tom Cuthbertson and John Horton, had a working model of the Hofsess DeBreather built and operational by June 25, 1998. Smith personally tested the debreather's effectiveness. "It takes only five minutes to drop the oxygen level from 21 percent to 5 percent. I stopped the test at this point," wrote Smith, "since I wasn't eager to be the first successful user."[19]

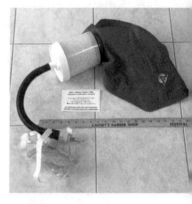

The Spartacus IIb DeBreather

Hofsess named his new invention Spartacus II. The name was, he said, "in honor of the legendary Roman slave who led a revolt against his oppressive masters. I believe that Spartacus II will set us free from patronizing politicians, doctors, ethicists, and all the other do-gooders or nay-sayers who have come to dominate the assisted-suicide field."[20]

Hofsess, Neils, and their technicians were not just avid mechanical tinkerers with too much time on their hands. They believed deeply in personal autonomy and in the right to death with dignity. Hofsess had personally tested the Spartacus II DeBreather, alternately playing the role of guinea pig and observer. As the former, he wrote:

> I placed a soft, pliable silicone mask over my nose and mouth.
> I continued to breathe normally. There was no odor. The air

---

*An asterisk indicates that a pseudonym has been used to protect the person's privacy.

seemed exactly the same (including its temperature) as that which I was accustomed to breathing. But it wasn't the same. A sensor connected to the mask measured the amount of oxygen in the system. Within minutes, the oxygen level declined sharply. There was no discomfort. I had no awareness of any significant change going on. . . . I felt momentarily light-headed but quickly recovered when the mask was removed.[21]

Neils stated that the Dying Well Network's debreather, which was being developed and patented, would be licensed only to groups using stringent psychological screening protocols. If any organization wishing to use his team's debreather refused to agree to safeguards, Neils would legally encumber the debreather "in such a way that it could never be used *unless it is used deliberately, safely, compassionately, efficiently and under guidance of overseeing committees.*"[22]

By 1998, however, Hofsess' Spartacus II DeBreather was already fully operational, leaving Neils, who had no finished and operable device, unable to regulate the use of carbon dioxide scrubbing debreather technology. As a result, the Dying Well Network abandoned its debreather work and began to develop another device.

Using Kevorkian's Mercitron as their inspiration, the network produced the Expirator. It was a simple device that consisted of a soft, inflatable face mask connected by flexible plastic tubing to a pressure-regulator-equipped tank of nitrogen gas. Like helium, nitrogen is inert and not potentially hazardous to bystanders. All of the components were legal and easy to obtain. Inhaling pure nitrogen, a gas to which the body is fully accustomed, produces, as does helium, a painless, nonviolent, and certain death in minutes by displacing oxygen in the breathing cycle.

In the Dying Well Network's website on June 25, 2001, Neils wrote, "We've now had more than 100 deaths due to the use of the inert gases nitrogen or helium.... In all cases death occurred within a few minutes with no apparent discomfort. The deathings went as predicted."[23]

At a later date, Neils, a veteran grief counselor, gave testimony to the governor of Montana at a meeting of Libby, Montana, residents. There, three hundred residents had already died and hundreds more would later die of mesothelioma, a lung cancer caused, in this case, by the mining of asbestos by the W.R. Grace mining company. Grace knew of the massive health threat and covered it up for years. Neils told the audience:

> I was raised in Libby through high school. Back then, no one knew to warn us kids not to breathe! Two or three percent of my lung lining is [now] coated with residue from breathing Grace-poisoned air. I didn't work for Grace nor did any of my family. I was just a kid like any other Libby kid who breathed the toxic dust…. Hundreds of Libbyites are dead from a slow, lingering, gasping, suffocating, terrifying death like my sisters'. . . .
>
> I can help my friends, neighbors, and loved ones die well. I am an international leader in the Right to Die movement. I created the Dying Well Network. I have developed a nitrogen delivery system which each of us victims can use to allow ourselves a more dignified death to happen at the time of our own choosing in the circumstances we create. More than three hundred persons throughout the United States and Canada have used this system to hasten death. None of us have to be the victim to a Nazi-like, Grace-induced horrible death.
>
> It is a felony in Montana to aid a person in controlling their own death even when that person is terminally ill, near death and even when loved ones support and are present at the hastened deathing. I am one of very few people who has been with persons as they hastened death. I will provide information to qualified Libbyites on how to hasten death if any so choose. The last hope of a terminally ill person is the hope to go peacefully…. A governor who would offer clemency or pardon to loved ones aiding a victim avoid a most horribly gruesome and lingering death would be appreciated…. I request the governor for clemency or pardon for those who aid their loved ones to die well.[24]

Neils' Dying Well Network, a no-fee, nonprofit organization, provided information and presence at deathings until the Hemlock Society created and developed its Caring Friends Program. Emotionally drained and exhausted from his exit guide work, and with professionally trained Hemlock exit counselors now available to fill the need, he closed down the network and returned to his practice as a full-time psychologist and grief counselor.

Late in 1999, Adam Smith perfected another version of the debreather, which Hofsess designated Spartacus III. Less than half the size of a shoebox, it had no face mask, weighed about five pounds, and was designed to be used inside one of Hofsess' plastic final exit bags after a barbiturate overdose was taken. Hofsess told me that the Spartacus III prototype pictured here, only one of which was ever constructed, was never released for use, although it would have been completely effective.

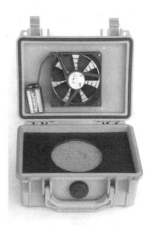

The Spartacus III DeBreather

Soon after the 1997 founding of NuTech, Hofsess contacted Derek Humphry. Now head of his privately financed Euthanasia Research and Guidance Organization (ERGO), Humphry agreed to sponsor NuTech's first official meeting in 1999. Humphry's enormous network of international contacts and his financial support were invaluable. A highly selective guest list was drawn up. The results of the auspicious get-together would change the international face of life and death forever.

The small research group met privately in Berkeley, California, from June 11-13, 1999, to explore ways to put right-to-die technology on the fast track. The attendees, who became known as "The Berkeley Ten," included most of the world's cutting-edge elective death researchers. This first formal conference was later designated NuTech I. Nine more would be held before the end of 2010.

The meeting was convened in the Queen-Anne-style home of Dr. Betty Noble, a retired physician and dedicated Hemlock Society member.[25] The group included three Canadians: Hofsess and his team members Adam Smith and Evelyn Martens. In addition to Dr. Noble and Derek Humphry, there were four other American attendees. Sylvia Gerhard, of Canton, Massachusetts, was a retired academic librarian and member of the board of the Greater Boston Hemlock chapter. She served as secretary for the Hemlock Society USA and became the confidential communications director for NuTech.[26] Dr. Charles E. "Chuck" Whitcher, an expert in the use of anesthetic gases, was a senior anesthesiologist then teaching at Stanford University. Reverend George Exoo and Josephine M. Koss, a psychologist and counselor, represented the Compassionate Chaplaincy Foundation, which they had cofounded.[27] The lone member from outside North America was Australia's Dr. Philip Nitschke.

Many of the attendees were meeting each other for the first time. Their fields of expertise varied greatly. Hofsess and Smith had designed and created working euthanasia devices. Humphry had studied hundreds of euthanasia cases and had been present at the assisted suicides of three relatives. Nitschke had developed sophisticated self-deliverance technology and used it for four legal physician-assisted deaths in Australia. Exoo and Koss were both experienced exit guides and had also been present at a number of deathings.

Martens had watched her brother die of cancer after terrible suffering and joined Hofsess' Right to Die Society, volunteering to help with office work. Soon she was managing their membership activities and helping Hofsess manufacture and distribute exit bags. She then became an exit guide herself. Whitcher, at seventy-eight, was the senior member of the group. An anesthetist but not an exit guide, he nevertheless had a long-standing interest in euthanasia that predated his graduation from the University of Buffalo Medical School in 1950. Exoo said of him, "Chuck was one of the most humble persons I ever met; a physician with no God complex at all."[28] Whitcher was extraordinarily valuable because he knew everything that could go wrong in the process of anesthetizing surgical patients and understood the importance of having a professionally trained person supervise the use of inert gases in any situation.

Hofsess was eager to demonstrate his operational Spartacus II DeBreather. It could be manufactured for $250 to $400 per unit, he estimated, and was extremely portable. He wanted to take the obvious next step and offer use of the device to suffering people. After its developers conducted non-lethal human tests on each other, the DeBreather was sent into the field for use.

Rather than sell his debreathers to users, Hofsess said he would make them available only to organizations he trusted. He named Philip Nitschke's Exit International and George Exoo's Compassionate Chaplaincy Foundation as the first to have access to them. They, he believed, would make sure that the equipment was used properly.[29] Nitschke thought the debreather had too many logistical limitations and never used it. Exoo, the most daring member of the group, volunteered his foundation as Hofsess' clinical field-testing arm.[30] He had an operational Spartacus IIa DeBreather and the necessary Sofnolime for it by April 1999.[31]

The group also considered the oral use of pentobarbital, a powerful, fast-acting barbiturate commonly used by veterinarians to euthanize animals and sold in North America under the trade name Nembutal. Possession of the drug, except

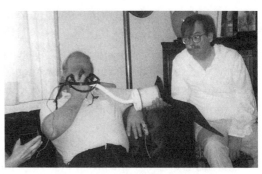

Demonstrating the Spartacus IIa DeBreather in Berkeley

for veterinary use, is prohibited in the Western world. Nembutal, however, is available without a prescription from veterinary supply stores in Mexico, Central and South America, and Asia, although importation for non-veterinary use was banned by most Western countries.[32] Although ingesting six to fifteen grams of Nembutal was guaranteed to produce a swift, painless, and certain death, the difficulty of obtaining it made it impractical for most people who wanted to die.

NuTech needed a new option, and it found it in the ideas of Dr. Bruce Dunn. In 1975, Dunn wrote of lethal gases then used to euthanize laboratory animals, "It would be relatively easy to arrange the apparatus so that the flow of inert gas could be initiated by opening a small valve or removing a hose clamp. This could be done by a terminally ill individual on his or her own, helping to preserve the ethical and legal distinction between a voluntary suicide and a death induced by another party."[33]

Dunn's prescience was profound, and his research resurfaced as the basis for one of NuTech's major new self-deliverance protocols, as the concept was already proven and his method did not require the participation of a physician or an illegal substance.[34]

John Hofsess was the technological pioneer to put this self-deliverance method into use. He and his technicians, Adam Smith and Tom Cuthbertson, had been working on the helium concept well before the Berkeley meeting. With a soft plastic exit bag enclosing the person's head and with nothing but helium to breathe, death would come quickly through anoxia. In addition, helium dissipates rapidly and is extremely difficult to detect in an autopsy unless its presence is suspected in advance.

The exact date that the helium method was first used in the field is not known, but Hofsess was advertising information about its existence in the spring 1998 issue of the Hemlock *Timelines.* After his team had initially experimented with a small tank of helium sold to divers, Hofsess discovered a much more widely available source by searching the internet. There he found that almost all large retail or party supply stores sell kits containing balloons and a tank of helium to inflate them. The party balloon kits come in two standard sizes and are generally sold without age or identification requirements. I found nine retail stores selling them within ten miles of my home in South Carolina. Realizing the potential of the gas, Hofsess reduced the size of his classic exit bag to make the most efficient use of it.

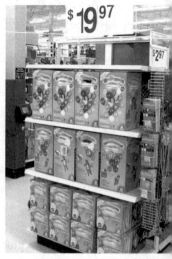

Helium party balloon kits

There was only one potential problem with Hofsess' method. Although the manufacturer offered kits for twenty-five or fifty balloons, the smaller kit was the most easily available. Each twenty-five-balloon kit contained only one relatively small, low-pressure tank, which might not supply enough gas to guarantee a successful suicide. One larger, fifty-balloon kit tank—harder to find—or two smaller tanks working together would definitely be more reliable, so Hofsess' technicians used short plastic hoses and a "T" connector to join two small tanks and ran a third plastic hose from the T-connector into an exit bag to complete the system.

The helium concept immediately captured NuTech's attention.[35] Whitcher, the expert on inert gases, strongly recommended incorporating a combination gas pressure gauge and flow meter between the tanks and the exit hood. This would ensure that the helium supply could be monitored by an observer and would not run out before the suicidal person died. However, if a second person controlled the flow of helium, a solo suicide, which is not a crime, became an assisted suicide, with the threat of possible arrest and imprisonment. To ensure that lack of sufficient gas did not botch a deathing, Exoo took Whitcher's advice and learned how to use the gauge.

Following the Berkeley meeting, the debreather was the first of the two promising NuTech technologies to be used in field trials. Exoo had a debreather and Sofnolime available for use by mid-April 1999. Between then and early 2000, five to ten clients in the United States, Canada, and France used debreathers to make peaceful final exits. Exoo and other exit guides from the Compassionate Chaplaincy Foundation were present at the majority of them. Each person died peacefully within ten to thirty minutes, without any significant discomfort or other problems.

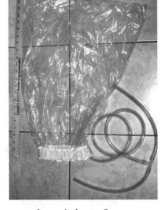

An exit bag for use with helium

Although the debreather worked well, it did not meet one of the criteria established by NuTech: it could not be used without assistance. Since the device was not sold, an exit guide had to provide it, and when the event was over, the guide had to take the unit back to refill it with fresh soda lime. If detected, the act could be classified as an assisted suicide.

An aesthetic consideration also emerged. Because the initial debreather face mask was made of inflexible plastic, air often leaked out around the bridge of the nose unless the elastic straps were kept quite snug. That tight a fit could leave marks on the face, which might be noticed by officials who found the body. People who choose self-deliverance often want the world to believe they died of natural causes, and would not want anything to indicate otherwise. The solution turned out to be a soft, inflatable partial face mask, which better conformed to the contours of the face both before and after death.

Another challenge was the cost and availability of the soda lime granules used to absorb the carbon dioxide. That product had to be purchased from a diving supply distributor, which, although legal, created a paper trail—a potential liability for the exit guide and the patient seeking privacy. In addition, at that time, the granules were available only in forty-four-pound (20 kg) containers—enough for more than forty deathings—for about $149 USD per container. After considering its use, supply, and cost drawbacks, the field testers concluded that the Hofsess Spartacus II DeBreather was unsuitable for widespread use. As a result, NuTech turned to inert gases.

The new helium method made a legal and dignified final exit

very affordable. Only two items were necessary, and each was legally available without a permit or prescription. The party balloon kits could be purchased for about $25 USD, but the purchase of two was suggested. In Canada, Hofsess' Last Rights Research Group manufactured and sold helium exit bags for $40 CAD each until 2002, when Evelyn Martens, who manufactured the bags, was arrested (and later vindicated) for aiding and abetting the suicides of two Canadian women. From 2002 to 2005, the supply of professionally manufactured bags was disrupted.

Rod Newman, a life member of the Hemlock Society and of its Caring Friends Program, took over the manufacture of the bags in 2005. Under the company name NuLife Products, he and his wife made the bags in Montana until 2009, when he was eighty years old and health problems intervened. That same year, Sharlotte Hydorn, a ninety-one-year-old California retired science teacher and great-grandmother, began producing the bags under the business name The Gladd Group, standing for "Good Life and Dignified Death." She made the bags with great care at home and sold them for $60 USD. Her production was shut down on May 25, 2011, when a team of FBI agents arrived at her door and confiscated all her supplies, her sewing machine, computer, and records. With scarcely a pause, the production of the exit bags, which remain in high demand, was quickly restarted elsewhere by others in the movement. In response to the loss of Hydorn's bags, Derek Humphry stepped in and offered anyone worldwide a $5.00 USD downloadable booklet detailing the precise directions on how to make their own exit bags at http://www.finalexit.org/ergo-store/.

The first helium deathings occurred in late August or early September 1999 and continued for several months. At least six NuTech-trained exit guides, generally working in teams of two, put the helium system into use, with no significant problems reported. The guides discovered that one tank of helium was generally sufficient for a rapid and peaceful death.

Whether or not a client qualified for a hastened death via the debreather or the helium system was left in the hands of the client and whatever exit guide he or she worked with. To some euthanasia advocates, the unfettered use of the new technology was the exercise of the ultimate civil right. Some outside the movement saw it as a threat to vulnerable people. What has never been in question is that in its early years, the entire self-deliverance movement was as unregulated as America's "Wild West."

NuTech pulled off another coup when it convened an international euthanasia technical conference in Seattle on November 13 and 14, 1999, just five months after the Berkeley meeting. The timing was no coincidence, as President George W. Bush's backers in the U.S. House of Representatives had just passed the Pain Relief Promotion Act (also known as the Hyde bill), which would have made it illegal for doctors to prescribe the lethal doses of prescription drugs used in Oregon's newly enacted Death With Dignity Law, thereby rendering it impotent. Although the Hyde bill never became law, it had an unintended effect: it lit a fire under the do-it-yourself self-deliverance boiler. By no coincidence, George Stone, a physician and euthanasia activist, published a comprehensive do-it-yourself book, *Suicide and Assisted Suicide*, that same year.

Attendance at the 1999 NuTech II conference was by invitation only. Canadian and American inventors presented an astounding array of self-deliverance equipment and techniques. Nitschke described the impetus that drove the group: "The feeling that death has nothing to do with doctors, that laws that involve the medical profession are flawed, that the political process will never free itself from religious interference and satisfactorily address this issue is leading to an increasing demand for technical, do-it-yourself solutions."[36]

In all, the meeting drew twenty-nine physicians, technicians, and other experts from right-to-die organizations worldwide. The conferees included Humphry, who funded the conference; Hofsess, the convener; Exoo and Koss; Whitcher; Neils; Nitschke; Dr. Faye Girsh, then president of the Hemlock Society; Dr. Pieter V. Admiraal, from the Netherlands; Russel D. Ogden, a Canadian criminology scholar; and Michael Bineau and Dr. Kurt F. Schobert, both of the Deutsche Gesellschaft Für Humanes Sterben (DGHS – the German Association for Humane Death). Save for Ogden, an academic, attendance at all sessions was restricted to those with direct experience in self-deliverance.[37]

One notable euthanasia activist was not invited: Dr. Jack Kevorkian. He was adamant that all deathings should take place only under the direct supervision of physicians, whereas the NuTech advocates wanted to totally cut the umbilical cord that tied dying people to the control of doctors. Even if he had wanted to attend, Kevorkian could

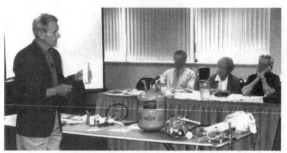

*Dr. Charles Whitcher explains
NuTech equipment in 1999.*

not have. Two months earlier, he had been convicted of the second-degree murder of Thomas Youk and was serving his prison sentence in Michigan.

NuTech's direct-action, do-it-yourself philosophy stirred up more controversy than naked pagans dancing at an Easter parade. Within the movement worldwide, many conservatives saw Humphry, Hofsess, Nitschke, and Exoo as dangerous radicals who would disrupt the delicate consensus-building process needed for state and national death-with-dignity laws to be enacted. Two Oregon right-to-die groups, Compassion in Dying and the Oregon Death With Dignity Legal Defense Center, were not invited to the Seattle meeting because they advocated only legally regulated physician aid-in-dying.[38]

After the Seattle meeting closed, Barbara Coombs Lee, then director of Compassion in Dying, a precursor of the present-day Compassion & Choices, accused NuTech members of being extremists. "Oregonians don't need this conference because they have a safe and well-regulated option for peaceful dying," she told a reporter. "Compassion chooses to keep working for aid-in-dying as one choice included in end-of-life medical care. It should be part of medical care."[39]

Three carefully chosen journalists and their photographers from the United States, Canada, and Australia were invited to a closed-door briefing and given descriptions and demonstrations of some of the new equipment. Based on his field experience, Exoo told a reporter that the use of helium was the "Cadillac of final exit methods at a Volkswagen price."[40]

When the *Seattle Times* and the *Vancouver Sun* ran the story a few days later, ferocious controversy erupted along predictable lines. Euthanasia supporters were delighted that the new technology was totally egalitarian and would take the sting out of death for suffering people, regardless of their ethnicity, nationality, religion, or income level.

Anti-euthanasia groups were appalled that "death merchants"

were using the media to brazenly promote immoral and unethical ways to kill people. Ted Gerk, of the Pro-Life Resource Centre in British Columbia, was angered that Hofsess, a fellow Canadian, had developed the debreather, and urged police to "investigate whether he [Hofsess] was involved in the deaths of those who use it."[41] The Mounties chose not to do so.

Wesley J. Smith, an attorney and frequent spokesman for the International Anti-Euthanasia Task Force and a prolific pro-life author and blogger, was incensed—but not surprised—that NuTech had been formed and had developed do-it-yourself suicide devices. Referring to NuTech's revelations at the Seattle conference, he wrote:

> As macabre and bizarre as this gathering was, it provided some badly needed truth in advertising about the assisted suicide movement. . . . as the Self Delivery Technology Conference [sic] illustrated, assisted suicide isn't all about health care or the proper treatment of illness or disability. Beneath the propaganda of compassion and the euphemisms, such as 'aid in dying,' assisted suicide is purely and simply about making people dead. . . . Killing devices are not akin to kidney dialysis machines, and poison is not medicine.[42]

As NuTech's devices and procedures rapidly came into more general use, those facing ghastly deaths saw NuTech methods as an answer to their most fervent prayers. Opponents regarded NuTech as the embodiment of the devil's work and claimed that the group would spark a huge slide down the ethical slippery slope, ending in devaluation of human life and a society that approved of death-on-demand for anyone who no longer wanted to live, regardless of their reasons.

Rob Neils framed the debate this way: "Would a person vehemently against the right to die ask for it? Not very likely, unless that person became terminally ill with no hope of recovery, no quality of life, no dignity left and no relief from pain. . . . The idea of controlling dying may offend persons with overly rigid beliefs against it but it is a reasonable and popular idea which now needs exploration."[43]

Despite its critics, the helium method began to make major waves. In 2001, Russel Ogden noted, "Roughly seventy out of one hundred people known to have killed themselves with NuTech [devices or procedures] over the last eighteen months have opted for the helium system."[44] By 2002, the helium system was the primary method recommended and used by most major right-to-die organizations in North America—whether they publicly admitted it or not.

NuTech III was held in Boston from September 1-3, 2000, in parallel with (but not part of) the World Conference on Assisted Dying. The main gathering was sponsored by the World Federation of Right to Die Societies and its host, Dying With Dignity (Canada). Because it was not a member of the more conservative World Federation, NuTech held its meetings separately—but concurrently—so any World Federation delegate who wished to do so could attend. The main conference attracted nearly five hundred participants who came to hear sixty-six speakers.

It was also greeted with a well-organized and highly vocal protest by Not Dead Yet (NDY), a grassroots U.S. disability rights organization formed in 1996 that opposed the legalization of assisted suicide and euthanasia because they perceived both as direct or indirect threats to disabled persons.

The protest was ignited by a seemingly innocuous event. Diane Coleman, a disability rights activist who is confined to a wheelchair, is the founder of NDY. An intelligent, articulate, and impassioned woman who earned a law degree and an MBA from UCLA, she was invited to participate in a panel discussion. The moderator of the session, Dr. Paul A. Spiers, an MIT neuropsychologist, a paraplegic, and a wheelchair user, was designated to offer NDY two places on the six-person panel to debate euthanasia issues. Spiers served on the Hemlock Society's board to provide a disabled person's viewpoint on elective death with dignity, but he wrote, "In spite of the fact that I am myself physically challenged, I find it difficult to understand their [Not Dead Yet's] perspective."[45] Not Dead Yet, on the other hand, considered him to be public relations window dressing to defuse criticism of the right-to-die movement by disability advocacy groups.

Coleman felt that her group was not being offered fair and equal representation. She made a counterproposal: an equal number of pro- and anti-euthanasia speakers would debate the issue in a neutral, public space. Her proposal was declined, and Coleman led her group into the streets.

On the cold, rainy first day of the conference, fifty NDY members, some in wheelchairs, some walking, circled across the street from the conference hotel, chanting slogans and carrying signs. One sign, held high by a smiling young woman, proclaimed, "Serial Killers: Bundy, Gacy, Kevorkian, Humphry."[46] Coleman called the right-to-die assembly "a wolf in sheep's clothing: the trappings of compassion, but the reality of corporate greed—and social contempt for ill and disabled people who are seen as expendable."[47] Referring to NuTech, Coleman added, "It's a little ghoulish. It shows how easy it is to commit suicide without someone's assistance and . . . how easy it is to disguise killing somebody."[48]

As a minivan emblazoned with hot pink "NOT DEAD YET" signs circled the hotel, several of the right-to-die delegates unsuccessfully tried to engage the protesters in meaningful dialogue. Ilene Kaplan, president of the Connecticut chapter of the Hemlock Society, recalled:

> I went over to a man in a wheelchair and wanted to ask him about the protest. I wanted to tell him that we were for the right to die, not the *duty* to die. I was wearing a Hemlock Society badge, so he knew I was a representative of 'the enemy.' He said to me, 'Just because I'm a cripple doesn't mean that I don't have a right to my life to the fullest.' I tried to tell him that we totally agreed with him; that he had an absolute right to his life, and that our issue was one of choice of when to die, not an obligation to. . . . but he refused to listen, and returned to yelling his slogans.[49]

On Sunday, the third and final day, thirteen people walking and rolling arm-in-arm on the street behind a bright pink banner that read "Not Dead Yet / We Want to Live" were arrested for blocking traffic. With no police vehicles equipped to accommodate wheelchairs, the authorities commandeered two lift-equipped city buses, emptied them of their bewildered paying passengers, and used the buses to transport the protesters to the police station. Once processed, the demonstrators were all quickly released and were never prosecuted.

Of NuTech's next meeting, held May 12-13, 2001 in Vancouver, Canada, Hofsess wrote:

> Forty-one people from seven countries brainstormed about ways and means of advancing non-medical means of creating 'a good death.' It appeared that . . . a creative ferment had been

activated and that NuTech was on a roll. . . . everyone was welcome to make suggestions, or better yet, work on creating practical applications of their ideas and testing them, reporting on the results at some future NuTech conference. It was deeply gratifying to me to see that we were liberated from the confining concept of 'physician-assisted suicide' and that we had [developed] practical means of non-medical suicide.[50]

One presentation made in Vancouver was unique: that of Georgene V. ("GiGi") Sandberg, seventy-four, a petite, determined, silver-haired woman from Mississippi, who had an extensive professional expertise in large-scale commercial hydroponic gardening. Her interest in the right-to-die movement stemmed from the agony of her mother's terminal illness. In unrelenting pain, her mother had repeatedly begged her daughter to help her die. Because Sandberg did not know how, her mother suffered through a prolonged, horrible death. Looking for ways to help people in similar situations, Sandberg joined the Hemlock Society and became their southeastern regional coordinator.

Through Hemlock Society newsletters, she learned of NuTech. John Hofsess, who always pushed for multiple channels of independent research, enthusiastically encouraged her ideas for developing lethal plant hybrids for self-deliverance. Within months, Sandberg and her husband developed a simple hydrogarden that anyone could build at home for less than $100. In her garden, tasty organic vegetables grew side by side with lethal plants such as yellow jessamine (the South Carolina state flower), dumbcane, monkshood, and coleus.

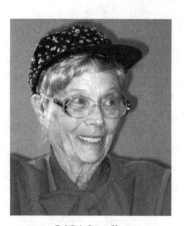

GiGi Sandberg

A tiny, tenacious woman with mischievous brown eyes, Sandberg was eighty-two years old when I interviewed her in December 2008. She was full of energy, sporting an outrageously decorated hat, and talking a mile a minute. She was also just two months away from dying of terminal cancer, but she gushed about the encouragement she had received from Hofsess and beamed while describing the hydrogarden she had created for her NuTech botanical experimentation. Her rapid success led to her presentation at the Vancouver conference. Hofsess said of her with pride, "When the flame of NuTech burned at its brightest, GiGi's research held great promise."[51]

Nevertheless, she was disappointed by the general response. "When I demonstrated the growing system in Vancouver in 2001, there was little interest. Growing toxic plants wasn't sexy enough."[52] She was baffled that using toxic plants for self-deliverance was thought odd, considering that Socrates, the patron saint of the euthanasia movement, had ended his life by drinking the sap of the poisonous hemlock tree.

Undaunted, she pursued her hydroponic ideas on her own. She also had a closet full of state-of-the-art NuTech deathing equipment ready for her personal use. But, like the majority of death-with-dignity activists, she had no intention of using any of it prematurely. Two days before her death, she insisted that her husband let her drive the 150-mile roundtrip to New Orleans for her chemotherapy. A bundle of energy until the end, she died a peaceful, unassisted death in her sleep on February 4, 2009, nine days short of her eighty-third birthday.[53]

At the fifth NuTech conference held January 9-12, 2003, in San Diego, Nitschke was scheduled to demonstrate a new deathing device. He had developed a simple carbon monoxide gas generator, nicknamed COGen, which could be manufactured from common items (mostly plastic pipes) readily available in hardware stores.[54] Nitschke ran into a major problem when he tried to bring the device to the United States. Australian customs officials confiscated it at the airport before they allowed him to depart. However, he found the basic parts he needed during a hasty shopping trip in San Diego and quickly constructed a mockup in his hotel room.[55] This was the last meeting that Hofsess attended, and the first one at which he was able to overcome stage fright and address a large group of people.[56]

NuTech met again in Seattle in January 2004, followed by meetings in Toronto in September 2006, in Paris in November 2008, and in Melbourne in October 2010. Each NuTech meeting was concurrent with the convention of the World Federation of Right to Die Societies. Despite these NuTech conferences, most surviving members of the original Berkeley Ten are disappointed with the lack of technological progress in the last decade.

Oddly enough, the scientific, medical, and forensic community remained virtually oblivious to the rapidly growing use of NuTech methods for a full decade after the headline-making newspaper coverage of the 1999 NuTech conference in Seattle. As late as 2007, by which time at least five thousand people worldwide had chosen a peaceful death by helium, and scores of public newspaper and magazine articles about the subject had been published, a peer-reviewed article in *The American Journal of Forensic Medicine and Pathology* nevertheless stated that the helium system "is a rarely described method of committing suicide."[57]

Because of the ready availability, low cost, and high reliability of the helium method, Hofsess believed little interest existed in exploring new techniques. "I used to say that Bolivian drug dealers were more enterprising in creating new versions of designer drugs than anyone in the right-to-die movement was in relieving the pain and distress of millions through our simple new methods. Now we tend to talk a lot, wring our hands a lot; but, when it comes to imaginatively transforming the deathing process, we have generally accepted the role of government and medical associations instead of creative defiance," he lamented.[58] Nevertheless, Hofsess is extremely proud of what he launched. As he stated in 2008, "Creating the NuTech movement was the apex of my life."[59]

Nitschke continued to develop deathing techniques, but both his COGen machine and his Peanut Project, an ongoing effort to synthesize Nembutal using homemade technology, got a cool reception at NuTech conferences. "The spirit of enquiry, openness to new ideas, and entrepreneurial spirit of John Hofsess typified in the early days had been lost," Nitschke wrote.[60]

NuTech is deliberately ephemeral. It has no officers, by-laws, constitution, dues, or fixed meeting schedules or meeting places. It does not even have a formal membership—just a floating, ever-changing pool of collaborators, linked by its senior members.

Nevertheless, NuTech has had a profound effect on the way that people now view their end-of-life choices. Dr. Margaret Pabst Battin, a distinguished professor of philosophy at the University of Utah, has been studying the ethics of death and dying for two decades. She believes that NuTech's methods could provide a compromise in the debate over voluntary euthanasia by enabling self-determination while avoiding the controversy of physician involvement. She foresees the possibility of a future where dying is no longer something that happens to us but is something we choose to do for ourselves.[61]

Currently, NuTech is focused on refining successful self-deliverance technologies, seeking new ones, sharing experiences, and educating law-enforcement authorities about the realities of legal self-deliverance. Although no one has found another concept that meets all twelve of NuTech's critical standards and is better or less expensive than the helium system, someone eventually will discover what Philip Nitschke refers to as "The Peaceful Pill," the ultimate painless, fast-acting, legal self-deliverance method.

One thing is certain. Whoever creates the better method will be building on the foundation of the radical pioneers who met in 1997 and, for the first time, defined how rational people, acting alone, could legally control the time, place, and quality of their own deaths.

Grandma Martens Makes Her Rounds

Enforced life, by any other name, would be called slavery. Forcing someone to stay alive when they believe that only death can release them from intolerable suffering is an unjustified restriction of individual freedom.
— Wanda Morris, Executive Director, Dying With Dignity-Canada

Until her brother Cornelius died of bone cancer in 1989, Evelyn Marie Martens had never thought a great deal about dying. But Cornelius' last two months, as the cancer metastasized, were excruciatingly painful. Watching him suffer, she and her family confronted his physicians and demanded more morphine to control his pain. They were told bluntly that if he had more sedation, it would hasten his death, and they would be responsible. They agreed to accept the responsibility. The dose was increased, and Cornelius died the following morning.[1]

Martens was born into a hard-working family in rural Swift Current, Saskatchewan, Canada, on January 10, 1931. She and her three siblings were left fatherless when she was six. After her mother remarried, Martens gained another brother and sister, and then her stepfather died, leaving the children fatherless again. "We've known poverty at its worst. We've always maintained that hardship builds character, and indeed our circumstances brought us closer together," she said.[2]

At the age of seventeen, Martens married Jack Batsch, but she soon suffered another catastrophe. Only a year after the birth of their first child, her husband became one of the first Canadian soldiers killed in the Korean War. She later married a Catholic man who turned abusive. She had five more children before she left him. Penniless and wondering how to make ends meet as her husband shut down their bank accounts, she was able to find a government job. The children provided financial help, and the family got by. Because of the church's position on family planning and other issues, Martens became disillusioned with Catholicism in particular and religion in general and found what she was looking for in humanist philosophy. After she retired in 1989, Martens and her daughter bought a home in Victoria, British Columbia.[3]

When John Hofsess launched the RTDS-C in 1991, Martens, then a vigorous sixty-year-old, was one of the first to join. She volunteered to stuff envelopes, run errands, and perform any odd jobs that needed to be done. Because of her willingness to work and her natural gift for supportive listening, she quickly became invaluable to Hofsess. She was assigned the job of manufacturing and shipping the Hofsess/Last Rights exit bags.

"The exit bags and literature on how to die were in great demand, keeping me busy mailing orders all over the world," she said. "I met many wonderful people. Some were desperate for information on end-of-life issues, for themselves or loved ones. I spent countless hours on the telephone. Sometimes all they wanted was for someone to really listen to them, without judgment."[4]

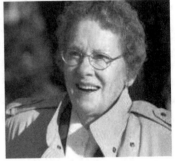

Evelyn Martens

The pain and frustration she heard while dealing with the society's members convinced her to go a step further and become an end-of-life counselor and exit guide. "I agreed to be present at the self-deliverance of some of our members. I wanted to give human comfort whenever I could. I empathized with these people, so ill, in pain, and having to make such difficult decisions at the ends of their lives. I can imagine the trauma they feel. It must also be so terribly lonely to have no one else with them at this time."[5]

Before becoming an active exit guide, Martens asked her oldest son what he thought of the idea. "If you don't have the courage of your convictions," he asked, "what good are your convictions? That's what you always taught us, isn't it?"[6]

"Around 1997 she sat for the first time at the bedside of an individual who decided to end their suffering by a carefully planned suicide," wrote Russel Ogden, a Kwantlen Polytechnic University criminologist and Canadian scholar who had focused his research on assisted suicides. "When there was nobody else to support a dying person, Evelyn, ever the compassionate one, was there."[7]

Exit guides put themselves at great legal risk when the telephone rings because they never know who is on the other end. Someone with a rational reason to consider self-deliverance? Someone suffering from treatable depression? Someone with treatable medical problems? A law enforcement officer seeking to entrap them? Martens was soon to run into the latter.

On January 2, 2002, Martens received a call from Monique Charest, a member of the RTDS-C. She lived in a small town eighty kilometers north of Victoria and had already been in contact with Martens.

Charest, whom Martens described as "a very precise little woman, warm-hearted," was in her sixties and suffered from a thyroid deficiency, reflux disease, and chronic back pain caused by a degenerative spinal disorder.[8] She also had acute intermittent porphyria, a group of potentially fatal disorders affecting the nervous system, and a pulmonary embolism for which she had been hospitalized.[9] Though Charest was not technically terminally ill, her physician had signed a DNR order for her because she was afraid that she would suffer a stroke and be unable to make her own decisions.[10]

Charest chose January 7, 2002, for her final exit. She asked Martens to be with her. Martens brought up the option of palliative care, but Charest was firm. She was ready to die. By previous agreement, Martens' colleague, Brenda Hurn, a fellow RTDS-C member, drove with her to Charest's home the following week. Charest had purchased all the necessary supplies: a Hofsess exit bag and two tanks of helium. She also had sufficient drugs to suppress her physical pain and permit her to proceed rationally. Charest had formerly been a Catholic nun and still had some sensitivity to the church's stance on suicide. She asked Martens to remove the helium tanks and exit bag after their use because she wanted her death to appear to be the natural result of her underlying illnesses.

Martens and Hurn arrived at her home at 1 p.m. Charest had already taken a double dose of morphine so that she could be a little more mobile. When Charest appeared to be reluctant to proceed, Martens strongly suggested that she and Hurn could come back another day and that it was perfectly okay for her to change her mind.

Charest became agitated, and insisted, "Now, today is the time.

I've had enough pain. I want you to know that I'm not frightened of dying, but I'm deathly afraid of living and having another seizure. If I were to become impaired and trapped [inside my own body], life would be intolerable for me."[11]

After she calmed down, Charest made her final preparations. Martens described her last minutes as purposeful and peaceful.

> After making herself comfortable on the couch, she swallowed the drugs with some wine. When she started to feel drowsy, she put the exit bag on her head as far as her forehead [and] opened the tank valves, filling the bag with helium. Her last words were 'My good Lord did not come for me, so I am going to Him.' Then she pulled the bag down over her face, and closed the Velcro neckband. She took several deep breaths, and quickly lost consciousness. Soon thereafter, she stopped breathing. When the tanks were completely empty, and I could find no pulse, we packed the items and left. It was almost 4 p.m.[12]

Charest's body was discovered by her apartment manager. The coroner, for lack of other evidence, ruled the death to have been from natural causes. Charest's friend and executrix, Wendy Hepburn, and her family cleaned out the apartment the following day. When going through Charest's papers, Hepburn found suspicious correspondence between Charest and Martens. She notified the police. The authorities questioned the apartment manager, who recalled seeing two women in the building on the relevant day.

Corporal Wilton, the investigating Royal Canadian Mounted Police (RCMP) officer, suspected that Charest's death might be part of a worldwide mercy killing organization. If so, cracking the case would be a major career-builder. His hunch was strengthened when he later received word from Irish authorities that they had uncovered evidence of a link between Martens and Rosemary Toole, whose sensational 2002 self-deliverance case engulfed George Exoo. Despite the fact that Martens had counseled Toole to consider alternatives to suicide and had refused to travel to Ireland to sit with her as she died, the presence of Marten's emails on Toole's computer was enough to implicate her.

Wilton set up an elaborate police sting operation. Corporal "Jane Smith" (a court order forbade the release of her real name), a twenty-year veteran of undercover operations, posed as Charest's goddaughter. She contacted Martens, telling her that she had found her name in correspondence with her godmother. Smith purported to be distressed by her godmother's death and asked if they could meet to help her cope with her feelings. "She was so smooth," Martens said. "I believed her story. She was so convincing."[13]

Martens told Smith that she had a meeting in Vancouver on June 26, 2002, but she would call her afterwards to arrange to talk. Martens was, in fact, going to be at the side of RTDS-C member Leyanne Burchell, who was in the final stages of stomach cancer, as she ended her life.

Burchell had been a vibrant, intelligent teacher who had traveled extensively until the disease made it impossible. The cancer had spread to her bowel, causing a growing obstruction that prevented her from eating, and by the summer of 2002, she had become severely emaciated. Morphine could no longer control her pain.[14] On the morning of June 26, with Martens at her side, Burchell ended her life with an overdose of prescription drugs.

Martens, then seventy-one, was unaware that she was now on an RCMP active watch list and had no idea that she had been shadowed that morning by three unmarked police cars. All had followed her from her home onto the ferry to Vancouver Island and then on to Burchell's home, where the authorities continued their surveillance until Martens went to meet Monique Charest's "grieving goddaughter."

The meeting was supposed to take place in a hotel room, which the police had wired to record their conversation. But Martens told the undercover officer that she was not familiar with that part of the city and offered to meet at The Grind, a popular coffee shop, instead. They talked at an outside table, on a main street, making it hard for the detective's concealed microphone to pick up the whole conversation clearly.

"I told her that Monique was adamant in her decision to end her life, and that all I did was offer her comfort," Martens said. "I really tried to console this poor girl. She seemed so darned sincere. She was feeling so guilty for not being with her godmother when she died. She cried bitter tears and could [have been] an award-winning actress! I felt so sorry for her."[15]

She talked with the "goddaughter" for more than an hour and then headed back to the ferry to return to Victoria. After she left, the police officers noticed that Martens' stay at Burchell's house had not taken very long. Becoming alarmed at what might have happened there, the authorities returned to the house and found Leyanne Burchell's body.

Martens had already driven her van onto the ferry and was headed home. The police at the station nearest the ferry terminal were notified and told to arrest Martens for aiding and abetting the suicides of two people. Consequently, her van was held back until all the other vehicles were unloaded. Two RCMP officers then arrested Martens, impounded her van, and locked her up in a holding cell. There she sat, with nothing to eat until 1 p.m. the next day. On the counsel of the Legal Aid Society, Martens refused to answer any questions, much to the displeasure of the police.

Three anxious days passed until she could see Catherine Tyhurst and Peter Firestone, the two attorneys her daughter had retained for her. She was transferred from one police detachment to the other and was eventually sent to a women's penitentiary on Vancouver Island, where the guards were civil and the inmates were kind to her. One of the older prisoners took her arm and assured her, "Grandma, if anybody gives you any trouble, you come and I'll look after it."[16] Martens, who had never gotten even a traffic ticket, was relieved.[17]

Evelyn Martens was the first and only right-to-die activist in Canada prosecuted for the offense of aiding a suicide. The two counts levied against her, one for Charest and one for Burchell, left her liable for imprisonment for up to twenty-eight years.[18] The prosecutors evidently thought Martens was part of an international death ring and wanted to keep her in jail until her trial, which could have been two years.

A petite woman with neatly curled gray hair and gold wire-rimmed glasses, she looked weary but composed as she sat in the prisoner's dock at her bail hearing seven days after her arrest. Thirteen members of her family sat in quiet support in the courthouse.

After considering letters of reference from all over Canada, Judge Keith Bracken granted her bail, with strict restrictions. These included allowing random searches of her home, observing a curfew from 10 p.m. to 6 a.m., reporting to her bail supervisor every two weeks, not leaving Vancouver without permission, not contacting anyone connected to the RTDS-C, and not having access to a computer. The last two conditions threw the RTDS-C into chaos.

In the late 1990s, John Hofsess had split the organization into two parts. Toronto native and long-time member Ruth von Fuchs became executive director, putting her in charge of making public appearances and giving interviews on the legal and political aspects of assisted suicide law reform. Hofsess ran NuTech and Last Rights Publications (LRP) from Vancouver. Both of his operations were essentially covert enterprises that skirted the law, and he did not want them to be associated with the society's more conventional right-to-die public outreach and political lobbying efforts.

Martens' arrest, however, jeopardized everything. As membership secretary, Martens maintained all of the RTDS-C's computer-based mailing lists. She also manufactured Hofsess' exit bags and was the shipping manager for both the bags and LRP. When the police seized her computer and all of her RTDS-C records, the society lost its membership and financial databases.

When Martens was charged with two counts of aiding and abetting a suicide, Hofsess was afraid that the police would swoop down on him because of their close working relationship. His attorney advised him to stand down immediately from all right-to-die activities and sever all contact with RTDS-C staff, volunteers, and members until after her trial was over.

"I knew that if I went on being too well known as spokesperson for the organization, my efforts to provide underground [counseling and exit guide] services would be compromised. Therefore, I sought to disappear like the Cheshire cat in *Alice in Wonderland*," he said.[19] Hofsess quickly vanished from public view in Canada and became known as the "Underground Man."

He sought to transfer his publishing and exit bag manufacturing businesses to the United States to maintain his income. "I tried twice in the years that followed—2004 in West Virginia and in 2005 in California—to rebuild LRP from within the United States, first by re-establishing a distribution source for Exit Bags," he wrote.[20] "None of our NuTech or right-to-die colleagues were supportive of LRP's survival, even to the smallest degree of letting their members know that our Exit Bags were available within the U.S. And so, LRP and its NuTech activities came to an end.... Personally, I feel that everything that was important in my life ended in 2002," Hofsess noted bitterly.[21]

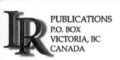

PUBLICATIONS
P.O. BOX
VICTORIA, BC
CANADA

EVELYN MARTENS
NuTech Consultant

Voice: 250-
Email: miled@   Fax: 250-

Evelyn Martens' business card

Although Martens' professional card carried the Last Rights Publications logo and the title, "NuTech Consultant," and it was she who manufactured and distributed the Hofsess exit bags worldwide, Hofsess claimed that he had no knowledge of the details of her work as an exit guide and, specifically, knew nothing of the Charest and Burchell cases.[22] Stating that he had run up $7,000 CAD in legal fees himself because of her activities, he did not contribute to the legal defense fund established by Martens' supporters. Martens felt abandoned and betrayed. Fortunately, right-to-die societies around the world, and hundreds of individuals, came forward and paid over $200,000 of Martens' estimated $250,000 in legal fees.

With Hofsess having fled Canada, and with a court order preventing Martens from having any contact with him or her legion of Canadian friends and supporters, the gentle grandmother spent two lonely years waiting for her trial. When it began on October 12, 2004, Martens was deeply moved to see so many supporters in the courtroom. They included Tom Horton, the Hofsess electrical engineer responsible for developing the Coleman air pump timer and other devices relating to the helium system. Because he was a man with no close family members nearby, Martens had frequently invited him to holiday dinners.[23] Martens also had the moral support of the humanists of Canada. Their president, Gary Bauslaugh, editor of the *Humanist Perspective*, attended the trial every day and published an extensive and insightful account of the proceedings. Canadian criminologist Russel Ogden, who had deep scholarly interests in the right-to-die underground, also attended. Many more demonstrated in front of the courthouse, and others held rallies in Victoria and Vancouver.

One observer hoping for Martens' conviction was Beverly Welsh, a member of the Euthanasia Prevention Coalition, whose newsletter had earlier stated, "death zealot kills two." She was quoted in the press as saying that she hoped Martens would go to jail.[24]

The much-vaunted covert tape recording of Martens' conversation with the undercover police officer in the coffee shop, which was seemingly the prosecution's most damning piece of evidence, proved to contain nothing that would incriminate her in Charest's suicide.

The prosecution sought to show that Martens had provided the drugs, the helium hood, and the helium that caused Monique Charest's death, but Martens' lawyers methodically unraveled the Crown's case. They showed that the prosecution had no proof that Martens had provided the drugs, that two locations near Charest's home sold helium tanks, and that the hood itself could be purchased from several other sources or made at home.

As for Leyanne Burchell, her condition was so severe that her physician stated that she would probably have died within thirty days even without Martens' visit. He also noted that she died of a mixture of several drugs that would have increased the lethality of the morphine overdose she had taken. No helium bags or tanks were found at Burchell's apartment, but Martens had two empty tanks and an exit bag in her van when she was arrested. That, however, did not prove that Burchell had used them, and no such evidence was ever provided by the prosecution.

Although facing a possible twenty-eight-year prison sentence, Martens remained calm and resolute. "I had steeled myself about going to jail and I was ready for it," she said. "I'd take courses, and do lots of things."[25]

Late in the afternoon of Thursday, November 24, 2004, the judge ordered all parties back into the courtroom. The jury had made its decision. Gary Bauslaugh wrote, "Everyone in the courtroom stood as the Judge entered. Evelyn stood up, with perfect calmness, seemingly unafraid…. The ending came suddenly. The Clerk read out the first of the two charges—the Charest charge, the problematic one. I glanced at Evelyn; she was perfectly steady. The jury Foreman said 'we find the defendant not guilty.' And in that one wonderful, terrifying instant, we knew that Evelyn had won. And we knew that, in a world where it is too rarely so, human decency and kindness had won."[26] She was also found not guilty of assisting the suicide of Leyanne Burchell.

Martens was deeply moved and very proud. "It is important to note that the enormous expenditure was not in vain. The trial has established that mere attendance at a suicide is not a criminal offence within the meaning of section 241(b) of the criminal code."[27]

After her ordeal, Martens retired from active duty in the death-with-dignity movement. She died of natural causes on January 2,

2011, while visiting family and grandchildren in Alberta, a week before her eightieth birthday.[28]

In the last years before she died, Martens must have been discouraged by the lack of memberships in her own and other Canadian right-to-die organizations. By 2010, more than 75 percent of Canada's thirty-four million people supported the right to die with dignity. But supporting the concept and joining organized right-to-die groups were two very different things. In that year, the two surviving groups—DWD, headed by its new executive director, Wanda Morris, and RTDS-C, still led by president Ruth von Fuchs—had a combined total of less than two thousand members. Both groups had spent the previous decade encouraging the use of advance directives and providing counseling and a compassionate bedside presence for their members, not actively seeking legislative change. The 1993 failure of Sue Rodriguez' court fight for the right to die led to years of relative inactivity in the attempt to amend Canada's assisted suicide law.

But as Canada's English-speaking majority lost its fervor for legislative change, its French-speaking countrymen and women more than picked up the slack. In the first decade of the twenty-first century, the most intensely fought battles for the legalization of death with dignity in Canada were being led by the residents of Québec.

Unlike the rest of Canada, which is largely a mixture of English-speaking Protestants and non-believers, the Québécois have deep roots in Catholicism. But, as their ancestors demonstrated with the French Revolution in 1789, they also oppose tyranny and support the *Declaration of the Rights of Man and of the Citizen* (*Déclaration des droits de l'Homme et du Citoyen*), which defined the individual and collective rights of all citizens. The Québécois form a distinct cultural bloc of people who started their own internal Canadian revolution in the 1980s by proposing that their French-speaking province separate itself politically from English-speaking Canada. When the subject of death with dignity came to the forefront of Canadian news stories via the Sue Rodriguez case, it sparked a special wave of interest among the liberty-minded Québécois.

On May 13, 2009, Francine Lalonde, a Bloc Québécois member of the Canadian Parliament and a cancer sufferer, introduced her second of three private members' bills, C-562, which would

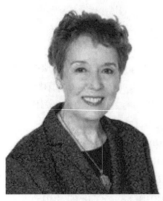

Francine Lalonde

have established the right of a terminally ill person to obtain physician aid-in-dying throughout Canada. It was opposed through a mass mail-in, ballot-box-stuffing postcard blitz conducted by Alex Schadenberg's Euthanasia Prevention Coalition. That same year, the Collège des médecins du Québec (Québec College of Physicians), the province's medical regulatory body, voted in favor of euthanasia "as appropriate care under certain circumstances when death is immediate and inevitable" and in favor of urging the national government to amend the criminal code to legalize euthanasia across Canada.[29]

The depth of public concern over the issue led to the formation of a provincial government committee, "Dying with Dignity," which scheduled eleven public forums in Québec in 2009 to determine what the Québécois thought about hastened death. During the committee hearings, Hélène Bolduc, president of the Association Québécoise pour le Droit de Mourir dans la Dignité (AQDMD—the Québec Right to Die with Dignity Association), testified that she was surprised by the opposition of palliative care doctors, who saw for themselves the misery caused when pain-control drugs were no longer effective. She noted that the death-with-dignity movement fully supported hospice and palliative care. But she also said that in some palliative care units, health professionals tried to delay an individual's death as long as possible for the sake of the family, who want to see the patient resigned and serene. "But they're not serene," Bolduc said, "They're simply drugged to ease the pain."[30]

The committee also received testimony from eighty-nine-year-old Sara Raphals, a retired schoolteacher and cancer survivor. Raphals explained that there is little dignity in the way the elderly are treated. She believed that self-deliverance should be a basic human right. "For the few of my peers who are still left, the first greeting is, 'I hope I go to sleep tonight and don't wake up in the morning.'"[31]

In November 2010, the Canadian Broadcasting Company (CBC) and Radio Canada engaged the Centre de recherche d'opinion publique, a professional polling firm, to explore the views of Québécois about physician-hastened death. This unbiased poll of 2,200 residents of Québec found that 83 percent favored physician aid-in-dying.[32] The CBC published the results of the poll on its website and provided another opinion poll, open to anyone. The question was, "Do you support the legalization of euthanasia?"

Professionally conducted polls are carefully designed to ask questions of a representative sample of the public, but online polls are very easy to manipulate via organized ballot-box stuffing by a small group of individuals with an agenda.

Canadian euthanasia opponent Alex Schadenberg immediately sent a mass email to his Euthanasia Prevention Coalition and the Catholic and fundamentalist Christian religious organizations who sponsor it. The subject line read, "Important poll - Vote NO." "This is the most important online poll we have ever seen in Canada," he stated. "VOTE NO and forward this to all of your contacts."

The results showed how effective his ballot-box-stuffing technique could be. In the professionally conducted poll, 83 percent of those interviewed agreed that euthanasia and physician-hastened death should be legalized. In the open-to-anyone poll Schadenberg had targeted, 83.47 percent of the voters cast their votes to *oppose* legalization.[33] Schadenberg also assisted his anti-euthanasia colleagues in England in a similar open-to-anyone poll, with the same effect. There, a professional poll taken in November 2010 showed 67 percent approval of the right-to-die. But with a massive push from Schadenberg's Canadian power base, an uncontrolled online British newspaper poll (which did not require voters to disclose their country of residence) showed predictably skewed results indicating massive public opposition.

To counteract the large majority of Québécois who support legalized euthanasia, Vivre dans la Dignité (Living with Dignity) was formed. A Catholic-based anti-euthanasia protest group promoted by the Euthanasia Prevention Coalition, it focused on motivating a grassroots religious opposition movement. Its director, Linda Couture, stated, "Euthanasia and assisted suicide are killing, plain and simple. We cannot allow killing to be confused with health care in Québec. The provincial government must direct its efforts and resources to offering Québécois the best possible end of life care, including ready access to palliative care."[34] And so, the battle continues.

Writing in Montreal's *The West Island Chronicle* in 2010, columnist Toula Foscolos summed up her reflections on the end-of-life dilemma in Canada.

> Just like it is our soul's obligation to seek happiness and fulfillment in life, it is perfectly reasonable to want a dignified death. We can philosophize all we want about the sanctity of life, but . . . if you were facing certain death from an incurable illness, while suffering intolerable pain, would you not want the option of ending it all, while you still had the capacity to? And wouldn't you see that as the ultimate act of compassion; not as a crime? I know I would.... Isn't it hypocritical and illogical that most current laws allow doctors to accelerate death by withholding a drug, but claim it illegal to administer a drug to achieve the same end?[35]

Nevertheless, Canadian legislators, like those in many otherwise progressive countries, doggedly refused to pass this law that the majority of their constituents demanded. Francine Lalonde's bill to permit assisted suicide under supervised conditions was rejected on April 21, 2010, by a vote of 228 to 59. Few of the members who voted against the measure had even taken the time to read it. But the fight for the right to death with dignity in Canada did not stop with the bill's defeat. Within a year, a new legal challenge to Canada's assisted suicide law would again spring up, demonstrating convincingly that Canadians would not rest until their right to die with dignity was enshrined in law. They were far from being alone. On the other side of the planet, the push for legislative change was being made just as strongly—and facing opposition no less entrenched— "down under" in Australia and New Zealand.

The Search for the Peaceful Pill

We may be old but we're not stupid. We have lived through war
and depression. We know a lot about life and death and we have every
right to hear this information
— A senior citizen, defending a Nitschke right-to-die workshop

O n the afternoon of Sunday, September 22, 1996, in Darwin, the capital of Australia's Northern Territory, Bob Dent calmly read the first screen of Dr. Philip Nitschke's laptop-driven euthanasia device. The screen displayed an unambiguous question in large, bold letters: "Are you aware that if you go ahead to the last screen and press the 'Yes' button, you will be given a lethal dose of medicine and die? Yes/No." He clicked on "Yes." The next screen asked: "Are you certain you understand that if you proceed and press the 'Yes' button on the next screen, that you will die? Yes/No." Again, he clicked on "Yes."

Then he faced the final question: "In 15 seconds, you will be given a lethal injection. Press 'Yes' to proceed. 'Yes/No.'"

Dent, sixty-six, a former carpenter, pilot, and lay minister with a missionary society, was in the terminal stage of prostate cancer and had endured a roller-coaster of pain for five years. He had no doubt about how he would answer the final question.[1]

Dent's decision occurred shortly after the Rights of the Terminally Ill (ROTI) Act was passed by the Northern Territory Legislative Assembly.[2] This law, the world's first physician aid-in-dying measure, was proposed in 1995 by Marshall Perron, the conservative chief minister of the Northern Territory. He noted that between 1995 and 1997, 439 Australians older than seventy-five had committed violent suicide.[3]

The act, which passed on May 25, 1995, by one vote, defined the procedure as follows: "A patient who, in the course of a terminal illness, is experiencing pain, suffering and/or distress to an extent unacceptable to the patient, may request the patient's medical practitioner to assist the patient to terminate the patient's life."[4] The law required that the applicant be at least eighteen years old and mentally competent. In addition, three doctors in the Northern Territory must concur in the decision, including a specialist in the condition from which the patient was dying and a psychiatrist to certify that the patient was not suffering from treatable depression. After completing the paperwork, a nine-day cooling-off period was required before the physician-assisted death could take place. The patient could change his or her mind at any time, and if so, the process would immediately end.[5]

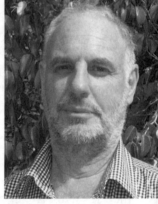

Dr. Philip Nitschke

At that time, Philip Nitschke was an obstetrician, working *pro bono* after hours to treat HIV-infected drug users and dying AIDS patients. He heard about Perron's proposed euthanasia law on the radio one morning. "I thought, *well, that's a good idea*, rolled over, and went back to sleep."[6]

Many of his colleagues agreed with Nitschke, but the Australian Medical Association (AMA) announced they would ensure that no such legislation would ever be passed in Australia. "I was really taken aback," Nitschke commented. "They were saying to the Territory population, 'you might think it's a good idea (and most Territorians did), but we [the doctors] know what's best for you.' And I thought, *doctors might know something about medicine, but dying is a fundamental issue.... You don't have to be a doctor to understand dying.*"[7]

When Dr. Chris Wake, president of the Northern Territory branch of the AMA and chairman of the Coalition Against Euthanasia, claimed that "no doctor would provide euthanasia under the proposed legislation,"[8] Nitschke was incensed. "I thought, *what an insufferably arrogant, paternalistic attitude.*"[9] To refute Wake's claim, he located twenty-two doctors in the Territory willing to have their names listed in a full-page ad in the *New Territory News* as supporting the legislation.[10] Almost overnight, Nitschke, who had been described as a "forthright, blunt-talking man of action," became the central figure in the drama.[11]

The act would not take effect until July 1, 1996, so Catholics, fundamentalist Protestants, and the AMA set out to derail it. Dr. Wake, a staunch Catholic, and Rev. Djiniyini Gondarra, an influential aboriginal Uniting Church minister, entered a lawsuit with the Territory Supreme Court challenging the act's legality. The challenge was eventually defeated by a 2 to 1 vote. While the act received strong support from the majority of Australians, it also elated right-to-die groups worldwide, who saw it as a model of the intelligent application of end-of-life compassion for the terminally ill and hoped it would lead to similar laws in other countries.

Ultimately, seven people sought to take advantage of the act, but only three were successful. The first to come forward was sixty-eight-year old Marta Alfonso-Bowes, a Hemlock Society USA member and teacher from Albuquerque, New Mexico, then living in Australia and suffering from bowel cancer. On Australian television, she declared that she would take her own life if the ROTI act was not soon activated. Unwilling to wait for the 1996 activation date, Alfonso-Bowes ended her life on September 24, 1995, by drinking Nembutal.[12]

The second applicant was Max Bell, a single man and former taxi driver, professional golfer, boxer, and bodyguard from Broken Hill, an isolated mining town in the far west of outback New South Wales. He was dying from stomach cancer and told Nitschke, "I'm just existing. I can't see the point anymore. I've seen my time. I'm ready for the sweet long sleep."[13]

Emaciated and ashen-faced, he set off in his ancient Holden Commodore taxicab for Darwin, about 3,000 kilometers (1,900 miles) across country. By then, he was living solely on milk and yoghurt, getting progressively weaker.[14] Nitschke had no doubt that Bell qualified for help in dying and had him admitted to Royal Darwin Hospital. There, he languished for three weeks.

Although the ROTI act was now in effect, Bell had made his arduous journey for nothing. "None of the [AMA] doctors would break ranks," said Nitschke. "I rang every specialist in the Northern Territory."[15] Two doctors who had previously agreed to examine Bell backed out. "At the end of three weeks, Max signed himself out of the hospital and drove all the way—vomited his way—back to Broken Hill," Nitschke related. "He was disgusted and angry at what he saw as the cowardice of the doctors. He was furious with me for not warning him that this could happen."[16]

Nitschke felt responsible for Bell's plight. He flew to Broken Hill at his own cost. "I stayed with him in his house for the remaining three weeks of his life," Nitschke said. "At Broken Hill Base Hospital, on August 2, 1996, Bell died precisely in the way he most dreaded, slowly and with the process out of his control."[17] In an egregious misrepresentation of the facts, to which Nitschke strenuously objected, Britain's most prestigious medical journal, *The Lancet*, stated, "The patient died peacefully whilst receiving good medical and nursing care at his local hospital."[18] Nothing could have been further from the truth.

"Today," Nitschke related, "Max's cab lives on as my car and, like his memory, travels with me around Australia."[19]

In the final months of Bell's life, ABC-TV produced *Road to Nowhere*, a documentary about Bell's futile trip. It convinced the first surgeon in Darwin to break ranks. Originally refusing to be part of Bell's quest for self-deliverance, Dr. John Wardell called Nitschke and said, "I've just seen Max Bell on television and I feel like shit. If it happens again, you ring me."[20] His actions motivated other surgeons to follow suit.[21]

Between the time the ROTI act was passed and implemented, Nitschke, with the aid of friend and computer programmer Des Carne, built the Deliverance Machine.[22] It was a computer-powered upgrade of Jack Kevorkian's 1989 Thanatron lethal injection machine.[23] The device consisted of Nitschke's three-year-old Toshiba laptop computer, a syringe system to deliver the lethal drugs into the patient's vein, and a software program written by Carne that required patients to confirm their intent to die three times before the machine would activate the system. Fifteen seconds after the last "yes" response, the drugs would start flowing. The patient would fall asleep within seconds and die while unconscious within five to ten minutes.

Nitschke built the machine to give the patient full autonomy over death.

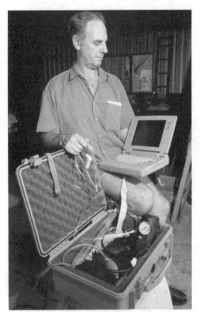

The Deliverance Machine

There was no way that an unscrupulous doctor could kill someone against his or her will because the machine required the patient—and the patient alone—to make the unequivocal choice to die. If the patient pressed the "no" button, or the wrong key, the program would immediately shut down and nothing would happen.[24]

Bob Dent, a Buddhist, was the next to contact Nitschke. Even though he had received palliative care for his pain, it was not working. "I'm going to die from this and I want to do this on my own terms. What do I have to do?" he asked.[25] Dent met all the legal requirements, but before he and Nitschke could proceed, they needed to work as allies in a highly publicized struggle to persuade two other doctors to support his request. After Nitschke located two other doctors to examine Dent and sign the paperwork, Dent was free to choose his date of death.

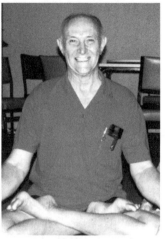

Bob Dent

When I interviewed her in Melbourne in October 2010, Judy Dent, his wife, told me, "Bob had been regularly visited by Philip on Wednesdays and Sundays. So Bob said, 'Aw hell, he's coming Sunday anyway; we'll make it Sunday.'"[26] Dent called and asked if Nitschke could join him for lunch on Sunday. On Saturday, he went, with great effort, to visit the Buddhist Temple to say good-bye to all the people there who had been so kind to him.[27]

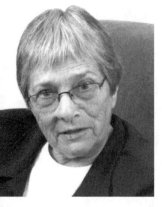

Judy Dent

Nitschke tested and retested the Deliverance Machine on Saturday. He wanted to be certain nothing would go wrong during its first use on an actual patient. "On Sunday, my mouth was so dry that I couldn't eat. . . . I just about choked on my ham sandwich. I was very, very anxious. [Bob Dent] spent a lot of time trying to calm me down, and I thought, *Great. You [have to] spend your last meal trying to pacify the doctor.*"[28]

After the meal, Dent, his wife, and Nitschke watched a soccer game. While Dent talked about the teams, Nitschke found it hard to carry on a coherent conversation. At two o'clock, Dent went to the back veranda of his house and lay down while Nitschke prepared his equipment. "He had to mix the drugs into an IV bag that was hanging from the stand and had to put the needle into Bob's arm," Judy told me. "And I could see that he [Nitschke] was nervous, sweating."

"Bob said to me, 'You are not to cry.'"

"I said, 'whatever you say,' but that was very difficult."

Nitschke then inserted an IV tube into a vein in Dent's arm, and told him, "It is all ready. It's up to you."[29]

Nitschke moved back to make room for Judy to be at his side. Bob and Judy hugged and then Dent reached for the laptop. He pushed the button, saying "yes" three times. Once the third question was answered, a signal was sent to an air compressor that pushed the plunger of the syringe, which contained two drugs. One was 100 ml of liquid Nembutal to rapidly render Dent unconscious. The other was vecuronium, a muscle relaxant derived from curare, which would stop Dent's heart while he was asleep.[30] After the pump injected the chemicals into Dent's arm, the computer screen went black, except for one final word: "Exit."

"Once he said, 'yes, yes, yes' to the computer," Judy told me, "I heard the pump start, and Bob heard it, too. And I could practically see the fluid go into his vein, and the pain and stress on his face just disappeared. He looked ten years younger. He had no wrinkles. He just looked at peace. And I thought, *What a lovely way to go.*"[31] As Judy held him, Dent gave one last sigh and fell into a deep sleep. Five minutes later, he died.

"The machine worked as was designed to," Nitschke recalled. "I remember thinking, 'Thank God it worked.' If it hadn't, I couldn't say, 'I'll come on back tomorrow.' It *had* to work."[32]

Judy Dent said, "The most painful aspect of [Bob's] illness was the inevitable erosion of his independence. He was so pleased that Philip had made the Deliverance Machine so that he could control his death himself. I shall forever admire and respect Philip for his commitment to Bob and to making ROTI work."[33]

The story of this first legal use of assisted suicide did not hit the media for three days. Then, Nitschke said, "All hell broke loose. I had calls coming in from journalists on every continent, all wanting interviews for radio, TV, and newspapers."[34]

The Vatican described Dent's death as "an absurd act of total cruelty." Edward Cardinal Clancy, head of the Catholic Church in Australia, said that Nitschke's reckless act would be widely condemned.[35] The positions of the Pope and the cardinal were rigidly doctrinal and showed no compassion for the dying man. Neither the Pope nor Clancy took into account the extent and duration of Dent's suffering or of his wishes. The Australian public reacted quite differently than the Catholic officials. After Dent's death, instead of condemnation, his case was viewed by the majority of people with both compassion and approval.

Dent left behind a letter that stated, "If you disagree with voluntary euthanasia, then don't use it, but don't deny to me the right to use it if and when I want to…. The Church and State must remain separate. What right does anyone have because of their own religious faith (to which I don't subscribe) to demand that I behave according to their rules until some omniscient doctor decides that I must have had enough and increases my morphine until I die?"[36]

In what had become a typical journalistic knee-jerk reaction, Nitschke was quickly branded as the latest "Doctor Death" by the media. "The labels come with the territory," he said. "But I don't enjoy being referred to as another 'Dr. Death' or having people attempt to make links between my German name and the Nazis."[37]

Former nurse Janet Mills was the second person to achieve a peaceful death under the ROTI act. The fifty-two-year-old woman from Naracoorte, South Australia, did not get the support that she was expecting from her medical colleagues. For nearly ten years, she had suffered from a rare form of lymphoma known as mycosis fungoides. Slowly, the cancer had broken down her skin, leaving extensive scarring, constant infection, and ever-present itching.[38]

"When she could not get that last signature from a doctor in the Northern Territory to allow her to use [the ROTI act], she went on television," wrote Sandra Kanck, a member of the South Australia parliament. "Janet was shown all over Australia appealing to get that last doctor, and the appeal ultimately succeeded. She was in the most appalling situation. . . . Her skin was peeling off. She felt like she had thousands of ants crawling under her skin. Palliative care can do nothing for that…. Every morning when she woke up her skin and the pus and the mucus were stuck to the bed sheets and every morning it had to be peeled off."[39] With her husband, Dave, and one of her sons at her side, Mills died via the Deliverance Machine on January 2, 1997.[40]

"Bill X," sixty-nine, who did not want his full name released, was the third ROTI assisted-suicide patient. A Darwin resident terminally ill from stomach cancer, he had already undergone extensive hospitalization, surgery, and palliative care. His surgeon confirmed that his condition was hopeless, but Bill had extreme difficulty finding a willing psychiatrist to complete the necessary paperwork and declare him mentally competent. Only two hours before his scheduled death, Bill finally found a psychiatrist who would see him if he would first answer a ten-page "new client" questionnaire and pay a $200 AUD consulting fee.

"He was in so much pain he had trouble sitting up, but had to try and appear happy in case the psychiatrist didn't give the go-ahead," Nitschke recalled. The psychiatrist consented. Bill answered "yes" three times on the laptop's keyboard and died on January 22, 1997.[41]

Disgusted by the hostile treatment he had received from the Australian press, Nitschke decided to beat them at their own game. Instead of holding a traditional press conference, he posted the news of Bill's death on his Deliverance homepage on the internet. In 1997, that was a radical concept. Within forty-eight hours, almost four thousand people had read about the event. Jon Casimir, writing for Melbourne's *The Age*, noted that by using the internet, Nitschke was spared a bombardment of questions, the answers to which could have been turned against him. The media was no longer something done to him; it had become something that Nitschke did for himself.[42]

The fourth successful applicant to use the act was Valerie P., a divorced Australian woman who flew into Darwin from outside the Northern Territory. At his mother's request, her son, Ray, first contacted Nitschke and gave him a full report of her condition: advanced carcinoma of the breast, which spread throughout her body. Her sister had recently died an excruciating death from breast cancer, including the indignity of double incontinence, and she feared the worst for herself. In great pain, the former amateur golfer was "frustrated at being house-bound and dependent on visits from friends and family" and was deeply troubled by her downward-spiraling loss of personal autonomy, which further fueled her wish to die.[43] Despite chemotherapy, the cancer spread. Palliative care did not relieve her will to die. Her children agreed with her choice to use the act, and flew with her to Darwin. A week after having been approved by doctors as compliant with the act, she moved into a hotel apartment. Surrounded by her five adult children, she died using Nitschke's Deliverance Machine.[44]

At the Tenth Anniversary Conference of the ROTI act in October 2006, her son, Ray, told the audience, "Philip helped my mum to die with dignity. For that I am eternally grateful.... I am here to speak on behalf of my mother and on behalf of the people who one day may need to confront a similar situation that my mother did. In the end their choices may be different to my mother's but I firmly believe that they must have the same opportunity as my mother."[45]

Australia's political makeup made it easier for the enemies of the ROTI act to have it nullified. Australia's six states have sovereign, co-equal levels of autonomy. However, the three self-governing territories (the Northern Territory, the Australian Capital Territory, and Norfolk Island) are different. Their legislative power is limited by Act 22 of the Constitution, which allows the Commonwealth to override their laws.

Kevin Andrews, a Liberal Party M.P., a devout Catholic, and a vehement opponent of the ROTI act, introduced a nullification bill into the Commonwealth Parliament on September 9, 1996. The church and a network of influential people pulled out all the stops to defeat the ground-breaking act, despite the fact that "Euthanasia No" proponents were greatly outnumbered by those who approved of the act.

Rick Bawden, a Northern Territory resident, spoke out against the nullification bill when a parliamentary committee gathered information there in 1997. He said, "Last time I saw it, 74 percent of Australians were in favour, 19 percent were against and 7 percent just did not know. Kim Beazley [leader of the Australian Labor Party] says that we have to get closer to the people, and yet he votes against it. [Prime Minister] John Howard is always spouting about mandates. This is a mandate that would give most politicians an orgasm."[46]

The politicians evidently did not care for voter-sponsored orgasms. The Euthanasia Laws Bill, nullifying the ROTI act, was passed by the House of Representatives 88 to 35 and by the Senate with the slender margin of 38 to 35 votes on March 25, 1997.

At the time the act was nullified, Esther Wild, a retired Darwin nurse suffering from terminal carcinoid syndrome, had her request for assistance in dying approved by four doctors, but she had not yet chosen her final exit date. Subsequently, a bill was introduced in the federal parliament to permit her to die using the ROTI procedures, but it was denied. Member of Parliament Sandra Kanck read into the official record, "Esther Wild, as part of her condition, was vomiting up her own stomach lining and her own feces, but I guess that is sanctity of life," she said, making a pointed reference to Kevin Andrews' ties to his religion's dogma.[47]

Unable to use the act, Wild agreed to have Nitschke put her into a coma to escape her agony. He moved into her house and slept on the floor of the room next to hers. Once she awoke in pain, which, Nitschke maintained, justified raising the dosage of medicines to deepen her coma. She died four days later, on April 17, 1997.[48] Paul Rofe, Australia's Director of Public Prosecutions, said Nitschke's description of Wild's death "amounted to a murder confession."[49]

Nitschke fired back, "It is considered to be good medical practice to allow a person to die over two days, and yet if you increase the infusion rate and they die in two hours it is considered to be murder!"[50]

In a dramatic gesture, he unveiled what he claimed to be the prototype of a computer-controlled device that would "keep the dying in a permanent state of unconsciousness." Nitschke said his new device "was designed to guarantee the terminally ill patient would never again regain consciousness after an infusion of painkillers." He stated the device "would expose the hypocrisy of current laws which allow doctors to induce death through drug overdoses under the guise of treating pain."[51] A working version of the device was never made.

This procedure—terminal sedation—makes it possible for a doctor to avoid prosecution if he or she can show that an increased dose of painkiller—typically morphine—prescribed to control pain had, as a side-effect, killed the patient. This medical legal defense is known as "the doctrine of double effect."

In normal palliative care practice, painkillers are routinely prescribed to relieve acute physical suffering, with the knowledge that death may sometimes result as a byproduct. If a patient dies of a drug overdose and the physician can prove that the lethal dose was used with the sole intent of relieving pain, rather than to kill the patient, the physician is not considered to have hastened the death.

The death record will list the cause of death only as the underlying disease. Nitschke fumed that this "wink-wink/we'll pretend" system was perfectly legal, but overtly helping the same patient die more quickly with less pain and suffering was illegal.[52]

When the repeal of the ROTI act took effect on March 25, 1997, Nitschke angrily crossed his personal Rubicon and irrevocably committed himself to working as a full-time euthanasia activist.

> I saw our piece of legislation that was, I think, very innovatively and wisely brought in the Northern Territory and it was a world first. And to watch it just destroyed by the federal system and the arguments that were run to try and undermine it and to discredit it. A law that actually by the time they did overturn it in 1997, eight months after it had started to be in operation, had worked well and four people had achieved a very humane and peaceful death and ended their suffering in the way they wanted.... and now since that time I've just been inundated with people who would've benefited from such a piece of legislation. Now they're trapped in this jungle out there, this legal jungle, with difficulties and we try to work out what we can do and I guess that would make anyone passionate about it.[53]

Nitschke's new goal was a radical break from supporting and enabling legislation to authorize physician aid-in-dying. He made a 180-degree turn, seeking ways to totally remove doctors and politicians from the deathing process by providing people with the information and do-it-yourself technology they needed to end their lives on their own terms. Their final acts would be perfectly legal simple suicides. This made the authority, opinion, or blessing of any government, medical, or religious authority irrelevant. To the AMA, Nitschke was now a dangerous renegade, but his supporters saw him as a compassionate, trailblazing hero. To his opponents within the right-to-die movement, he was seen as a threat to achieving legalized physician-hastened death.

Crusading for unpopular causes began early for Nitschke. The youngest of three children of rural schoolteachers, Gwen and Harold Nitschke, he was born on August 8, 1947, in Ardrossan, a small town about ninety miles northeast of Adelaide.[54] Always a bright student, Nitschke created one of Australia's first holograms and earned a Ph.D. in laser physics from Flinders University in Adelaide. But his interests lay elsewhere.

"I was deeply interested in politics and the causes that were raging at that time," he said. Not just [protesting] the Vietnam War but the Aboriginal land rights issue."[55] After hearing an elder of the Gurindji aboriginal people speak about land rights protests at Wave Hill, he was inspired to join them.[56]

Wave Hill, one of Baron William Vestey's cattle stations (ranches) in the Northern Territory, was established on aboriginal land in 1883. Shortly after the white colonists arrived, the Gurindji found the newcomers fencing off their land. Soon, water sources—few and far between in the Outback—were fouled by cattle. The livestock also trampled the fragile plant life that indigenous people depended on. Cattle station managers shot the aborigines' invaluable hunting dogs and killed kangaroos, a vital source of meat.

The Gurindji had only two choices: move onto the cattle stations to get menial work as stockmen and domestic help or die of starvation. Formerly free to roam the land, they were reduced to the level of virtual slavery. In 1966, led by Vincent Lingiari, the aboriginal workers and their families walked away from their jobs at Wave Hill, demanded the return of their land, and asked for higher wages. As a result, for seven years they were brutalized and nearly starved to death.

During their struggle for recognition, Nitschke came to Wave Hill to act as a community advisor for the aborigines. He was welcomed by the elders, who were desperate to have someone help them communicate with government officials. Nitschke found the unpaid job of translating correspondence for Lingiari extremely fulfilling. He and his girlfriend, Jenny Thiele, spent two years at the station, living in a corrugated tin hut with no running water or personal privacy, surrounded by people who were barely scraping by, a significant percentage of whom had leprosy. "It was the hardest job I've ever done," he said.[57]

Eventually, Thiele could no longer tolerate the social isolation and deprivation. Nitschke described her departure: "She met a drifting American fella, said 'Bugger this, I'm out of here,' and rode off into the sunset with him on his Honda 450 V-twin."[58] Shortly after that, Nitschke, a historical motorcycle aficionado, bought a legendary Russian Cossack twin 650 driveshaft bike, which he rides to this day.

The loss of Thiele's companionship left him emotionally bereft. He left the Gurindji and spent the next year drifting around Melbourne. But the call of the Outback lured him back, and he took a job as a ranger with the National Parks and Wildlife Department in Alice Springs in the Northern Territory. There, he came under fire for his support of the Gurindji people and for his protests against Australia's large-scale uranium mining. After six years as a ranger, an accident left him with a crushed heel, and he had to quit. He moved to Sydney, where, at the age of thirty-five, he was accepted by the University of Sydney as the oldest student ever to start the study of medicine.

During an anesthesia internship, Nitschke came into contact with people seeking death as a release from a spiraling tailspin of pain and loss of autonomy. This was his introduction to the concept that accelerating the process of death could be viewed as compassion. In 1990, while a resident at the Royal Darwin Hospital, he met Tristan Pawsey, a bright, attractive pediatrician whose conservative and traditional background was the polar opposite of his own. They fell in love and moved in together. She stood by him during some of the most arduous years of his life.

On March 26, 1993, the accident-plagued USS *Houston*, a Los Angeles-class, nuclear-powered fast-attack submarine, arrived in Darwin for a six-day visit.[59] In addition to its nuclear reactor, the sub also carried nuclear-tipped Tomahawk cruise missiles.

Every port open to U.S. nuclear-powered ships was supposed to have a nuclear disaster response plan in place, but Darwin and its hospital had none. Nitschke, the hospital's quickly appointed radiation safety officer, complained publicly about the city's unpreparedness for a nuclear accident, but the government and the hospital both heatedly denied his claim. Privately, the hospital director said to confidants that he would not renew Nitschke's contract when it expired in December 1993, even though most of the other residents came to his defense.

The whistle-blowing stink that Nitschke raised about the Royal Darwin Hospital's incompetence became so bad that on April 15, 1993, the hospital's management, the Royal Medical Officers' Association, and the Northern Territory Health Department issued an astounding joint news release. The hospital admitted that it was unprepared for a nuclear accident and noted that Nitschke's advice had been ignored.[60] Behind the scenes, the hospital's management wanted Nitschke's head on a platter. Nitschke watched with disbelief as he was marginalized, ostracized, and finally demonized.

In a final blow, unable to endure any further turmoil from his crusades, which were severely damaging her own medical practice, Tristan Pawsey parted company with Nitschke after the USS *Houston* incident. "There is little doubt that the experience at the Royal Darwin Hospital prepared me well for the onslaught as the euthanasia issue broke," Nitschke said.[61]

After the ROTI legislation was overturned in 1996, Nitschke started to search for the Holy Grail of do-it-yourself dying: the "Peaceful Pill." This "pill" has widely and erroneously been assumed to be a specific instant death pill or potion, like the cyanide pills and toxin-coated death needles that emerged from the World War II and Cold War espionage years. It is neither of those two things. The term is Nitschke's generic metaphor for an effective, painless, lethal do-it-yourself means to a peaceful, accomplice-free self-deliverance, rather than any specific pill, product, or method.

His goal was to develop a way for the average person, with no special skills or training, to legally obtain or create a substance or use a method to end his or her life with dignity and without assistance. That, in 1997, was a strong reason for him to join forces with euthanasia activists John Hofsess of Canada and Rob Neils of the United States to launch NuTech, the radical euthanasia think tank, which focused on this concept.

The peaceful pill theory was first proposed in 1991 by Huibert Drion, a former Dutch Supreme Court justice and vigorous proponent of voluntary euthanasia. Drion argued that "people aged seventy-five or over, living alone, should have the choice of being provided by a doctor with the means to end their lives at a time and manner which was acceptable to them." Such a right would "offer older people the knowledge that they could choose to die before experiencing the final stages of decline and dependence."[62] Drion's philosophy had a profound influence on Nitschke's development of a succession of do-it-yourself deathing technologies.

Nitschke's goals for his Peaceful Pill concept were well defined:

- It should lead to a gentle death for all people, preferably through a steadily deepening sleep.

- It should be able to be ingested or inhaled orally by patients, eliminating the need for skilled medical assistance from someone else.
- It should have an unequivocal effect, with no chance for failure or resuscitation.
- It did not need to be in the form of a pill—a drink or a gas would do just as well.
- Most important, it should be able to be obtained or assembled and used by the patient without assistance. It must, therefore, be easily accessible and unpoliceable.[63]

Nitschke's initial Peaceful Pill announcement was a masterful publicity event: a "shot across the bow" of the medical and political establishments to signal that they had better pay attention to what the *people* wanted, not what *they* wanted. As soon as the "death pill" story broke in 1998, the British Medical Association expressed alarm over the idea, seeing it as a major threat to at-risk groups. Nitschke's lifelong confrontation with medical orthodoxy was now underway.

On May 5, 1998, fourteen months after the annulment of the ROTI act, Nitschke formed the Voluntary Euthanasia Research Foundation, a private membership organization dedicated to developing technologies that would make dignified, elective death accessible. As it evolved in size and scope, the group's name was changed to Exit Australia and then, as it expanded abroad, to Exit International.

One of the group's first goals was to hold euthanasia clinics throughout the nation. After small-scale trial versions were held in Brisbane and Sydney, Nitschke launched the first full-blown clinics in Melbourne. There, he met privately with sixteen terminally ill patients who wanted information on how to end their lives. Nitschke had to be extremely careful. Australia's assisted-suicide law stated that "assisting" might be interpreted to include stating which drugs would be lethal. If so, the information provider might be found guilty of a felony and could be imprisoned for up to fourteen years.

Despite the risks, by the end of 2000, Nitschke had operated underground clinics in Sydney and Brisbane, with plans for eight more in other cities. In a typical clinic, Nitschke examined patients, reviewed their medical records, and developed recommended strategies for the last period of their lives.[64] Nitschke felt safe going that far, for such consultations fell within the guidelines for the doctor-patient relationship published in the Australian *Ethics Manual for Consultant Physicians* in 1999.

Nevertheless, Nitschke's euthanasia clinics were fiercely opposed by right-to-life groups. In addition, the AMA was quick to accuse him of encouraging patients to illegally obtain life-ending drugs. Nitschke's response was pragmatic: if they could not find gentle ways to die, they would have to use the "traditional" violent ones. Providing accurate, specific information now forms the backbone of Nitschke's power-to-the-people campaign, where he offers, in a face-to-face setting, virtually everything there is to know about self-deliverance options.

Today, the "Exitorials" typically attract fifty to one hundred people. They are held in two parts to avoid legal problems. The first is open without charge to anyone who is over fifty or who has a terminal or debilitating condition. It covers uncontroversial end-of-life-options in general, including living wills, advance medical directives, the legal right to self-deliverance, and the legal dangers posed for anyone who assists a suicide. The second part is open only to Exit International members, who can join on the spot. Here, Nitschke answers specific questions about peaceful self-deliverance and demonstrates specific methods.

In the early years of the twenty-first century, Nitschke's fertile brain latched onto several imaginative ideas. First, he proposed to operate a floating euthanasia facility in international waters. The concept briefly found support from the West Australia Voluntary Euthanasia Society, but when Nitschke's lawyers looked at the plan, they spotted its flaw. Even if the suicides took place in international waters, the ship's staff would still be bound by the laws of the country that licensed it.[65] The "euthanasia ship" idea sank quickly.

Another idea was a home-made carbon monoxide (CO) generator called the COGen or COGenie Machine. Like Nitschke's Deliverance Machine, the COGenie was loosely based on the research work of Jack Kevorkian.[66] The chief difference was that Nitschke's device could be made and used by laypersons to produce lethal carbon monoxide gas by themselves, making its use an act of simple suicide. Kevorkian's Mercitron required a commercially supplied tank of carbon monoxide and was designed for use by a physician assisting a suicide.

The COGen could be constructed out of inexpensive materials available in any hardware store and could be built at home in a single day. The basic idea was to combine formic acid with sulfuric acid, cool the mixture, and pass it through caustic soda (lye), producing a high-concentration, single-use supply of carbon monoxide gas. A person who inhaled the gas through tubing held on with two small nasal prongs (or who locked themselves into a small car with it) would die quickly. The downside was that the gas is explosive and toxic and could harm anyone who was accidently exposed to it. The device went through several design improvements over the years, but no use of the COGen for self-deliverance has yet come to light.

On a 2001 Australian speaking tour, Wesley J. Smith, a high-profile U.S. anti-euthanasia campaigner, focused his fire on Nitschke. "First, I busted him with a press release, timed to explode as I was landing in Melbourne, stating that he had told *National Review Online* he believed that 'troubled teens' should have access to the Peaceful Pill."[67]

The question put to Nitschke by the conservative online publication was essentially, "Who should or should not have access to the 'Peaceful Pill,' if it were ever to be produced?" Speaking as an intellectual defending an intellectual concept, and failing to remember that he was being interviewed by a philosophically hostile right-wing reporter, Nitschke voiced a damaging opinion.

> I do not believe that telling people they have a right to life while denying them the means, manner, or information necessary for them to give this life away has any ethical consistency. So all people qualify, not just those with the training, knowledge, or resources to find out how to 'give away' their life. And someone needs to provide this knowledge, training, or recourse necessary to anyone who wants it, including the depressed, the elderly bereaved, [and] the troubled teen. If we are to remain consistent and we believe that the individual has the right to dispose of their life, we should not erect artificial barriers in the way of sub-groups who don't meet our criteria.[68]

The "troubled teen" statement, which he has since renounced on many occasions, continues to haunt him to this day.

Next, Smith exposed the importation of the Canadian exit bags. "The Exit Bag story ran on the front page in *The Age*, Australia's largest national newspaper . . . under a banner headline, complete with an above-the-fold photo of me holding an Exit Bag in one hand and the instructions on its use in the other."[69] His action prompted the Australian government to ban the importation of the Canadian bags and impound them at the border.

But Smith's attempt to stem the availability of the bags was a failure, as the bags can easily and legally be made at home in thirty minutes from $15 worth of readily obtainable materials. To ensure that those who needed them could obtain them, Nitschke not only

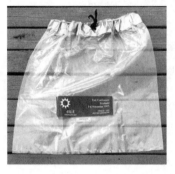

A 2006 Aussie Exit Bag

made the instructions widely available but also included them and the needed materials in the "welcome kit" at his 2005 Exit International conference in Brisbane, where attendees could—and did—learn how to make their own hoods on the spot.

One of the most humane methods of bringing about peaceful death ever devised was the drug pentobarbital, a fast-acting barbiturate commonly referred to by its North American trade name, Nembutal. Voluntary euthanasia of humans was not its intended use. In the United States in the 1950s, Nembutal was sold either by prescription or was dispensed over-the-counter as a sedative and sleeping aid for both adults and infants. In the 1960s and 1970s, its abuse started to peak among the jet-setters and celebrities, who used "uppers"—generally amphetamines—to stay awake and alert as long as the party was going on, and then gulped "downers"—such as Nembutal or other barbiturates—to relax them quickly. The dangerous upper/downer combination led to the deaths of many high-flying celebrities, including Marilyn Monroe. Nembutal is now restricted chiefly to veterinary use. However, its ability to bring about a fast, peaceful, and certain death quickly made it the international drug of choice for self-deliverance. Although illegal for human use and extremely difficult and to obtain today, Nembutal remains the most sought-after final exit drug.

In November 2005, Nitschke gathered a group of Exit International volunteers at a secret location to work on making Nembutal. The attempt came to be known as "The Peanut Project." At the first workshop, the average age of the participants was over seventy years, and each had contributed $2,000 AUD to cover the cost of the sophisticated equipment and supplies. If all went well, each attendee would leave with a one-person dose of the lethal drug. Because of potential legal liability issues, Nitschke's senior design engineer, John Edge, ran the on-scene trial. Ultimately, the participants produced a mixed barbiturate substance, but its level of purity could not be determined and it could not be used.

During this period of controversy and experimentation, three cases added extra dimension to Australia's death-with-dignity debate. In 2002, Nitschke received a call from Nancy Crick, sixty-nine, a widowed native of Melbourne. She had been through three operations for bowel cancer and was burdened with a colostomy bag. As she told Nitschke "I spend most of my day in the smallest room of the house."[70] A feisty, outspoken ex-barmaid with a wide circle of devoted friends, Crick joined Exit International to find out how to end her life. Although she was in intense pain, she was not terminally ill. Nitschke urged her to pursue a variety of curative and palliative care options, which she did, but her condition worsened. A militant campaigner for voluntary euthanasia, she attracted great attention through the media and obtained Nembutal over the internet.[71]

Crick wanted to die at home, surrounded by friends and family, but the assisted suicide law in Queensland could have made the presence of her loved ones a criminal act, subject to arrest and imprisonment. Nitschke suggested a strategy that had worked to help end racial segregation in the United States in the 1960s: mass civil disobedience. He told Crick that she should include many elderly people among her witnesses. It would be a public relations nightmare for any public prosecutor to bring criminal charges against them.

On May 21, 2002, those who loved her arrived from several parts of Australia, and Crick provided them with tea and cake. Nitschke was absent, by design. At about 8:00 p.m., Crick drank a dose of Nembutal and washed it down with a small glass of Bailey's liqueur. She smoked a last cigarette, joined hands with those around her, fell asleep, and died peacefully after about twenty minutes.[72] The authorities were notified the next morning.

Crick's home was immediately declared a crime scene, and her body was autopsied. It was determined that the source of her excruciating pain was extensive adhesions of the bowel following her cancer surgeries, not the cancer itself. Anti-euthanasia groups cried

foul when the story was published. Because Crick was not terminally ill, Nitschke's involvement with her case was unacceptable,
some charged.[73] Nitschke dismissed the protests, maintaining that
that intolerable pain and suffering alone justified rational self-deliverance.[74]

Soon after Crick's death, Nitschke's offices in Darwin, Adelaide,
and New South Wales were raided by police. Two hundred and fifty
client files, 90 percent of which were unrelated to Crick's death,
were confiscated. The authorities' fishing expedition was later found
to be unjustifiable, and Nitschke was awarded $40,000 AUD in com-
pensation.[75]

On a warm, sunny day in the third week of November 2002,
with her Mont Blanc fountain pen filled with indigo ink, Mademoiselle Lisette Gabrielle Nigot, brilliant and healthy, began writing on
a sheet of watermarked ecru linen station-
ery. With a clear and steady hand, the highly accomplished literary resident of Perth
told why she did not want to live to see her
next birthday. "After 80 years of a good life
I have had enough of it," she wrote. "I want
it to stop before it gets bad."[76]

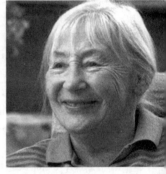

She pinned the note over her bed, made
herself comfortable, drank a fatal dose of
Nembutal, which she had acquired several
years earlier, fell asleep, and quickly died.

Mlle. Lisette Nigot

Her clear, studied decision—that she had finished everything meaningful in life and now wanted to end it before she began slipping into
decline—was a striking new twist in the classic who-owns-my-body
debate. It drew an entirely new line in the sand. Self-deliverance
under these circumstances came to be known as the *completed life
syndrome.*

Nitschke had visited Nigot many times, seeking to dissuade her
from suicide. He later wrote, "Lisette was . . . the first person to call
my bluff. . . . She told me to 'stop patronizing' her. I was mortified to
hear her allegation that I had become the type of doctor I despised.
Lisette noted that I preached one thing in theory…and another in
practice.… I stopped trying to thwart her plans."[77]

In 2004, Richard, a seventy-six-year-old Australian dying from
advanced emphysema, wanted the "Mexican option": buying Nem-

butal in Mexico. He made the grueling trip from Australia to California with a wheelchair, an oxygen tank, and Nitschke. From San Diego, the two men took a tourist bus across the border to Tijuana's main shopping district on the Avenida Revolución, where Nitschke quickly located a veterinary pharmacy.

"As Richard sat in his wheelchair, I ventured in and returned in five minutes with the required bottle [of Nembutal]," Nitschke wrote. He was not asked for identification or any kind of prescription. Purchasing Nembutal in Mexico did not violate any Mexican laws, but importing it into the United States or Australia is illegal. Richard put the Nembutal in his shopping bags. "At the [U.S.] border, we passed through the metal detector and our bags were checked. We said nothing about the bottle and no questions were asked," Nitschke wrote.[78] There were also no problems with customs when they entered Australia. Two days after they arrived home, Richard chose to die. "He drank down the Nembutal. As advised, he followed that drink with the smallest sip of his favorite Port. I held and kissed him and cried, and within a few minutes he had slipped into a deep sleep," Nitschke recalled.[79]

By 2007, thousands of people were flooding Mexican border towns from Tijuana to Matamoros. For a while, the huge influx of "Nembutal tourism," and the adverse publicity it generated, goaded Mexican law enforcement officials into clamping down on the sale of the drug. To fill this void, the internet was soon buzzing with offers to sell or ship Nembutal anywhere in the world—at highly inflated prices. A large percentage of internet "dealers" were rip-off artists, who took the money but never sent the goods. Nevertheless, the flow of Nembutal shipped or personally imported from Mexico, Peru, Bolivia, China, and Thailand continues to flourish. As Nitschke stated in 2010, "Never was Australia more awash in Nembutal than now."[80]

In 2005, with his Exit International colleague, Dr. Fiona Stewart, a public health sociologist, Nitschke launched another broadside salvo into the hull of organized medicine. He and Stewart had met during a debate at the 2002 Brisbane Festival of Ideas, debating (on different sides) the concept that "there's no such thing as a new idea." Together, they published *Killing Me Softly: Voluntary Euthanasia and the Road to the Peaceful Pill*, an end-of-life planning and self-deliverance manual. "*Killing Me Softly* is about my shift in thinking away from legislation towards the DIY Peaceful Pill," Nitschke said.[81]

The book, extensively featured by the Australian media, immediately brought the traditional howls of outrage from the religious right and medical officials. The public, however, bought it by the thousands.

In 2006, Nitschke followed his earlier best-seller with *The Peaceful Pill Handbook*, an explicit self-deliverance guide. In addition to revealing the specific doses of those drugs best suited for self-deliverance, it gave complete instructions and illustrations on how to make a plastic exit bag at home and use it with a helium tank. It also described in detail other self-deliverance methods, including Nitschke's fourth-generation COGenie, which could be built at home in about fifteen minutes, and explained how to obtain Nembutal from foreign sources. The handbook quickly became more controversial than Humphry's *Final Exit* had been when it was released in 1991.

The Australian Office of Film and Literature allowed *The Peaceful Pill Handbook* to be sold only to those over eighteen as an RC (Refused Classification) book. But within weeks, the Australian attorney general and a fundamentalist Christian group, Right to Life Australia, challenged the RC classification as being too mild. Caving in to their pressure, the authorities reclassified the handbook as completely objectionable, and its sale was banned throughout Australia. However, Australians could easily order it from Amazon. com, where the handbook rose to number sixty on the list of the best-selling books in its 2.3-million-title inventory. When Nitschke launched it as an eBook, *The Peaceful Pill Handbook* became available to anyone anywhere in the world who had a mailing address, an internet connection, and a credit card.

Government officials were not the only ones who opposed the book. Dr. Rodney Syme, a former president of Dying With Dignity-Victoria, and a bold, pioneering advocate for physician-hastened death, was one of the book's opponents. He wrote, "I am totally opposed to the development of a 'peaceful pill,' a 'make-it-yourself' recipe that would inevitably escape into public knowledge and websites and, without the influence of any medical assessment or advice, become a pathway to disaster."[82]

Nitschke, however, had no tolerance whatsoever for censorship and turned the handbook into a downloadable, multimedia ebook over which governments had virtually no control. *The Peaceful Pill eHandbook's* new online version uses high-end internet publishing technology and includes over seventy embedded instructional videos. Purchasers pay $75 USD and receive monthly state-of-the-art, internet-delivered updates for two years. Because the ebook is downloaded from an Exit International internet server in the United States, anyone with internet access and a credit card can obtain the latest edition.

The book was publicized worldwide via short videos posted on youtube.com. One such video, "Do It Yourself with Betty," turned retired nurse-educator Betty Peters, a bubbly seventy-eight-year-old Exit International volunteer from Melbourne, into an international media celebrity. The quirky video with its bouncy 1950s music went viral and became a runaway hit. When discussing the exit bag, which is placed over the head, Betty tells the viewer with a cheerful smile, "Now if you want to look nice [when you die], you better go and get your hair done, because this [bag] does mess your hair up." The video was deleted after YouTube was swamped with complaints from right-to-life activists, but as of 2010 it could be viewed at www.veoh.com, a similar free video website.

Faced with an increasing deluge of right-to-die information, all freely available via electronic means, Nitschke's Australian political and clerical opponents resorted to a level of censorship unprecedented in any modern democratic country. They crafted the federal Suicide-Related Materials [Communications] Offences Act, which made it a crime for any Australian citizen to use a telephone, fax, or email or the internet to seek, send, or discuss information about suicide. The fines are up to $110,000 AUD for individuals and $500,000 for organizations. Unlike most Western democracies, there is no legislative right to freedom of speech in Australia, so using an electronic method of communication to counsel suicidal people or incite suicide became a criminal offense. Until then, this level of censorship was only used by despotic regimes such as those in China, North Korea, Myanmar, and Cuba.

The censorship bill went into effect on January 7, 2006. Knowing that his Australian website would probably be shut down, Nitschke moved its content to the server of the Voluntary Euthanasia Society of New Zealand. He also advised members who shared information via email to use free email privacy software known as Pretty Good

Privacy (PGP). Euthanasia information transmitted via face-to-face meetings (including at Exit International workshops) and by the public mail service was not affected.

In 2008, the Australian government announced plans to install a mandatory internet filter to block websites worldwide that provided "inappropriate material" deemed harmful to the public. This included child pornography, racist hate speech, and right-to-die information. When the blacklist of internet sites to be blocked was revealed through Wikileaks in 2009, it was learned that the filter would specifically block sites providing information about euthanasia and abortion. Nitschke's website was on the list. To counter the threatened ban, Nitschke startled his opponents in 2010 when he and an anti-censorship organization, The Pirate Party, established internet-hacking master classes. There, elderly Exit International members were taught how to set up virtual private networks (VPNs) and internet tunnels that could easily bypass the "Great Firewall Down Under" to legally access any website they wanted. The "Great Firewall" was reduced to a censorship method as solid as Swiss cheese.

Faced with ongoing opposition in Australia, Nitschke set out to extend his influence to the British Isles in 2008. He knew that the London-based National Centre for Social Research had found that 80 percent of Britons approved of legalizing physician-hastened death for a patient with a painful terminal illness. On his first foray into the Mother Country, however, Nitschke was shocked to learn that, although the majority of the natives were friendly to his ideas, their chiefs were decidedly hostile. Indeed, the established voluntary euthanasia groups, including Dignity in Dying and Friends at the End, were as strongly opposed to his do-it-yourself philosophy as the Catholic Church and Christian fundamentalists. Nitschke was refused meeting space in several locations, and a lecture he had been invited to present at Queens University, Belfast, was abruptly canceled.

Jo Cartwright of Dignity in Dying severely criticized Nitschke's handbook, stating, "We would not object to banning the book because we don't encourage suicide without safeguards."[83]

Derek Humphry pointed out Dignity in Dying's morphing, relativist views of political correctness. Not only had its predecessor, the (U.K.) Voluntary Euthanasia Society, compiled the world's first comprehensive do-it-yourself suicide manual, but, said Humphry,

"In its bygone days, Dignity in Dying sold hundreds of copies of [my book] *Final Exit.*"[84]

Dignity in Dying was making a special case of Nitschke and his book because they felt his "in-your-face" tactics threatened to undermine their methods for achieving legislative change. Ultimately, when it came to outsiders, the actions of the U.K. death-with-dignity groups amounted to an amazingly vicious display of ideological and turf-war fratricide, with the elder, more conservative right-to-die groups turning out in force to confront one of their young, unruly offspring.

Bruised but far from beaten, Nitschke decided to return the next year. This time, when he and Fiona Stewart, who had become an indispensible part of his support team, arrived at Heathrow Airport, London, on May 2, 2009, they were searched, fingerprinted, interviewed, and warned that his teachings could be in breach of British law. After nine hours, they were released. The frosty reception did not end there.

"Nitschke is an extremist and a self-publicist," said Peter Saunders, director of Care Not Killing, an anti-euthanasia group in London. "He will prey upon vulnerable people with these kits, and as a result they won't get the medical treatment and proper palliative care that they really need."[85]

Across the ideological street, the internecine warfare continued. Dr. Michael Irwin, former chairman of Britain's Voluntary Euthanasia Society, fired off his remarks to the *Sunday Telegraph*, stating that he believed in freedom of speech but totally disagreed with Nitschke's promotion of veterinary Nembutal. Another colleague, Dr. Libby Wilson, a retired Glasgow physician and cofounder of Friends at the End, said Nitschke had done great harm to the movement because he was so confrontational.

In another slap in the face, the Oxford Union Society, Britain's second-oldest debating society, withdrew Nitschke's invitation to an assisted suicide debate in March 2009. Three pro- and three anti-euthanasia speakers were slated to speak, but because two other pro-euthanasia representatives, including Dr. Michael Irwin, were unwilling to appear alongside him, their withdrawal made a balanced debate impossible.

Overall, Nitschke considered the grueling British tour to be a success because he was able to reach large numbers of people in person and through the media. Perhaps the best support was Joan Bakewell's open-minded feature article in *The Times*, Britain's premier newspaper. "Why Dr. Death Should Have Been Given a Welcome in Britain," closed with

> Death defeats us: we cannot ultimately do anything to change it. It will come what may. In the end our destiny will claim us. We can tamper with the details, we can minimise the pain, but we cannot turn death aside. What we need is the compassion to collaborate with it, to ease its coming, to smooth the path. Laws can frame the conditions for such care, but they are not the care itself. For that, each of us must be free to find his or her own way.[86]

Although Nitschke had made numerous specialized trips to the United States and Canada, his first North American lecture/seminar tour did not get underway until November 2009. He hoped that greater freedom of speech in North America would make his reception warmer than in Britain. In Canada, whose laws are based on English common law, he soon found out otherwise. The Vancouver, B.C., public library canceled his first event because of allegations that letting a voluntary euthanasia proponent describe means of self-deliverance could be a violation of Canadian law.

The cancellation seemed bizarre to Nitschke because the library already owned multiple copies of his handbook. The venue was quickly changed to the Unitarian Church in Vancouver, where about one hundred and fifty people and no protesters attended. Ironically, the following week, the Vancouver library, which had slammed its doors in his face, sent Exit International a large order for *The Peaceful Pill Handbook* because of the huge demand from its patrons.

At a November 7, 2009, meeting in Bellingham, Washington, attendees were outnumbered three-to-one by a large, highly organized crowd of yelling, poster-carrying "protect the elderly" protesters from a pro-life, anti-euthanasia group called True Compassion Advocates.

The San Francisco meeting, held at (but not affiliated with) the Buddhist Center, was preceded by an op-ed article in the *San Francisco Chronicle* titled "Australia's Dr. Death Comes to San Francisco," written by anti-euthanasia activist Wesley J. Smith.[87] Unlike some of Nitschke's previous destinations, the San Francisco Bay area had a long history of openness to intellectual freedom of thought and expression. Indeed, just a few miles across the Bay lay Berkeley, where Nitschke and nine colleagues had held the first NuTech working meeting in 1999, a decade earlier. In that liberal hotbed of freethinkers, Nitschke's views were about as controversial as chicken soup. The only protesters who showed up were disability rights activists allied with Not Dead Yet.

When the final North American meeting, in Anaheim, California, was over, Nitschke and Fiona Stewart breathed a sigh of relief and decided to take a few days off in Las Vegas. They found it as bizarrely different from Darwin as the fictional Mick "Crocodile" Dundee found Manhattan from the Outback. Nevertheless, they decided to take advantage of their location. "Fiona and I got there and, well, you can't *not* get married when you get to Vegas," Nitschke said with a chuckle.

Outside the Clark County Marriage License Bureau, "spruikers" (hawkers) were handing out discount marriage chapel coupons. "Please take one," a spruiker implored nervously as she pressed a coupon into Nitschke's hand. "My boss is watching." The brochure announced, "Fifty dollar special today at The Stained Glass Wedding Chapel on East Ogden Street, just moments from The Strip." A few hours later, after a five-minute civil ceremony, Philip Haig Nitschke, sixty-two, and Fiona Joy Stewart, forty-three, were married, each for the first time.[88]

Nitschke spent the next two years living in the eye of a hurricane. His 2010 North American "Safe Exit" tour drew good turnouts in Vancouver and Toronto and a small group at a brief, last-minute stop in Québec. The U.S. segment had quite a different outcome. The programs scheduled in San Francisco, New York, and Orlando, Florida, were canceled on short notice, when, for unknown reasons, the U.S. government refused to grant Nitschke a visa to enter the country. I was especially disappointed, for Orlando was the place I was planning to interview him in person for the first time.

"It would be a great pity indeed if the Land of the Free, where freedom of speech is enshrined in the Constitution, were to forbid Dr. Nitschke entry, simply because of the views he holds," commented Exit International in its *e-Deliverance* newsletter. Nevertheless, he was barred. The reasons were never made public.

Nitschke returned to Dublin in February 2011 and was greeted by about fifty Catholic-based Life Institute protesters, carrying signs reading "Suicide 'workshop' illegal and sick," and "Lock up your grannies, Dr. Death is here."[89] Although Irish officials chose not to intervene, only twenty people came to his presentation, a dozen of whom were with the press.

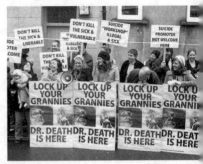

Undaunted, Nitschke now uses internet technology to spread his message where distance, cost, or extreme opposition frustrate his work. In addition to Australia and New Zealand, he continues to make annual tours of England, Wales, Ireland, and Scot-

Dublin protesters in 2011

land. He has also started making initial visits in Southern Asia and plans to visit India. Using video-equipped laptop computers, he also conducts webinars (interactive internet web seminars) using Skype software to hold meetings throughout the English-speaking world without the high cost of travel.

Condemned as he is by Catholics, fundamentalist Protestants, and many conservatives within the right-to-die-movement itself, Nitschke knows that he has intense support from his large and growing group of members and followers. His goal of telling people exactly how they can end their lives peacefully is grasped instinctively by people from widely diverse backgrounds. His position is simple and direct: those who are dying or beyond their ability to cope with their pain do not have to take anyone's side but their own. One may agree or disagree with him, but his answer to the classic Sue Rodriguez question, "Who owns my life?" is unequivocal: the person, and not any governmental, medical, or religious authority.

Nitschke's intense commitment to the concept of total autonomy at the end of life strikes a loud and responsive chord worldwide, as witnessed by his 100,000-plus newsletter mailing list, the euthanasia world's largest. And his flamboyant tactics attract immense amounts of international attention to the death-with-dignity cause. But Nitschke's blunt, contentious public image and do-it-yourself deathing philosophy does not sit well with the conservative/legislative change wing of the death-with-dignity community around the world—or in his native Australia. There, all the state-based voluntary euthanasia groups except Nitschke's have recently banded together to form a unified, single-minded coalition to enact death-with-dignity laws at the state and national level. And the man chiefly responsible for this alliance is none other than Nitschke's former close friend and widely respected medical colleague from the ROTI era: Dr. Rodney Syme of Melbourne.

– 9 –

Death Down Under

The next sixteen years became a roller-coaster ride that thoroughly tested my conscience. It involved years of helping patients to die in order to relieve their suffering, potentially breaking the law and confronting authority in the process.

— Dr. Rodney Syme, 1992

It was a beautiful fall day in Melbourne, Australia; warm and mild, with a gentle breeze and blue skies. Had it not been for the task that lay before him, forty-year-old Rodney Syme, for fifteen years a urological surgeon, would have walked briskly into the hospital with his trademark smile and a warm greeting to his colleagues. But his mind was not peaceful that day, and deep concern had replaced his smile with a somber face. Nothing cheerful faced him or his patient. He was on his way to visit Betty,* who suffered from spinal cancer. Despite the best surgical care, her life had become a vicious, harsh reality. Far down the corridor from her room, he could already hear her screams of pain as nurses tried to move her onto a bedpan.

Before he decided to specialize, Syme had spent many years in hospitals, seeing numerous patients, most of whom received treatment and got better and a much smaller group who died from acute illnesses. In that setting, he was seldom exposed to slowly dying patients.

In 1972, he had removed Betty's right kidney, which contained a large cancer. He and his patient were pleased with the results of the procedure, but in 1974, she returned, complaining of severe pain in her lower back. The cancer had spread with a vengeance into her upper lumbar vertebrae, causing the bone to collapse and creating intense pain.

From Dr. Michael Ashby, a professor of palliative care at

Monash University, Syme learned that there were several syndromes that are particularly difficult to treat: nerve pain, bone pain, and pain that is largely psychological.[1] Palliative care was barely in its infancy in Melbourne in 1974, and Syme knew of only two doctors who specialized in pain management. When one of them consulted with Betty, he concluded that the only effective therapy was the use of powerful narcotic drugs—typically morphine.

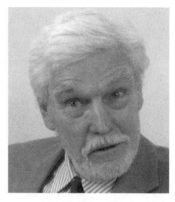

Dr. Rodney Syme

Betty's worst problem was the excruciating "incident" pain, which flared up immediately whenever her spine moved, which happened constantly. The cause was acute nerve pressure, not unlike the lightning bolt of pain that comes when a dentist accidently drills into an unanesthetized nerve in your tooth. Morphine does not control incident pain well.

Physicians have long been hesitant to use heavy doses of morphine for end-stage pain because most patients develop a tolerance for the drug. The patients then need progressively higher doses of the painkiller until a point is reached where the dosage itself may kill them, not the disease. In the past, doctors often claimed that dying patients might become addicted after progressively larger doses of painkillers. But today, it is clear that the risk of addiction to a painkiller is a relatively small concern considering the painkiller's palliative value to a terminally ill person.

Like Philip Nitschke, Syme knew that this situation often resulted in medicine's doctrine of double effect. The legitimate aim to alleviate pain may, as a byproduct, hasten a patient's death. Every doctor who deals with end-of-life cases at least theoretically faces the possibility of being charged with a mercy killing when it comes to choosing the painkilling dose for a terminally ill patient in extreme pain. But if such a charge is made, the outcome depends on a judge or jury deciding whether the doctor increased the medication to reduce the pain or to end the patient's life. If the former, the action is generally considered to be appropriate medical practice. If the latter, it might be considered a serious crime.

The doctrine of double effect is derived from the writings of St. Thomas Aquinas (1225-1274), who set out four conditions that would morally sanction actions that have both good and bad effects:

1. The action must be good in itself.
2. The person must intend only the good or beneficial effect and not the evil effect.
3. The good effect must not be achieved through the bad effect. The good and evil effects must follow immediately from the same action.
4. There must be sufficient reason to permit the bad effect. That is, there must be a favorable balance between the good and evil effects of the action.[2]

In 1957, British judge Lord Justice Patrick Devlin first established the doctrine of double effect as a doctor's legal defense against malpractice. An English general practitioner, Dr. John Bodkin Adams, had been charged with murder when a number of his elderly patients died after he prescribed high dosages of painkillers for them. Focusing on the doctor's intent, Lord Devlin ruled that "a physician…is entitled to do all that is proper and necessary to relieve pain and suffering, even if the measures he takes may incidentally shorten life."[3]

Decades after Devlin's decision, doctors were still struggling with its implications, and the threat of prosecution still hung over their heads. Syme noted that "it needs only one person with a moral objection to hastening death in any circumstances to make an official complaint for a criminal or Medical Board investigation to become a reality."[4] Even today, he says, "the fear of regulatory scrutiny or disapproval of professional colleagues exists, despite the guidelines of the American Geriatrics Society who say 'it is the responsibility of physicians to relieve pain, especially when the prognosis is poor, pain relief may be the most important thing physicians can offer their patients.'"[5]

"In 1974, the idea of delivering continuous high-dose analgesics and sedatives to control such pain was unknown," Syme wrote. "In the climate of those times, doctors and nurses (and to a lesser extent today) were fearful that if they delivered large doses of narcotics, which could hasten death through their side effects, they might be hauled before the law. They did not understand that, in this situation, the dose required is the dose that *works*, not the dose that is *safe*."[6]

When Betty's husband could no longer tolerate his wife's suffering, he asked Syme if there was anything else the doctor could do. Syme wrote of the question, "I did not recognize that as a signal to begin a dialogue about hastening death (if indeed it was), but today I would certainly do so…. Doctors need to be alert to the subtle signals that indicate a particular person is ready to develop a dialogue about their future…. I was simply not prepared by experience, understanding, or education to be open to such a signal, even though I was now acutely aware that a society that would not allow an animal to suffer such pain would allow a sentient human being to do so."[7]

Afraid of being charged with malpractice if he aggressively treated Betty with painkillers and thereby hastened her death, Syme did not increase her dosage. Helpless, Betty lingered on and ultimately died an excruciating death. Syme later wrote, "I felt an enormous sense of failure as I had been unable to have any impact on her problem. My reaction was wrong but natural because there was almost nothing that anybody could have done in these circumstances at that time."[8]

In retrospect, Syme realized that his inability to help Betty more effectively "was not because of any lack of caring or of compassion . . . . It was because the law inhibited a dialogue of any substance to develop between us about alternative ways of treatment to relieve her of this profound and intolerable suffering."[9] He sought answers to why the law prevented such humane assistance and wondered if religion was at least partially responsible.

The Catholic Church claimed salvational value in suffering while dying, as though suffering in unimaginable pain until the last gasp of air left the lungs would somehow bring one closer to God. *What kind of allegedly beneficent deity would inflict unnecessary, avoidable, and incomprehensible torture?* Syme wondered. *None*, he decided.

When he compared Betty's situation to his own, he realized that he would not have permitted himself to suffer as she had. "I am absolutely certain that in the same circumstances I would have taken the opportunity to end my own life."[10] But as a physician, he had relatively easy access to the means of a peaceful death; means almost completely unavailable to the majority of patients themselves. The result, he quickly realized, was a hypocritical, two-tiered system: tortured deaths for the unlucky patients versus gentle, elective deaths for certain doctors and their patients.

I could not help thinking how grossly unfair this was for others who did not have my advantages as a doctor. Many people with terminal illnesses do take their own lives in order to end their suffering, but lacking knowledge and opportunity, do so in the most horrific circumstances. Shooting, hanging, cutting of wrists or throat, jumping from heights, or in front of trains, deliberate motor accidents, or gassing and corrosive poisoning are the commonly employed methods and often occur without discussion with relatives, leaving an appalling and indelible memory…. Gradually, I came to the firm conclusion that people with hopeless and incurable illnesses should have the right to assistance to end their lives if their suffering was unrelievable and intolerable. I also realised that it was wrong to feel guilt and shame at being unable to help patients in this situation, for it was not I who was at fault but the law that created this situation. I also gradually realised, over the following years, however, that I would continue to feel diminished if I did not try to do something to help people in the future. It would have weighed too heavily on my conscience to do otherwise.[11]

Syme was a junior registrar (medical specialty trainee) in London in the 1960s when he came to understand firsthand the types of moral choices that doctors must make. A woman in her late eighties had been run over by a car and was brought into the casualty department. "She was comatose, she was shocked, and she had obviously very severe injuries. I said, 'Quickly, get me a drip, see if we've got matching blood, get an X-ray, blah, blah, blah.' Then a hand came down my shoulder from behind. It was my senior registrar, a forty-eight-year-old surgeon, very experienced. He said, 'Don't worry, son, there's nothing we can do.'"[12]

"My training was to jump in and do everything. But this eighty-eight-year-old woman, if we had got her to survive the injuries, [we] would have left her shockingly impaired. I accepted what he said without question but later thought more about why he should say that."[13]

The shock that struck Syme, a sheltered, privileged young Melbourne man, the son of a surgeon and a former Anglican whose beliefs had evolved into those of an agnostic humanist, was the first sign that his career would be filled with powerful moral questions, the answers to which had no clear guidelines.[14]

Soon after his experiences with Betty, Syme's conclusions were put to the test when Ken,* a member of his wife's family, was battling a variety of health problems. As Ken aged, his heart began to fail. In earlier days, Syme had the opportunity to talk extensively with him about his end-of-life wishes. Ken agreed with the philosophy of hastening death to relieve intolerable suffering—and his heart problems were steadily getting worse. When Syme visited him in the hospital after a particularly bad attack, he found his friend blue in the face from a lack of oxygen. Even though he was receiving all of the appropriate treatment, Ken was in the last stage of heart failure. Between heaving breaths, he gasped, "Help me!" It was a case of immediate need, and he had clearly and unequivocally made his wishes known to Syme in advance.

Ken's primary physician had authorized large amounts of pain-killers, but the nurses were reluctant to administer them, afraid of being held liable for Ken's death. "I determined to give the injection of morphine myself," Syme wrote, and he asked the nurse to draw up the ordered dose. "I gave it to Ken intravenously, for rapid and maximal effect, and recall his almost immediate relief and his mumbled thanks. He passed into a coma as the dose of morphine suppressed respiratory drive and slowed his respiration, the direct effect of the injection. His suffering relieved, he remained asleep until he died about two hours later."[15] By hastening Ken's death, Syme had just taken his first step in becoming a right-to-die activist.

The death-with-dignity movement has deep roots in Australia. The newsletter of Dying With Dignity-New South Wales observed that the nation's profound attachment to the issue was grounded in its enormous size, thinly spread population, and the vast distances between doctors and patients in rural areas. "Families and others were obliged to care for the dying, experiencing the realities of the suffering inherent in dying without the pain relief and treatment more readily available to people in the cities."[16]

The first Australian voluntary euthanasia organization was formed in Victoria in 1973, followed by New South Wales in 1974, Western Australia in 1980, South Australia in 1983, Queensland in 1985, Tasmania in 1992, and the Northern Territory in 1995. Philip Nitschke's Exit International began in 1996, and Christians Supporting Choice for Voluntary Euthanasia was founded in 2009.[17] With the exception of Nitschke's organization, the voluntary euthanasia groups focused on providing information about advance medical directives and achieving legislative change to legalize euthanasia and physician aid-in-dying.

Syme eventually defined six medical "givens," or unarguable positions about dying:

- Dying may be associated with intolerable suffering.
- The doctor's duty is to relieve suffering.
- Some suffering will only be relieved by death.
- The doctor's duty is to respect his patient's autonomy.
- Some patients rationally and persistently request assistance to die.
- Palliative care cannot relieve all the pain and suffering of dying patients.

After pondering these ideas, Syme remarked, "It became clear that my duty as a doctor, taken seriously in conscience, put me in direct conflict with the law, which did not recognise consent (i.e., request) as a defence, and regarded hastening death intentionally, or aiding suicide (quite the wrong word in the circumstances) as a serious crime. As I saw it, there were circumstances where there was a necessity for a doctor to break the law."[18]

He also found a new ally in the quest for gentle death when a man with motor neurone disease wanted his assistance. "For the first time I provided somebody with barbiturates, which are the ultimate medication, because if you take a dose of barbiturates of an appropriate nature, you can just go to sleep in the most beautiful, peaceful, calm manner, and don't wake up, and die relatively quickly."[19]

In 1992, after years of research and personal experience with helping terminally ill patients die, Syme publicly admitted that he had purposely hastened a dying patient's death at the patient's repeated request. He deliberately made his action public to bring the doctrine of double effect out of the shadows. In an attempt to initiate legal reform, Syme repeatedly asked the Victoria Coroner's Office to tell him if a doctor who prescribed doses of painkillers that eventually led to the death of the patient via "terminal sedation" was a reportable case (suspicious death) under the law. The coroner refused to make a ruling.

"After a four-year investigation of Syme's case, the coroner ruled that his actions in honouring a cancer patient's desire to die by sedating her into a coma, without intravenous fluids or other support, was a natural death that was not reportable. This is consistent with Syme's thesis that a benign conspiracy exists to ignore physician-assisted dying in all but the most flagrant cases," an article in *The Australian* stated.[20]

Four years after the coroner refused to rule on Syme's efforts to clarify the boundaries of deliberately hastened death, it was clear to Syme that the government did not want to open a hornet's nest of rage from the medical community, which preferred the "wink, wink, nod, nod" *status quo*. When he found that formal applications were useless, he took to the press. In 2005, he and six other Australian doctors triggered a front-page story in *The Age*, Australia's largest newspaper, when the physicians—quickly dubbed "The Melbourne Seven"—went public. Admitting that they had deliberately hastened the deaths of some of their patients, they called for legal change. There was no response from the government.[21]

In 1995, two decades after Syme had hastened Ken's death, the first Australian laws for legal physician aid-in-dying were drafted. That year, the State of South Australia's first Voluntary Euthanasia Bill was presented by John Quirke but was rejected without a full debate.[22]

The first such law to be passed anywhere in the world was the Rights of the Terminally Ill (ROTI) Act, a visionary excursion into uncharted legal and medical waters. It was the brainchild of Marshall Perron, the Northern Territory's Chief Minister (head of government), who was finishing his last year in office. A vigorous supporter of the right to die, he saw the act as the crowning jewel of his socially progressive career. The act was based on a simple principle: "If there are terminally ill patients who wish to end their suffering by accelerating inevitable death, and there are sympathetic doctors who are willing to help them die with dignity, then the law should not forbid it."[23] Because the act was proposed by a territorial legislature, not the national parliament, it only applied within the territory itself, and only territorians could vote on it.

The first place Perron turned to for guidance was the Voluntary Euthanasia Society of Victoria (VES-V), which had been founded to educate the public about the need for living wills and advance healthcare directives. By the early 1990s, the society was developing

a prototype national bill to legalize voluntary euthanasia and physician-hastened death. Its chief architects included Rodney Syme,
then vice president of the society; Dr. Helga Kuhse, a pioneering
Australian philosopher, bioethicist, and supporter of the legalization of voluntary assisted euthanasia; and Professor David Kelly,
the former chair of the Law Reform Commission.[24]

At Perron's invitation, Syme traveled to the Northern Territory to talk to the parliamentary committee that was considering
the legislation and to support the act by dealing with the media. He
provided Perron and his ministers with extensive information, and
the bill passed. Although he was a strong advocate for the act, Syme
was not licensed to practice medicine in the Northern Territory and
could not treat any of the seven patients who ultimately sought to
take advantage of its provisions. When federal lawmakers set out to
overturn the act, Syme and his organization communicated actively
with lawmakers in the national parliament to no avail. The act was
nullified in 1997.

Terminally ill patients with unrelenting pain, many with little
or no access to palliative care, were once again forced to die in agony.
Australia's physicians, many of whom supported the law but feared
public censure, were denied the ability to afford patients the right to
death with dignity that veterinarians could provide to any dog, cat,
or horse. The only beneficiaries were the politicians who, by voting
for the repeal, dodged controversy and avoided taking a stand against
their formidable Catholic and fundamentalist Christian constituents.
The latter were pleased that yet again, their religious beliefs could
be imposed upon the non-concurring Australian majority.

"What Kevin Andrews and his colleagues in the Federal Parliament did was barbaric," said Marshall Perron. "It is clear that many
of the speakers in the House of Representatives and the Senate did
not even casually peruse the Northern Territory *Rights of the Terminally Ill Act* they were about to overturn."[25]

The repeal of the act polarized the Australian death-with-dignity movement. The conservatives, led by Syme, encouraged supporters in each state and territory to regroup and renew the fight for
passage of right-to-die laws in their legislatures.

Philip Nitschke, the only Australian doctor to personally help
the four dying people who were able to use the law, was outraged
when the act was overruled. Watching a well-planned right-to-die

law yanked out from under the feet of those who desperately needed it led him to renounce the legislative change approach altogether. It was the impetus for his future "in-your-face" career as a voluntary euthanasia renegade.

"When the law was overturned, Philip was beside himself," Syme said. "It was a tragedy, to be sure. But there are limits as to what we could do. In retrospect, I have no doubt that we should have done more to try and prevent that, although to this day I don't know what more we could have done.... But it didn't make me turn away from legislative reform. That's always been for me the only way in which one could possibly proceed. But it turned Philip in a different direction."[26]

Prior to the repeal of the ROTI act, Australia's right-to-die groups had been brought together by the 1996 biennial congress of the World Federation of Right to Die Societies, which was held in Melbourne. It was a significant meeting because the far-flung Australian and New Zealand voluntary euthanasia and Exit chapter members got a rare opportunity to interact, and it provided the first forum for Australian, Asian, American, and European right-to-die group members to exchange ideas face to face.

However, the next meeting was not as convivial. In August 2001, on the fifth anniversary of the nightmarish death of heroic cab driver Max Bell, whose attempt to die under the ROTI act failed, Philip Nitschke held the Inaugural National Congress, "Dying in Australia—Taking Control," in Broken Hill, New South Wales. Representatives from all voluntary euthanasia groups in Australia and abroad were invited. One hundred delegates, including Marshall Perron, the keynote speaker; Derek Humphry, past-president of the Hemlock Society; and Faye Girsh, then Hemlock's president, also attended.

Prior to the conference, Nitschke had proposed creating his "Peaceful Pill." He had visited Rodney Syme and the leaders of VES-V seeking financial support for the project. Syme was president of the group at the time and strongly opposed Nitschke's idea.

> I believed that the development of a "Peaceful Pill" which would be made available to anybody to make in their own kitchen or back yard, to put that sort of information out into the community so that it could be accessed by anybody who

had a notion of ending their life, was highly irresponsible. I knew from my own counseling of people who came to me for advice, that not an insignificant number of them were misguided. The point was that somebody had told them that they had cancer, and like that first woman in the ROTI segment [Marta Alfonso-Bowes], they flipped their bloody lid and decided that that was it. Life was done and go ahead and get it over with. And that was totally the wrong decision. What a person in that circumstance needs is to be able to sit down with an empathic doctor and talk about it and have it explained what the circumstances are, that they've got a small cancer that can be treated, that they can be cured and that even if they're not cured, they've got some years of good life ahead of them. That's just an irrational response. Then you've got another whole group of people who are situationally depressed, and if they can just go to an email site and pick up a lethal cocktail prescription and make it themselves, well they're going to end their lives unnecessarily.[27]

Syme was emphatic. He thought the basic concept of a peaceful pill was dangerous and irresponsible. He did not want a do-it-your-self system that had no safeguards against misuse by juveniles and those suffering from overwhelming but temporary mental distress or clinical depression. He also felt that Derek Humphry's how-to book, *Final Exit*, which was available to almost anyone, anywhere, fell into the same category.

"To have carte blanche to go and toss yourself [commit suicide] without any interface, I think, is just bloody stupid. It's not only stupid, it's irresponsible. And that's where Philip and I come apart [part ways]. I can understand why he does it, but I just don't think it's the right way for us to go and to advocate because you harm some people. You may help others, a lot of people, but you harm a lot of others." But Syme admitted that he had no good answer to the question, "What are the people who are suffering to do in the meantime until we change the law?"[28]

Nevertheless, before the Broken Hill conference, Syme's group invited Nitschke to its annual general meeting to advocate for his Peaceful Pill. Syme and a member of his board would argue against it. The meeting was a fiasco for Syme's group. Nitschke contacted the media in advance, saying that he was attending to advocate for his cause. Syme considered that an act of unconscionable sabotage. After both sides had spoken in the debate, Syme took a straw poll of the attendees. "How many of you would like to have a Peaceful Pill?" he asked. Almost 100 percent of those present raised their hands.

Undeterred he said, "Alright, you want to have a Peaceful Pill. What if I explained to you that if those who argue for a peaceful pill will effectively have to give up any advocacy for law reform because the two are in conflict. You can't logically argue for one and the other." He continued, "Who amongst you thinks it is imperative that we support law reform?" [29]

When 100 percent of the attendees indicated their support for legal change, Syme continued, "Well, if you want law reform, you can't have advocacy for a peaceful pill. We have to have one or the other, and your Committee believes that we should have law reform. You support that, so that's the position of the Society." [30]

When subsequently interviewed by the media, Syme said that the decision of the meeting was to support legal reform. Nitschke was incensed, exclaiming, "You can't say that!"

Syme retorted, "Well, that's the bloody conclusion, mate." He later explained, "At any rate, we [he and Nitschke] really parted ways at that point. I could only see the concept of the Peaceful Pill being real poison for legislative reform in Australia."[31]

Despite the feud with Syme, Nitschke's Broken Hill conference went on as planned. The first event was a speech by Marshall Perron about the tragedy of the repeal of the ROTI act. Next came the surprise announcement that the Hemlock Society USA had granted Nitschke $25,000 to aid in developing his Peaceful Pill.[32] The final event, which earned Nitschke enormous respect from everyone attending, was the dedication of a formal headstone and burial plot enclosure that Nitschke's group had erected in honor of Max Bell, who had been buried in an unmarked grave in 1996. Even though the atmosphere of the conference was posi-

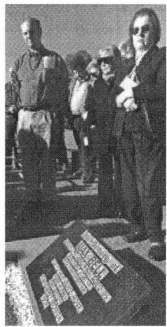

Max Bell's tombstone at Broken Hill

tive, too much enmity had been created between Nitschke and the conservatives. The two sides never came to any agreement over their differences.

As recently as 2011, Nitschke angered conservatives again. Voluntary euthanasia supporters in South Australia and Tasmania had convinced their legislators to seriously consider right-to-die bills. This was no mean feat, given all the other state-level bills that had failed. If any of these proposals became formal bills, they had a fair chance of being passed. Best of all, on November 1, 2011, the Federal Parliament passed an historic law significantly strengthening the rights of the Australian Capital Territory and the Northern Territory, meaning that individual federal ministers no longer have the power to veto territory laws, and those laws can now only be overturned if both houses of the Federal Parliament agree.[33]

Then, as Syme explained, "Out of the woodwork comes Philip to say that if the legislation is passed, he would set up [suicide] clinics there [in Adelaide and Tasmania]. He could have waited till the bloody bill was passed [and then say] 'I'm going to help.' But no. He may have had the best intentions, but his strategic sense is appalling, and he did a lot of damage to the prospects of that legislation."[34]

Despite their profound differences of opinion, Rodney Syme and Philip Nitschke would collaborate one more time. On Monday morning, June 11, 2005, Syme had his car radio tuned to 774 ABC radio in Melbourne to listen to the end of Jon Faine's erudite call-in show on the right to die. He was only able to catch the talk-back section, but he sensed that the topic had fueled serious debate. That night, he discovered the debate would get personal.

After he returned home, he received a call from one of the talk show's callers, fifty-eight-year-old Steve Guest, who sought his help to die. Guest told Syme that he had called the show to talk about those like himself with incurable cancer and to "express his anger at those religious people who prevented him from receiving the same compassionate help to die as his canine companion had and to advocate for a change in the law."[35]

On call-in shows, the caller normally gets no more than a minute or two to express an opinion. Guest got ten minutes of air time, and the lines were swamped with sympathetic responses. "Steve's message was that he had no control over his death, and he believed that

government, in thrall to the religious hierarchy, denied him that control."[36] Syme
agreed to meet Guest the next day.

He found Guest suffering from inoperable esophageal cancer, which blocked
swallowing and required the insertion
of a feeding tube in his stomach. Neither
radiotherapy nor chemotherapy had any
positive effect. Guest had lost more than
seventy-seven pounds in nine months,

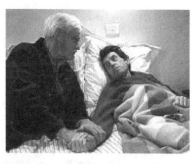

Rodney Syme and Steve Guest

had withered to little more than skin and bones, and suffered from a
profound lack of physical energy.

He had an extremely good relationship with his doctor and was
receiving excellent care, including large doses of morphine to dull
the pain, but that also dulled his mind. His greatest distress came
from not being able to do much for himself. He had irretrievably lost
the simplest pleasures of life: tasting food, drinking, and exercising his muscles. He was dying, and nothing could control his ever-
increasing pain. "Formal palliative care had nothing to offer him,"
Syme found.[37]

Guest had attended one of Philip Nitschke's workshops in early 2005. Because he was unable to attend the follow-up workshop,
Nitschke visited him at his home several times. Five days before he
died, Guest had planned to address an Exit public meeting. Too ill to
attend, he instead recorded a heartfelt speech that was played to the
packed room of more than one hundred fifty people.[38]

In Guest's last weeks, Syme and Nitschke visited him separately
and counseled him about his end-of-life options. Syme knew that it
was highly unlikely that the legislature of Victoria, of which Melbourne is the capital, "had the moral courage to address the issue
of choice in dying with dignity. They were more concerned about
retaining or gaining office to risk adopting this issue for legislative
reform, even if a majority of them personally believed that it was a
proper thing to do."[39]

Syme's medical colleague and friend, Professor Peter Baume,
thought that the law was more likely to change because of a legal
precedent than legislation. "It was obvious that there was a reluctance to proceed with prosecution or apply penalty on laypersons
accused of, or admitting to, 'mercy killing.'"[40] Syme's experience had

led him to believe that there was a wholesale reluctance on the part of the police and prosecutors to pursue these matters.[41] *Would a medical test case change the course of practice in physician-assisted dying?* he asked himself. *What would be necessary for a test case to have a chance of success?*[42]

Guest agreed to make his death a legal test case. In return, Syme and Nitschke would admit that they had told Guest how to die, and they were prepared to risk their medical licenses to test Victoria's assisted suicide law. Both doctors believed that the state government did not want the case to come to trial, for if it did, and the doctors prevailed, the precedent would effectively make the law unenforceable.

Steve Guest spent the last weeks of his life contacting the media to decry the lack of human decency afforded to the dying who did not want to live until the last agonized breath of life stopped. He ended his life with a self-administered lethal dose of Nembutal in his home on July 26, 2005.

Before Guest died, Syme stated that he had given him information about barbiturates, their lethal dosages, and their effects. He also said that he gave him unnamed "medication." Both Syme and Nitschke confessed to police that they had given him advice and medication to alleviate his pain, but neither disclosed the medication or dose. Guest, however, pre-empted the attempt to prosecute either doctor because he left a written statement testifying that neither physician gave him the Nembutal.[43]

Ultimately, Syme's prediction was accurate. After homicide detectives investigated Syme and Nitschke, and the State Coroner's Office and Victoria's Director of Public Prosecutions completed their deliberations, neither doctor was charged with any offense. Even after the 2008 publication of Syme's book, *A Good Death*, where he confessed that he had given Guest the Nembutal he used to end his life, no charges were ever brought against him. "I'm told they believe there is insufficient evidence to lay charges…. It seems like nobody's particularly interested in dealing with the issue. It's patently absurd if the law says one thing and yet the matter is being brushed under the carpet."[44]

Inch by painful inch, in state-level increments, Australians were slowly able to convince their courts to grant small advances in the right to die with dignity, even though their legislatures would not.

In a landmark decision on August 14, 2009, Western Australia's Supreme Court granted a quadriplegic in Perth the right to die by voluntary refusal of food and fluids. Christian Rossiter, forty-nine, formerly an avid hiker, rock climber, and cyclist, had developed spastic quadriplegia over several years after being hit by a car. Like Steve Guest, Rossiter was being fed through a tube in his stomach and experienced extreme physical discomfort. He referred to his life as a living hell.

"I'm Christian Rossiter and I'd like to die," he told the court. "I am a prisoner in my own body. I can't move. I can't even wipe the tears from my eyes," he said. "I have no fear of death—just pain."

He asked his caregiver, the Brightwater Nursing Home, to remove the feeding tube. Fearing the possibility of a wrongful death case, the home refused and sought a court ruling that it would not be a criminal offense to withdraw feeding via his tube as he had requested.

New South Wales Supreme Court Chief Justice Martin ultimately ruled that "If after Mr. Rossiter has been given advice by an appropriately qualified medical practitioner as to the consequences which would flow from the cessation of the administration of nutrition and hydration .... Mr. Rossiter requests that Brightwater cease administering such nutrition and hydration, then Brightwater may not lawfully continue administering nutrition and hydration unless Mr. Rossiter revokes that direction, and Brightwater would not be criminally responsible for any consequences to the life or health of Mr. Rossiter caused by ceasing to administer such nutrition and hydration to him."[45]

The feeding tube was removed soon after the court's ruling, and Rossiter died on September 21, 2009. His brother, Tim, said, "I think Christian will be remembered as someone who was very brave and took up a fight which will give a lot of people comfort.... He set a means where people could exit life with dignity. Essentially he won the right to refuse food and medication so he could die if he wanted to."[46]

In 2010, the Supreme Court of South Australia made a similar ruling in the case of a seventy-year-old, wheelchair-bound woman with post-polio syndrome and diabetes. Identified in court papers only as "J," she requested to be allowed to refuse food and fluid orally (not by tube) and to refuse insulin injections. Knowing that the result would be her death, she had signed an advance medical directive to that effect. The court determined that "there was no common law duty on providers of residential care services to provide nourishment to residents who refuse." South Australian Supreme Court Justice Chris Kourakis did not consider her refusal to be suicide, ruling that the nursing home "will not be assisting a suicide nor committing other crimes if it complies with her desires."[47] This decision took the right to die in Australia a step beyond that of the case of Christian Rossiter, as it extended the right of refusal of food and fluid from that delivered by tube to also include nourishment and medication taken orally.[48]

That same year, as it had fourteen years earlier, the World Federation of Right to Die Societies set the stage for a major meeting of the minds when its conference returned to Melbourne. When Neil Francis, president and CEO of Dying with Dignity-Victoria, stepped up to the microphone in front of two hundred and fifty attendees, he had history-making news to announce. After working quietly and diligently for two years, all of Australia's legal-reform-based death-with-dignity groups had agreed to unify their voices

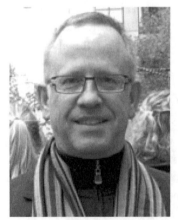

Neil Francis

and work on a common strategy to change the country's death-with-dignity laws.

The result was the formation of YourLastRight.com (YLR), a national alliance and umbrella organization that would promote a unified message of the need to reform Australia's assisted suicide laws. It would also produce legal models for these laws for both local and national levels. Francis became its chairman and CEO. The only group not included was Philip Nitschke's Exit International. Although, from his own experience, Nitschke had seen the enormous benefits of legislative change when the ROTI act was passed, his primary focus, after it was annulled, was to provide self-deliverance information directly to those who needed it.

The YLR alliance was funded by an $850,000 AUD grant from the estate of the late Clem Jones, a successful real estate investor and Brisbane's longest-serving lord mayor. After his death in 2008 at the age of eighty-nine, he left $5 million in grants to a number of charities, including one to promote the legalization of euthanasia. The trustees of the estate deliberated carefully before disbursing the grant to YLR, and provided the money only after determining that it was the best possible vehicle to achieve the grant's purpose of accelerating legislative change.

The YLR alliance campaign consists of a main website; websites for its member groups; television commercials (the first of which was banned but is available on YouTube); online social media interfaces, including Facebook, Twitter, and an eNewsletter; and relationship-building efforts to reach key groups, including political, religious, hospice, and medical organizations. Within weeks, Francis had sent out news releases to every media outlet in Australia and had been interviewed by numerous radio, television, and print reporters.

By 2011, the Australians had finally achieved substantial unity in their fight for the right to die with dignity. However, in New Zealand, a three-hour flight across the Tasman Sea, southeast of Melbourne, the fight for more humane end-of-life choices continues to be controversial.

Death-with-dignity authors beware: what you write may well be used against you in court. Derek Humphry discovered this after he published *Jean's Way*, describing how he helped his terminally ill wife die. The police came calling. After four months, the prosecutor ruled that there was insufficient evidence to prosecute him, and the case ended. New Zealand's Lesley Martin would face a grimmer outcome.

Martin, a dedicated, hard-working, purpose-driven woman, was born in Luton, England. In 1966, when she was three, she and her older brother, Michael, emigrated with their parents, Joy and Charles Martin, to Wanganui, a small city on the west coast of New Zealand's North Island. Soon after they reached their new home, her sister, Louise, was born. After studying nursing in her teens, Martin married and became a mother at the age of twenty. The marriage failed within a year. In 1986, she took her son to England where she trained as a midwife. She then worked in England, Cyprus, and France, returning to Wanganui in 1987. There she took flying lessons, qualified as a commercial pilot, and simultaneously worked at a local hospital. By 1991, she was working in Queensland, Australia's Gold Coast, as a seaplane pilot during the week and as a hospital nurse on the night shift.

A chilling phone call from her mother, Joy, with whom she was extremely close, came at Christmastime in 1998. Joy had been diagnosed with rectal cancer. She underwent surgery on January 21, 1999, but complications set in, along with infection. After two more operations, she was released, then re-hospitalized twice.

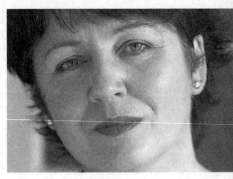

Lesley Martin

During a subsequent CAT scan, Joy found out that she also had terminal liver cancer. Declining further surgery, she went home to be with her children. Martin assisted her. Her brother Michael lived with his mother, and an intensive care nurse also provided medical assistance. Martin's mother said that she did not want to die inch by inch, as her own parents had. Martin promised to never let that happen.

Joy's doctor had prescribed sufficient morphine to deliver ten milligrams every twenty-four hours. By the time the authorized morphine drip had been set up, however, Martin had already given Joy forty milligrams over the previous eighteen hours, and on the evening of May 27, 1999, she gave her mother an additional sixty milligrams—a huge overdose. Joy died in her sleep the next day.

Despite suspicious toxicology evidence found during the autopsy and Martin's "off the record" statement to police that she had delivered a sixty-milligram morphine dose and held a pillow over her mother's head until she stopped breathing, the police closed the investigation after ten months and did not charge Martin with any crime.

New Zealand's laws on assisted suicide and voluntary euthanasia mirror those of Australia and the other former British colonies, including the subtle "wink, wink, nod, nod" attitude toward what might be perceived as mercy killing. However, if the assisted suicide is publicly rubbed in the faces of the authorities, the full force of the law may be unleashed.

When Martin published her memoir, *To Die Like a Dog*, in 2002, she reaffirmed the morphine dosages she had administered to her mother. This time, the police could not ignore her, and they reopened the case. In March 2003, she was arrested, charged with attempted murder, and released on bail. A gag order denied her the option of media interviews that would let her explain her case to the public in her own words.

Philip Nitschke publicly defended her, stating, "I totally agree with her [but] unless these things do go to trial there's less likelihood there will ever be change in the rather oppressive legislation both your country [New Zealand] and mine are saddled with."[49] In gratitude, Martin allied with Nitschke and formed Exit New Zealand as an arm of his Exit International organization.

She went to trial on March 15, 2004. Each member of the jury was given a copy of Martin's book, and the presiding judge invited them to read it. Sixteen days later, the jury retired to pass judgment on the case. After six hours of deliberation, they found her guilty of attempting to murder her mother by morphine overdose but not guilty of attempting to suffocate her with a pillow.

Martin cried out, "This is unjust" as her verdict was read, and she urged the public to fight to change the law. Then she burst into tears.[50] Outside the court, she told the press, "I don't know what else I can do to get New Zealanders off their bums and start taking part in the push towards humane legislation."[51]

She faced a maximum sentence of fourteen years in jail but was sentenced to fifteen months imprisonment on April 30, 2004. She ultimately served half of the sentence, with the other half credited as time off for good behavior. She was released on December 13, 2004, and vowed to return to her work campaigning for changes in New Zealand's euthanasia law.

Martin severed her ties to Nitschke in 2005, saying that she could no longer support his increasingly controversial self-deliverance methods. "I've come to realize that he is a product of the failure of the Northern Territory's legislation and is so marginalized now within the medical profession that he has to continually repackage do-it-yourself options for end-of-life decisions to maintain a profile and attract funds. To be constantly 'cleaning up' after him with people who have found his proposals cumbersome and unworkable has only reinforced for me that legislative reform is our best option."[52] She renamed her organization Dignity New Zealand Trust, which is now a registered charitable group dedicated to education on issues related to end-of-life decisions.[53]

In 2006, she published her second book, *To Cry Inside: Love, Death, and Prison*, which described the evolution of her thinking about euthanasia. Despite all the *sturm und drang* of her turbulent personal life, career, and imprisonment, Martin was able to do something no one else has done. She rose above her personal history and synthesized a brilliant and progressive view of end-of-life care.

Based on her nursing experiences and the aftermath of assisting the death of her mother, Martin put together a revolutionary, ground-breaking plan to merge hospice and its palliative care resources with what she called Dignity Havens: facilities where terminally ill patients could transition from hospice care to voluntary euthanasia or physician aid-in-dying without changing care locations. By 2008, she started working with a rest home towards the concept of setting up dedicated Dignity Haven beds, which would be properly stocked and ready if and when legislation enabling physician aid-in-dying was passed.

On October 31, 2008, I listened as she introduced the Dignity Haven concept to a worldwide audience of approximately three hundred delegates of the World Federation of Right to Die Societies at their biennial congress in Paris. I spoke with Martin after her speech, having noted that her concept and proposal had been very warmly greeted, based as they were on the principles of personal autonomy and end-of-life care.

A year earlier, Martin had demonstrated her integrity as a principled death-with-dignity leader following the death of Audrey Monica Wallis, forty-nine, in August 2007. The Auckland, New Zealand, woman had withdrawn $12,000 NZD from her bank account shortly before she died. The New Zealand police considered Wallis' death to be suspicious, and an analysis of her computer showed that—not unlike Ireland's Rosemary Toole five years earlier—she had conducted extensive self-deliverance fact-finding worldwide prior to her death. One email was directed to Lesley Martin, whom she had contacted for information. Martin had quickly concluded that Wallis was not terminally ill but was probably depressed and suffering from an addiction to prescribed medications. She declined to counsel or otherwise consult with her.

When contacted by the Auckland police on May 15, 2008, Martin had no reservation about telling them what she knew about the case. She told them that a mysterious American woman calling herself "Susan Wilson" (an undercover alias for her real name, Cassandra E. Mae) had contacted her in 2007 to recruit clients for her underground suicide guide service. Martin found her proposal to be totally unprofessional and offensive and shunned further contact with Mae. Mae had also solicited clients from Philip Nitschke in Australia. He, too, refused to send her referrals and, when asked, furnished the New Zealand police with the information he had about Mae.

If the Auckland authorities charged Mae with a felony offense in Wallis' death, they would seek her extradition to stand trial in New Zealand.[54] If convicted of assisting a suicide, she could VES a sentence of up to fourteen years in a New Zealand prison.

When I heard about the Wallis case and Cassandra Mae's alleged involvement, I put together what I had learned about her from George Exoo, along with my own interactions with her during Exoo's imprisonment. I contacted Lesley Martin for additional information.

About the same time, New Zealand Detective Sergeant Scott Armstrong contacted me about the case, as I had been George Exoo's volunteer international media representative while he was jailed awaiting his Irish extradition ruling. Armstrong assumed that I might be hostile to his inquiries because Cassandra Mae had been an Exoo understudy. But I assured him that I was a social historian and journalist, not a right-to-die zealot, and would be happy to tell him whatever I could about anyone who was running what appeared to be a reprehensible, covert euthanasia-for-hire operation.

Cassandra Mae had been interviewed as part of a five-year documentary film project titled *Reverend Death* by Jon Ronson, an independent British filmmaker. In the film, Mae admits to providing a euthanasia-for-hire service, stating on camera that she went to New Zealand, was with Wallis when she died, and collected money for her travel and end-of-life services.[55]

Using her alias, "Susan Wilson," Mae explicitly told Ronson on camera that she had surreptitiously taken over George Exoo's independent exit guide calling after becoming his volunteer assistant in 2007. Mae, speaking as "Susan Wilson," stated that she had set up her own solo assisted suicide business and would help practically anyone if the price was right.

"He [Exoo] doesn't know that I have been other places doing

this," she said as Ronson's camera continued to roll. "He thinks I haven't done it on my own yet. I see this as a business. He sees it as a calling. There's a big difference in [our] operations. With me, it's a business. No cash, no help," Mae told Ronson.[56] "I think that he [Exoo] will do it [end his own life] soon," Mae said. "And that's why I've been pressing him to give me a list of his current clients."[57]

"Susan says her price is $7,000," Ronson said in the film. "I'm beginning to see her as a monster of George's creation. She said she's about to do a solo job no other right-to-die group would touch."[58] That job turned out to be the Audrey Wallis assisted suicide.

"We're the people of last resort," Mae told Ronson.[59]

By the spring of 2007, she was already familiar with both the helium and Nembutal final exit procedures. And while Exoo was imprisoned that fall awaiting his extradition verdict, Mae was free to strike out on her own. And she did.

Audrey Wallis had attracted Mae's attention with a statement that she posted on Derek Humphry's ERGO internet newslist, which is read by nearly two thousand people worldwide who are interested in right-to-die issues. Although Wallis, who was seeking help for her assisted suicide, foolishly provided her full name and email address, Humphry always deletes contact information of those seeking suicide help to protect them from being misled or taken advantage of.

Wallis had written to the newslist on April 30, 2007, saying, "Well done to the lady who successfully gained entry to Mexico to obtain the necessary medication [Nembutal] to make her final exit more dignified. How I wish I had the strength to get there but my illness keeps me indoors and has so for 7 years. Ironically I have the funds for such a trip but not the health to get there. Good luck to others who may try. Kind regards Audrey Wallis, residing in New Zealand."[60]

Derek Humphry told me, "Susan Wilson asked me for Ms. Wallis' [email] address but I refused to give it to her because she sounded suspicious. I want nothing to do with such people." But "Wilson" searched it out by herself, befriended Wallis via emails, and flew to New Zealand.

Because it was an open case, the police could not divulge the cause of death, which I guessed would have been either been Nembutal or the helium bag system. In a telephone conversation with me in October 2011, "Wilson" confirmed that she had indeed been with Wallis when she died and that she obtained the helium supply for Wallis from a local party supply store.[61] She also stated that she had only received $2,000 USD for travel costs—which conflicted with her statement of her fee to Jon Ronson ($7,000) and with the amount of Wallis' bank withdrawal ($12,000 AUD). Actually providing the means of death (such as buying and delivering the helium tanks) would likely have led to the arrest and trial of Mae for aiding or abetting a suicide in New Zealand—but by the time the police discovered the details of Wallis' death, Mae was already safely back in the United States.

I was personally aware that Mae had offered to help Karen Stern, a talented, humorous, but socially isolated and desperate fifty-one-year-old American musician, end her life via helium, in trade for Stern's supply of Nembutal. For years, Stern had been tortured by multiple environmental illnesses, as well as Morgellons disease. That mysterious affliction causes open sores with string-like fibers poking out of the skin.

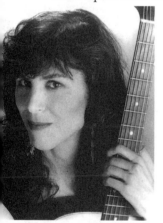

Over a period of several months, I corresponded and talked with Stern to learn why she so desperately wanted to end her life and to do whatever I could to help her avoid suicide. She had attempted and aborted several suicide attempts already. Six months before her death, she wrote to me, "I am scheduled to do the exit Wednesday night [April 11, 2007] with Susan Wilson [Cassandra Mae]. I have agreed to surrender my Nembutal dose as payment. I would rather have it to take, but I have no more resources."[62] Stern called off the plan at the last moment but ultimately chose a helium final exit six months later.

Karen Stern

The police report showed that someone had been with Stern when she died in a hotel room in Kingman, Arizona. Who that person was will probably never be known.

On March 26, 2010, New Zealand police formally charged Mae with assisting a suicide in the Audrey Wallis case and issued a warrant for her arrest. Mae was notified of the warrant but refused an offer to return to New Zealand voluntarily to face the charge. In a bizarre twist of fate, because of the ruling in George Exoo's extradition case, which determined that assisting a suicide is not a felony under U.S. federal law, New Zealand's desired extradition of Mae was unenforceable, and it is unlikely that she will ever face a judge in New Zealand.

Many of the end-of-life stories that played out in Australia and New Zealand and appeared in the media were full-blown tragedies. And, although the right-to-die efforts in those countries seem to be gaining traction, there is still formidable opposition.

However, in the United States, a beacon of hope was lit for a while when the Hemlock Society created the most comprehensive, compassionate end-of-life counseling and support system ever developed. Guided by a tiny staff in Denver, Colorado, a small group of Hemlock's Caring Friends Program volunteers brought an unparalleled level of information, support, and comfort to several thousand dying Hemlock members between its inception in 1998 and its evisceration in 2004.

Caring Friends and Hemlock's End

Compassion & Choices is the Hemlock Society, decaf version. Yes, they did acquire the society's membership rolls and engineered the take-over, but they did not hold the same principles as Hemlock did.
— Earl Wettstein, former Hemlock Society board member

G raduation day is a magical, energy-charged event for any student, but it was also a historic one for the twenty-eight men and women who made up the November 8, 1998, graduating class of the Hemlock Society's newly minted Caring Friends Program. Lois Schafer, the program coordinator, was euphoric and gave a small party for the leadership to celebrate how well the three-day session in San Diego had gone. A celebration was in order, for the program was the first of its kind in the world.

Caring Friends was conceived by Faye J. Girsh, a Harvard-trained clinical and forensic psychologist, who had become Hemlock's executive director in September 1996. "[The program] will not provide the means for hastening death nor will we actively help," she said. "But the law is clear that conveying information that is readily available through published sources and sitting with a person who has chosen to hasten his or her death are legally protected activities."[1]

The faculty for the first class featured ten seasoned end-of-life counseling professionals, including Dr. Richard MacDonald, already the world's most experienced exit guide; Dr. Stanley Terman, a noted psychiatrist and death-with-dignity advocate; and Ruth von Fuchs, president of the Right to Die Society of Canada.[2]

Attendees had come from all over the United States for this ground-breaking training session. Never before had a course been given to volunteer end-of-life counselors who, after formal training, would counsel dying people about the entire range of end-of-life issues.

Topics included using client selection criteria, reviewing an applicant's medical records, recognizing signs of depression, finding ways to encourage an applicant's dialogue with family members and physicians, and explaining other alternatives to hastened death. Comprehensive information about living wills, durable powers of attorney, POLST and MOLST orders, hospice care, palliative medication options, and the most painless methods of self-deliverance were all available to members accepted into the Caring Friends Program.

At the time, even though Hemlock had been in existence for sixteen years, general access to a self-chosen gentle death seemed unattainable for most people, except for those who had read *Final Exit*. With the inception of Hemlock's new program, however, members could finally discuss this vital subject with a trained, sympathetic counselor who could also be there with them if they were considering or had chosen a hastened death.

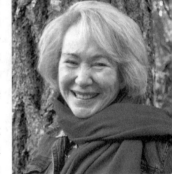

Modern medicine was saving lives, but it was also lengthening the time a patient took to die. It could not offer solutions to all pain and indignity problems and brought few significant advances in end-of-life palliative

Faye J. Girsh, Ed.D.

care. In the United States, countless people were suffering needlessly, anticipating or finding themselves warehoused in nursing homes or lying in hospital beds, attached to machines, and cared for by medical personnel who would not discuss the most vital end-of-life option with them: how to die well.

A major impetus for Hemlock to add a benefit for its members arose when *Washington v. Glucksberg*, a major right-to-die case, was heard by the U.S. Supreme Court in 1997. The court ruled that the right to an assisted suicide was not protected by the due process clause of the Constitution. States could legalize it, but federal law did not establish it as a civil right.[3]

This ruling was a great disappointment to the right-to-die movement, but Hemlock quickly adapted its strategy to the new rules. It would still push for legislative change at every opportunity, but it realized that the time had come for more assertive direct action for desperate people who were calling Hemlock every day, seeking help to die with dignity.

"At least for our own Hemlock members, we had to provide compassionate and well-trained volunteer experts who could see eligible people through their decisions to end their lives," Girsh said.

Hemlock's first attempt at directly helping terminally ill members who had no one to speak for them was its Patient Advocacy Program. It was created in response to a $28-million national investigation of more than nine thousand dying patients in five major U.S. teaching hospitals. It found that people were dying in pain, and their advance directives and durable healthcare powers of attorney were often being ignored.

The first of its kind, Hemlock's Patient Advocacy Program was launched on July 15, 1997.[4] An outgrowth of a pioneering program established in 1987 by Faye Girsh's San Diego chapter of Hemlock, it provided advocates for members whose wishes were being ignored and who had no friends or family to help them get the medical attention they needed or to block medical intervention they did not want. However, the program did not catch on because it started too late in the dying process. The people who needed its help were often too ill to apply for and make use of it.

After analyzing the performance of its first attempt to help its members, Hemlock made major modifications. The result was the development of the Caring Friends Program, whose core concepts were outgrowths of Rev. Ralph Mero's highly effective, Seattle-based group, Compassion in Dying.

Mero founded it in April 1993, two years after the failed 1991 attempt in Washington State to pass an initiative that would provide physician-hastened death for terminally ill patients who chose to end their lives after medical therapy could no longer help them.[5] Mero, a Unitarian-Universalist minister, had extensive experience with gruesome deaths, having spent years dealing with dying AIDS patients as executive director of Hemlock of Washington State. At that time, few effective medical treatments were available for HIV-positive people. Many were treated like lepers, and many medical personnel refused to care for them, fearing that they might contract the disease by contact.

In its first thirteen months, Compassion in Dying received over three hundred requests for counseling from patients in the Seattle area who expressed a desire for rational suicide. After extensive screening, the group ultimately counseled forty-six terminally ill patients who died within that period, twenty-four of whom hastened their deaths at home with prescription drugs.

Compassion's method of facilitating elective death was based on a medical model. If the patient could not obtain prescription drugs from a physician or through friends, he or she was out of luck. However, "In twenty of the twenty-four cases, the patients' personal physicians prescribed the drugs with the explicit knowledge of the patients' intention to use them to end life. In the remaining four cases the patients did not state their intention explicitly, and their physicians did not ask, but prescribed the medicines.... Members of Compassion did not supply drugs, and no physician associated with the organization wrote a prescription for or altered the medical care of any of these persons," Mero wrote.[6]

Inspired by Mero's intelligent blend of compassion and safeguards, Caring Friends was created to educate and inform Hemlock's thousands of members about the full range of end-of-life options while they still had the ability to make and carry out rational choices for themselves. "Prior to its inception, all Hemlock could say to members who wanted to self-deliver was 'read *Final Exit* and call us in the morning,'" Girsh said. "That just wasn't good enough. These were very sick people, old people, many living alone. They deserved better. They needed someone to explain things, and someone to be at their bedside offering comfort when they died."[7]

Hemlock's Caring Friends Program was ambitious from the start. Mero's program was designed primarily to serve the Seattle area; Caring Friends was envisioned to provide national coverage. Like Mero's program, there would be no cost to those served, and all the caregivers would be trained volunteers. In addition, Caring Friends would work both with the terminally ill and with members who were suffering from chronic and degenerative medical conditions where there was no acceptable treatment, such as Alzheimer's disease. Finally, it would not rely on the medical model: physician-prescribed drugs and/or assistance, both of which were extremely difficult to obtain. Instead, if members qualified for help and chose self-deliverance, Caring Friends would instruct them in the new and effective non-medical paths to a peaceful death developed by Hemlock's colleagues in the NuTech Group.

Not all of Hemlock's board members were convinced that creating the program was a wise move. When Hemlock's legal counsel reviewed its procedures, he noted grimly, "If you want me to keep you out of trouble, don't even think about doing this." Undaunted, Girsh did some lawyer shopping. "Lois Schafer and I had lunch with a well-known ACLU volunteer attorney in Denver, and he said, 'These are some precautions I would take, but I understand that you're trying to help people, so do it.'"[8]

A forceful personality, Girsh was passionate about the causes she supported. Unlike many death-with-dignity activists/leaders, Girsh's involvement with the movement was not triggered by the suffering of a close friend or family member. In 1983, in her professional capacity as a forensic psychologist, she was called in to evaluate the mental competence of Elizabeth Bouvia, a twenty-six-year-old paraplegic woman. In declining health and unable to care for herself, Bouvia checked into a hospital in Riverside, California. There, she refused food and fluids in order to die, but the hospital force-fed her to keep her alive.

Impressed by the woman's courage, Girsh accepted the ACLU's request to evaluate Bouvia's competence to make such a decision. Ultimately, a California appeals court overturned a lower court's decision on June 5, 1986, ruling that a patient who is mentally competent and understands the risks involved has a right to refuse treatment and that the state's interest in preserving life does not outweigh this right. Bouvia's feeding tube was removed, but she ended her attempts to starve herself, finding this process too painful.

The Bouvia case led Girsh to become deeply involved with end-of-life issues. "I discovered this was an issue that many families face and which often becomes a tragedy and a trauma when the person involved either takes their own life by shooting or suffers a long and agonizing death," she noted.[9] Girsh believed that "we could have a program for Hemlock members, who, we knew, found a hastened death consistent with their beliefs and values, and who were physically capable of self-deliverance."[10] Training Hemlock volunteers as end-of-life counselors to help other members explore all alternatives to a hastened death would create "a national program of community-supported dying which could bypass the medical profession, though health care professionals would be involved."[11]

To get the Caring Friends Program rolling, Hemlock needed funds. In 1997, Girsh gave a talk to a congenial group of about sixty people in Sun City West, an affluent retirement community in Arizona.[12] Shortly after her speech, a check for $40,000 arrived in Hemlock's mailbox with a note from Kay Milner, who had been in the audience. Girsh was stunned. Many people had remembered Hemlock with significant bequests in their wills—one bequest was for over $1 million—but only one gift of Milner's magnitude had ever come from a living person.

Girsh immediately called to thank her and asked if Hemlock could send someone to take her photograph for its newsletter. Milner declined. "I don't look very good now," she said, but she sent Girsh a two-page letter in January 1998. The first page contained a short handwritten note to explain the accompanying letter. The second page was a generic letter, directed to Milner's friends.

"It said, very eloquently, that she was suffering from lung cancer, that she never saw the virtue of senseless suffering, and had always believed in self-determination—so she took her own life."[13] Girsh called Sun City West to find out how Milner had died. She was dismayed by the answer. Milner had gotten into her car alone, driven to the edge of town, put a gun to her head, and pulled the trigger. Her body was found the next day by a young woman going to her job as a waitress.

Kay Milner's needlessly gruesome death stunned Hemlock's leadership. "Clearly, if our members were dying alone, violently, and having their deaths traumatize another person, we were not doing enough," Girsh explained. "It is obviously too much to ask someone who is very sick, frequently quite debilitated, maybe not thinking clearly, often alone, and usually very frightened, to read a book for instructions on how to die. They deserve to have someone see them through the whole process—and a planned death is a process, not just a matter of a few seconds—and to be there with them if they did choose to end their lives. The person who provides this service *should* be a doctor but it was obvious that doctors would not be able to provide that kind of help."[14]

Shortly after Milner's death, Hemlock's board of directors gave its formal approval, and the Caring Friends Program was launched with funding from Milner's gift.[15] A few months later, a gift of $80,000 arrived, this time from a healthy, active woman, Lois Crowell, who felt that Caring Friends was, "the crown jewel of Hemlock."[16]

The question of who would be eligible for Caring Friends' support was critical to the success of the program and the survival of Hemlock. Girsh and the board members knew that their key assets were the idealism, vision, and knowledge of their volunteers, but they also knew that providing end-of-life education and a compassionate bedside presence at the time of death were legally risky activities, where just one mistake could seriously wound or even cripple the entire organization.

In the early stages, more than one senior Hemlock official thought the plan was impractical, believing that Caring Friends' volunteer counselors "are not going to drive over mountains and rivers to go to people's houses. That's just a crazy program."[17] They were wrong. After the program was established, volunteers frequently drove or flew long distances, at no cost to the person being helped, to provide information and emotional support. Hemlock did not have the money to pay for travel expenses, but loyal Hemlock members always stepped forward to cover these costs. The ongoing costs of running the program were derived from Hemlock's operating income, voluntary contributions, and bequests. Ultimately, more than 150 volunteers were trained, and by early 2002, 119 volunteers were active in 33 states and Canada.[18]

When Hemlock announced the program to its membership, it was eagerly received. The promise of a "friend at the end" to talk to about dying quickly and gently when death was close or the pain grew unbearable made it a major success. In its first year, program coordinator Lois Schafer talked to more than three hundred people who were considering a hastened death.[19] Willing, altruistic volunteers, mostly older people, stepped up to become friends and counselors, and Hemlock's membership surged.

Girsh made it clear that the program was available to any Hemlock member who was either terminally ill or suffering intolerably from an irreversible physical condition that severely compromised his or her quality of life. The program would accept early stage Alzheimer's patients while they still had full mental capacity to make rational decisions. If those patients lost that ability and could not carry out the procedures without help, Caring Friends would, regrettably, no longer be able to work with them.[20]

From the start, Hemlock made sure that its members knew the program was not a death-on-demand service but instead one that would inform them of all their end-of-life options, not just those that would help them end their lives, and that there was no pressure on them to make the choice for death. Hemlock's *Agreement with Volunteers*, a legal contract, made this explicit. Its first two rules stipulated that volunteers were required to apply specific guidelines in screening prospective patients:

1. One of the major goals of the Program is to help the Member explore all alternatives to a hastened death. Hospice care is stressed for Members with terminal illnesses. The Volunteer should be acquainted with social services, pain management, hospice services, and other community resources that the Member might utilize.

2. If a hastened death is still being considered, the responsibility for learning about death-hastening options and methods lies with the applicant. The Volunteer should be familiar with books, pamphlets, tapes, and other written resources to provide this information.[21]

Hemlock had to strike a delicate balance between compassion and self-preservation. If its eligibility requirements for the program were too restrictive, members might be forced to suffer needless pain, indignity, and loss of control during a protracted death. If it was too liberal, Caring Friends might end up with problematic clients who could put the entire organization at severe legal risk.

Schafer commented:

As a result, if the family didn't like the idea, we weren't going to be involved. Blabber-mouthing was also a potential problem. Members had to understand that once they had consulted their immediate family members, and had decided on a hastened death, they could not talk about a planned exit with anyone outside their immediate family. In one case, we found out that the woman was talking about the event to all the people in her living complex. She was hysterical when we told her we had to drop her from the program, but she posed far too great a risk to Hemlock. If the organization didn't survive, it couldn't help anyone.[22]

Lois Schafer, head of the Caring Friends Program, held a master's degree in clinical psychology and had already run Hemlock's Patient Advocacy Program, which was still available to members. A calm, compassionate woman with a clear head, strong organizational skills, an effervescent personality, and boundless devotion to mitigating the suffering of others, she was the first person to interview any Hemlock member wishing to use the program.

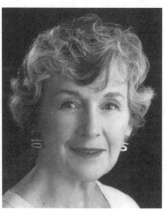

Lois Schafer

"One of the main things I did was help people write their durable power of attorney for health care, as well as their living will, because there was so much confusion and ignorance about that at the time. Although it was different in every state, I could quickly look it up on my computer and give them accurate information."[23] If the member was considering a hastened death, Schafer would discuss the person's situation in detail and request his or her medical records. Her report and the member's medical information were then passed along to a four-person medical advisory committee. The committee's responsibility was to ensure that the applicant was eligible for assistance, mentally capable, and emotionally stable and did not represent an unacceptable security risk to the Caring Friends team.

The head of the medical advisory committee was Dr. Richard "Dick" MacDonald, Hemlock's first and only medical director. A

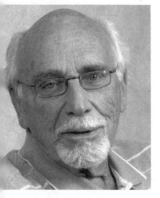

warm-hearted, insightful, and understanding man, he was present at the bedside of most members' self-deliverances. Others who served on the committee or on the training faculty roster included Dr. Stanley Terman, a psychiatrist; Sallie Troy, a clinical social worker; Mary Bennett Hudson, a retired hospice nurse; and Rev. Andrew Short, a Methodist minister. San Diego attorney and social worker Michael Evans was a frequent consultant.

Dr. Richard MacDonald

All four committee members had to agree before an applicant could be approved for the program. A Caring

Friends volunteer would then have one or more face-to-face meetings to learn the details of the case and assess the member's health, mental capacity, and any possible security issues, such as dissent within the family over the member's wish to die.

"The main thing we were looking for was mental and physical competence—the ability to make a rational choice to die and the ability carry out their death themselves, unassisted," Schafer explained.[24]

The volunteer's assessment then went to the committee for a final review. If the case was approved, the volunteer became the member's "Caring Friend," helping him or her with planning and paperwork and, if relevant, information about end-of-life procedures and bedside companionship at the end. Many Caring Friends volunteers genuinely bonded with the people they helped.

MacDonald explained that those who applied for help from Caring Friends often lived longer than people in similar circumstances who did not seek help. He found that having solid information on how to end their lives peacefully gave people the freedom to *not* end them prematurely, and not to choose pre-emptive suicide, born of fears of impending future loss of dignity and autonomy. MacDonald noted that after terminally ill people understood their options for controlling the manner and time of dying, they often postponed their final exit, feeling at peace after realizing that they had some choice. Many died from their diseases, rather than by self-deliverance, and had more peaceful, less painful deaths than they would have without Caring Friends.[25]

Five to ten percent of the applicants were judged to be too high a security risk for the program or were not physically capable of self-deliverance. Occasionally, Hemlock discreetly referred some of these members to non-Hemlock exit counselors who might be willing to take on higher-risk cases. The latter included Rev. George Exoo of the Compassionate Chaplaincy Foundation and Dr. Georges Reding, one of the five independent members of Dr. Jack Kevorkian's Physicians for Mercy group.[26]

The program's basic goal, service to any Hemlock member anywhere in the United States, was achieved within its first four years. Hemlock hoped that one day, every American would be able to choose a peaceful death under careful safeguards with the guidance of a trained volunteer.

Caring Friends quickly became a model for a carefully run, non-medical, person-to-person program providing end-of-life information and support. Despite the hundreds of members that it counseled, Hemlock was never confronted with a single family complaint or lawsuit stemming from the program. Caring Friends could have continued to demonstrate its success, but, in a way, it made Hemlock too successful, and its board became overly protective of its new-found assets.

Derek Humphry's resignation as director of the Hemlock Society in early 1992 left large shoes to fill. Having cofounded Hemlock in 1980 and built it up to 57,000 members and 86 chapters at its peak (during which time it was virtually the only assertive death-with-dignity group in the country), Humphry left the society in robust health. By the time he stepped down, several other right-to-die organizations and causes had wooed away some of its members. Yet Hemlock still had 40,000 members, 60 active chapters, and more than $1 million in the bank. The year after Humphry left, Hemlock's membership plummeted to 18,000 because no one could replicate his straight-talking, vigorous leadership.[27]

Following Humphry's departure, Hemlock's legal director, Cheryl K. Smith, served ably as interim director until a permanent replacement could be found. In1992, Hemlock's newly elected board chairman, New York attorney Sidney Rosoff, announced the appointment of John A. Pridonoff, as the new executive director.[28]

Faye Girsh, who was on Hemlock's board at the time, knew Pridonoff. She also knew two of the other applicants, but none of the other applicants were discussed. When she asked Rosoff, a strong-willed man, "Why Pridonoff?" he answered, "It's none of your business."[29]

Pridonoff had earned a bachelor's degree in psychology from California State University, Los Angeles, and a master's in theology and a doctorate in thanatology from the Colgate Rochester Divinity School in New York. He was also a minister in the Metropolitan Community Church, which had a focused outreach to lesbian, gay, bisexual, and transgendered people. Because effective medications were not available to treat AIDS in the early 1990s, the gay community had been actively involved in do-it-yourself suicides for some time, and their support for Hemlock was strong.[30]

Reversing Humphry's position, Pridonoff worked actively to forge a bond with Dr. Jack Kevorkian and urged Hemlock members to support the doctor's fight to modify Michigan's constitution to permit physician aid-in-dying. In a January 31, 1994, interview, Kevorkian thanked Pridonoff for Hemlock's support, noting, "I'm glad I can get a working relationship going with Hemlock, which, unfortunately, I couldn't do with the prior executive director [Humphry]."[31]

During his tenure, Pridonoff gave his new role his full attention, but he did not flourish as the leader of America's largest right-to-die organization. Dr. Dick MacDonald was one of several who found Pridonoff's managerial style problematic.

"In 1994 I attended the World Federation of Right to Die Societies meeting in Bath, England, and Pridonoff also attended," MacDonald said. "He stayed in an upscale hotel in town, flew first class, and generally treated himself very well. It became apparent that the board was unhappy with his personal expenses, which Hemlock had to pay. I stayed in a small hotel and flew in economy class," said MacDonald. The board found Pridonoff's tastes too expensive, and the general membership thought him too conservative. He lasted less than three years.[32]

After Pridonoff's ouster, Helen Voorhis of Denver, who had been executive director of the Colorado Epilepsy Association for thirteen years, was tapped as Hemlock's interim director in 1995. She persuaded the board to move Hemlock's corporate headquarters to Denver in January 1996 because she believed that she could obtain more volunteers there than in rural Eugene, Oregon, where Humphry lived and had assembled Hemlock's original staff.

None of the veteran Oregon staff was willing to move to Denver, so new staffers had to be recruited and trained. The board offered Voorhis the permanent position as executive director. Aware of the wearing schedule of public speaking and media interviews she would have to shoulder, she declined.

Without a dedicated, charismatic Humphry clone at the helm, Hemlock's membership and finances plummeted.[33] In addition, the quantity of hoped-for volunteers never materialized in Denver. John Westover became chairman of the board in 1996 and invited three candidates to be interviewed for the position of executive director. The board offered the position to Faye Girsh, who had founded Hemlock's highly successful San Diego chapter and had served on the board of directors during the Humphry era. Girsh, whose husband had recently died, reluctantly closed her practice as a psychologist in San Diego to move to Denver in August 1996, serving as executive director until 2000.

During her era, Girsh focused on her strongest characteristics: a passion for making dying a better experience and a talent for public speaking. "The main point about me is that I am very dedicated to the idea that people should be able to have a choice in how they die, and that they should be able to die well," she said.[34]

Although she was not, by her own admission, a strong administrator, she organized and ran the World Federation of Right to Die Societies' biennial congress in 2000. It was one of the best in its history, featuring 66 speakers and attracting 483 international attendees to Boston. Nevertheless, her role in Hemlock was debated in a special board meeting in Chicago after the congress, and Girsh recalled it as "very bitter, mean-spirited, and difficult." After the meeting, she was demoted to executive vice president and was asked to work from home, rather than in the Denver corporate office. The board, whose membership had changed substantially since Humphry's era, wanted her out of sight and out of mind. An administrator with little knowledge of the right-to-die movement was hired to replace her, but he lasted scarcely a year.

In 2003, after months of agonizing debate, focus groups were held around the country to discover why Hemlock was not attracting more support. The board concluded that the word *hemlock*, a poison, carried too much negative baggage—even though the society had thrived for twenty-three years and reached its peak under that name. Based on the focus group studies, the board changed Hemlock's name to End-of-Life Choices, an ambiguous and unwieldy mouthful. Long-time Hemlock members were aghast.

After the name change, Hemlock's ubiquitous and instantly recognizable symbol, the delicate Hemlock flower and the words "Good life, good death" also disappeared from its publications. The newsletter title morphed from the straightforward *Hemlock Quarterly* to the ambiguous *Timelines* in 1994. "For over two thousand years, Socrates personified the drinking of hemlock as a symbol of rational suicide," Humphry wrote. But by the 1990s, few people could even identify who Socrates was.[35]

Ilene Kaplan, a Connecticut Hemlock chapter president who served on the Hemlock board from 1993 to 1999, wrote, "I never supported the change, knowing the importance of name recognition. The name 'Hemlock' was perceived [by some board members] as toxic because founder Derek Humphry had the courage to use a name that didn't waffle about what the organization was all about: self-deliverance. It had instant name recognition," Kaplan said. She noted that at the time, few people recognized the names of any other right-to-die groups, including the newly rebranded End-of-Life Choices, "but mention the name 'Hemlock' and their eyes lit up," she wrote. "That name recognition lives on even today."[36]

Dr. Paul A. Spiers, a clinical neuropsychologist, a paraplegic, and a highly articulate man, became president of the board in 2003. He was intimately involved with the evolution and mainstreaming of the Hemlock Society, including the name change, and helped oversee a fundamental organizational restructuring.[37]

One of his critical acts was replacing Caring Friends' legal advisor, Michael Evans, who understood Hemlock's original mission and goals. "[The new lawyer] spent a whole board meeting telling us the consequences of breaking the law, and going to jail, and what would happen to us," Faye Girsh noted.[38] They had heard all those predictions of gloom and doom many times before, but Caring Friends had always operated on the assumption that it was within the law and that the envelope of assisted dying had to be pushed to include non-terminal patients and non-medical solutions. Case law on the subject being virtually nonexistent, the program pushed on. Having worked for years under a "no guts, no glory" assumption, the program's long-time supporters were neither impressed nor deterred by the new lawyer's dire warnings.

One dark morning in Denver, however, a cold, damp shroud fell over the Caring Friends Program. Spiers directed that, to lessen risk, the group would only work with members who had a terminal diagnosis. Girsh, Schafer, and their volunteers recoiled from what they saw as a spineless retreat, but they were essentially powerless. Lois Schafer remarked, "I considered it a 'chicken-shit' operation if we couldn't work with people who had MS or Parkinson's or those horrible, neurological degenerative diseases. I felt that those people had years of going downhill to look forward to, whereas the person who has a terminal diagnosis, maybe six months, didn't have as long to suffer."[39]

Many of the Caring Friends staff and volunteers were shocked to discover that their program was being castrated. Earl Wettstein, who was on the national board of Hemlock for three years, resigned when the board "changed the wording in our bylaws from will help (the dying) to may help. Five other board members resigned shortly afterward."[40] Hemlock's heart had just been cut out.

In November 2004, the boards of End-of-Life Choices, then led by Marsha Temple, and Compassion in Dying, led by Barbara Coombs Lee, agreed to merge the two groups to give both greater clout. On January 1, 2005, Coombs Lee took the helm as CEO of the new organization, named Compassion & Choices (C&C), which had offices in both Denver and Portland. Temple would head the Denver office. Lee, who had been a nurse and a physician's assistant for twenty-five years before becoming an attorney and gravitating to end-of-life-choices advocacy, would run the former Compassion in Dying office in Portland. Each would draw a handsome annual salary of $105,000.[41]

To reassure rattled ex-Hemlock members who revered the unique Caring Friends Program, C&C said that it would continue providing services to members "who seek peaceful and humane choices at the end of life," as well as promoting legislative reform. Board president Paul Spiers told long-term staffers, "This is not a takeover or a sellout. Caring Friends will not cease to exist under unification. On the contrary, it will thrive."[42] The truth, however, quickly surfaced.

On December 9, 2004, three weeks before the merger, Marsha Temple told Faye Girsh that her position would be terminated on December 31.[43] Lois Schafer, the director of Caring Friends, had already gotten the boot in October. It was a cruel slap in the face to Girsh who, during her term as executive director, had rescued Hemlock from its downward spiral, building the organization back up to 33,000 members and increasing its available funds to more than $4 million.

Compassion & Choices wanted to present a less radical face to the world than had Hemlock. Its chief focus would be on changing the law to permit physician aid-in-dying for terminally ill people. Hemlock's Caring Friends/non-medical model had become unwanted extra baggage—a public relations liability to pursuing C&C's new primary objective. They wanted a group led by someone with a corporate management background who was less of a controversial public figure.

Between January and June 2005, Dr. Dick MacDonald was retained as medical advisor of C&C after the merger, and he trained or retrained all volunteers from both the preceding organizations in six sessions across the country. However, once that critical role was completed, he, too, was terminated. MacDonald's close attachment to the widespread use of non-medical, NuTech procedures to facilitate peaceful self-deliverances was not compatible with the new, squeaky clean corporate image that C&C wanted to project.

"I was called by Barbara Coombs Lee on July 1, 2005," MacDonald said. "She informed me that she no longer wished to have a medical director for the organization, and that my contract would not be renewed."[44] The truncated remains of the Caring Friends Program was now known by the sterile title, "Client Services."

Dubbed "The Hemlock Society, decaf version" by former Hemlock board member Earl Wettstein, C&C wanted to distance itself from the Wild West table manners of its predecessor. Hemlock did not represent the politically correct face that it wanted to show to the world.[45] By summer 2005, C&C had purged itself of the few remaining Hemlock Society leaders and activists and was well on the way to carrying out an extensive corporate and public relations facelift. The takeover left a bitter taste in the mouths of many of the surviving ex-Hemlock staff members and volunteers.

The Hemlock Society and its flagship dying-member assistance program might itself be dead and buried, but the idealism and ideas

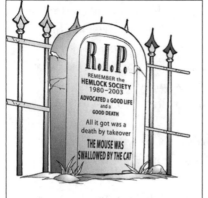

"The death of the Hemlock Society"

that had ignited and fueled both were unquenchable. Unknown at the time to C&C, Girsh and other key Hemlock activists had already predicted that the curtain would drop on the feisty, dedicated, maverick organization they had founded and built. She, Derek Humphry, Ted Goodwin, Earl Wettstein, and other ardent former Hemlock leaders formed the core of a gutsy new upstart group.

On September 16, 2004, the torchbearers of the original Hemlock philosophy founded the Final Exit Network. Its goal was to carry on the original vision of Hemlock and the unique model of the original Caring Friends group: to provide to its members free, comprehensive end-of-life-options counseling and, if requested, a bedside presence at their deaths. They, and many dedicated, like-minded Hemlock activists, carried with them the sparks of compassion and controversy that would soon attract the world's attention once again.

– 11 –

Going Dutch

If I were asked, 'Do you think that it is right for a doctor to end the life of a patient, from a medical and ethical point of view?' I would counter with another question: 'Do you really think it is right to let a patient live in unbearable suffering?'
— Dr. Pieter V. Admiraal

During the 1992 World Humanist Congress in Amsterdam, Sanal Edamaruku, a native of Kerala, India, and founder of Rationalist International, listened to one of the most moving speeches he had ever heard. Dr. Pieter V. Admiraal, a noted Dutch anesthetist and pioneer in the field of voluntary euthanasia, described the last months of one of his favorite patients, an elderly man suffering from the final stages of terminal cancer, whom he had helped to die.

"He told us about the last evening his patient spent with his family, the farewell, and finally, his peaceful death," Edamaruku said. "And after ending his speech, Admiraal revealed to his moved audience that he had told us of the story of his own father."[1]

Unlike other Western countries, where many of the physicians of the post-WWII generation dug in their heels in opposition to physician-hastened death, Dutch doctors led the development of humane strategies to help people to end their lives if they were dominated by terminal or incurable illness, extreme existential pain, or unacceptable loss of dignity.

Medical professionals who advocated for the right to a self-determined "good death" have created a unique climate of acceptance of voluntary euthanasia in the Netherlands. The Dutch public debate on the legitimacy of prolonging life and the permissibility of terminating it began about 1969, when Dr. Jan Hendrik van den Berg, a psychiatrist and neurologist, wrote a provocative book, *Medical Power and Medical Ethics*. The book explored critical issues, particularly those resulting from the case of Mia Versluis.[2]

Versluis, a twenty-one-year-old woman, lapsed into an irreversible coma after surgery in 1966. During the operation, she probably had a cardiac arrest. She was resuscitated but remained in a coma, and it was evident that she had suffered severe brain damage. A breathing tube was inserted to provide artificial respiration. After her physicians concluded that recovery from her extensive brain damage was extremely unlikely, the anesthetist proposed to have her breathing tube removed, which was likely to lead to her death. Her distraught father was vigorously opposed and took the matter to the medical board and the court. In 1969, the anesthetist was ultimately found guilty of "undermining the confidence in the medical profession" and fined 1,000 NL guilders, a heavy punishment for the times.[3]

The question of whether such a patient should be considered dead or alive was widely discussed in the Dutch media. "Many commentators tried to imagine whether they would want their own treatment to be continued in such a case or if they would prefer having an end put to their life."[4]

Van den Berg argued that medical ethics must adjust to changes in medical technology; that the doctor was no longer the sole determinant of what medical practices should be used and for how long; and that the patient had the right to make autonomous medical choices. He maintained that the motto of the new ethical code must be: "It is the doctor's duty to preserve, spare, and prolong human life whenever doing so has any sense." He concluded that a doctor "may passively or actively shorten life that is no longer 'meaningful.'"[5]

Two other noted Dutch authors contributed supporting philosophies. In 1969, Catholic ethicist Paul Sporken dealt with the permissibility of shortening a patient's dying process, arguing that active intervention leading to termination of life and non-intervention when a life-threatening complication occurs are not significantly different. Both can be justified from a moral standpoint.[6] The next year, lawyer H.A.H. van Till-d'Aulnis de Bourouill wrote, "Medical actions necessary to assure the humane end of a person's life can be justified from a medical-ethical and from a legal point of view."[7] Within two years, the theories of Van den Berg, Sporken, and van Till would all be put to the acid test.

Dutch physician Geertruida E. Postma was appalled when she visited her terminally ill, seventy-eight-year-old mother in October 1971. Dr. Postma, a *huisarts* (general practitioner), knew that her mother was close to death.

A cerebral hemorrhage had left the woman in a coma. After awakening, she was partially paralyzed, nearly deaf, almost speechless, and had pneumonia,

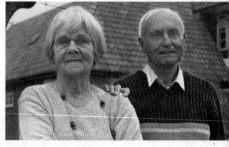

Drs. Geertruida and Andries Postma

although she still had a clear mind. Frustrated by her helplessness, Postma's mother attempted suicide by throwing herself from a high bed. The dying woman repeatedly begged her daughter, "I want to leave this life. Please help me."[8]

Postma wrote later, "When I watched my mother, a human wreck . . . I couldn't stand it any more. So I shouted in her ear, 'It's all right, Mother! I will take care of you.'"[9] The next day, she gave her mother an injection of morphine, a painkiller, and curare, which stops the heart. The elderly woman became unconscious almost instantly and died within a minute.

Given her mother's condition, the death might not have evoked any suspicion. However, being a principled professional, Postma told the director of her mother's care facility what had happened and asked him to sign the death certificate. Despite Postma's widely known reputation for integrity, the director promptly called the police. When they failed to act, he contacted Gerard Nubé, the provincial public prosecutor. Nubé reluctantly charged Postma with mercy killing, which carried a penalty of up to twelve years in prison.

A landslide of support for Postma immediately followed. Many other doctors in the province signed a letter to the Dutch Minister of Justice, stating that they had done the same thing at least once. Two thousand residents of Noordwolde, Postma's home town, signed a statement of support. And when an old man in an Amsterdam nursing home called for the formation of a foundation for voluntary euthanasia, three thousand people responded in the first week.

Postma's lawyer argued that rational, physician-assisted suicide should be a legal defense, but the judge rejected the concept and directed the prosecution to proceed. Prosecutor Nubé conceded that he saw no problem with passive euthanasia, that is, withholding medicine and life support for hopelessly ill people who request it, but he could not accept the blanket legal sanction of mercy killing. *Where*, he pondered, *would that lead? Would people kill off relatives who were obnoxious or had property to inherit? Or would a chronically ill or profoundly disabled patient be killed because his hospital bed was needed by someone else?* He asked Postma if her mother's physical suffering had become unbearable.

She replied forthrightly, "No, it was not unbearable. Her physical suffering was serious, no more. But the mental suffering became unbearable. That was what was most important to me. Now, after all these months, I am convinced that I should have done it much earlier."[10]

In 1973, after a panel of three judges agreed, Dr. Postma was convicted, receiving a month's suspended sentence and two years' probation. Her supporters, who flocked around the courthouse, considered the lenient sentence a defeat, and each handed her a flower in sympathy as she departed.[11]

That same year, the Royal Dutch Medical Association relaxed its condemnation of mercy killing. While stating that euthanasia by request should still be a crime, it urged that courts should decide whether physicians could be justified in doing so in particular cases.[12]

After the ruling, when a reporter for the *Radio Times* asked Postma and her husband, also a physician, how they now viewed mercy killing, they outlined their new mission. "Our object is to encourage doctors to talk about euthanasia and to declare their practice openly. Then the law would be changed straight away. The old medical laws are not fitted to modern medical science, where we can keep life going beyond its human limits, where we can continue physical life when the brain has ceased to function, when life has no dignity or personal meaning. . . .We must make the way clear for patients so that they are able to discuss their situations and make a rational choice about their death."[13]

Postma proposed three conditions that must govern euthanasia: (1) The patient must be obviously and unmistakably dying, with only days or weeks to live; (2) the patient must ask for death; and (3) the doctor must acknowledge what he or she has done so that there can be no question of, for example, murder for gain. She added that death certificates should be quite clear, saying, for instance, "Patient with secondary cancer, euthanasia performed."[14]

The Postmas also became early proponents of healthy people making a "testament of life" (an advance medical directive now known as a living will) to make sure that they would receive specific treatments, no treatment, or euthanasia if they were injured and lost the use of their rational minds, for example, in an automobile accident.[15]

In response to the spontaneous upwelling of support that followed Postma's trial, three vigorous Dutch right-to-die societies quickly sprang up. The Nederlandse Vereniging voor een Vrijwillig Levenseinde (NVVE, the Dutch Association for Voluntary Euthanasia) was founded in 1973, and its constitution was approved in 1977. It is currently the largest Dutch euthanasia group. The NVVE does not prescribe medications and does not have doctors to help members die. Its mission is to explain the Dutch laws about end-of-life choices, encourage public discussion about the right to die, and provide members with key legal documents.[16]

Euthanasia supporters Jaap and Klazien Sybrandy founded the Informatie Centrum Vrijwillige Euthanasie (Information Center for Voluntary Euthanasia) in 1975 because they wanted more activism. In 1980, the Sybrandys were investigated for having allegedly promoted several suicides, which they denied. The precedent-setting legal ruling in their case came in 1981 and was the first component in the modern Dutch legal position on euthanasia. The Dutch Ministry of Justice ruled, "In the cases investigated there is no question of persuasion to commit suicide. . . . 'Aiding' in the sense of the Article [294 of the Dutch Penal Code] requires more than the giving of information in rather general terms. . . . [T]he deceased had bought abroad the means [to accomplish the suicides] recommended by this couple." Based on this information, the decision was not to prosecute.[17]

Most recently, Thom Thallheimer and like-minded friends formed the Stichting De Einder (The Horizon Foundation) in 1995. A formal member of the Humanist Alliance, it was granted membership in the World Federation of Right to Die Societies in 2008. It offers professional guidance to people who wish to end their lives and ask for help.[18]

The Dutch are known for their fierce independence, practicality, free thought, defense of civil liberties, and moral integrity.[19] Dutch public opinion in favor of euthanasia has led the rest of the world since the 1970s. In 1973, the year the NVVE was formed, a formal poll in the Netherlands asked, "Do you think that someone always has the right to have his life terminated when he is in an unacceptable position without any prospect of recovery?"

In contrast to other European countries and the United Kingdom, where the approval rate ran about 50 to 55 percent, the results in the Netherlands were overwhelmingly favorable. Seventy-eight percent of respondents agreed. Ten percent disagreed, and 12 percent had no opinion. When the Dutch results were broken down further, other interesting trends appeared. Ninety-three percent of those who professed no religious faith approved; 74 percent of Roman Catholics approved; 60 percent of the Dutch Reformed Church (Protestant) approved; and 48 percent of those professing other religions approved.[20]

The moral integrity of Dutch doctors cannot be assailed, for when their nation was overrun by the Germans in May 1940, Dutch physicians refused to cooperate with the invaders—unlike their colleagues in some other Nazi-occupied countries. Even after one hundred Dutch physicians were arrested for refusing to divulge the names of their patients and were shipped off to concentration camps, the rest never broke ranks. Instead, they simply stopped signing official birth and death records, operated out of their homes, and quietly continued to provide all medical services still possible. The NVVE maintains that this is one of the factors that established a high level of trust between doctors and patients, a much higher level than in most countries.

In the 1970s, because of his compassion for the plight of his dying patients, Dutch euthanasia pioneer Pieter V. Admiraal, whose moving speech would inspire the World Humanist Congress in 1992, began cooperating with terminally ill people who asked for final relief from unendurable pain.[21]

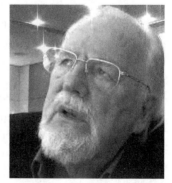

For most of his medical career, Admiraal focused on developing methods to provide patients with the right of a self-determined good death. He became an international figure through his comprehensive research and his personal humility. Derek Humphry considered him "the outstanding medical

Dr. Pieter V. Admiraal

man and campaigner in the Netherlands. Since the mid-1970s, he has been telling the world about euthanasia in an elegant, accessible way. He never held any office, but was so respected that he didn't need titles."[22]

Born in 1929, Admiraal earned his medical degree from the University of Utrecht and a Ph.D. from Erasmus University, Rotterdam. "I was working in Delft General Hospital when we officially started a Terminal Care Team in 1973," he wrote. "It was one of the first in the world. From the beginning we learned to accept and not to deny the fact that we cannot stop suffering or make it bearable in all cases. We accepted the possibility of euthanasia only as the last dignified act of terminal care. It is equally true that one cannot practice terminal care without the possibility of euthanasia."[23]

Admiraal ultimately became president of the Dutch Society of Anesthesiology and was the founder and first president of the Dutch Society for the Study of Pain. In 1994, he was named Officier in de Orde van Oranje-Nassau for his service to the nation. In 2000, he was awarded the Janet Good Memorial Award by the Hemlock Society.

Although thoughtful and reflective, Admiraal has never been timid. He listens and absorbs what others have to say and then speaks out forcefully and authoritatively, based on his extensive research and experience. Colleagues describe him as confident, assertive, righteous, sometimes temperamental, and occasionally derisive of those making statements that seem grounded in opinion or myth rather than fact.

He travels extensively, attending and speaking to medical and death-with-dignity conferences. He is frequently photographed leaning back in his chair, listening closely, with one hand on his chin, which sports a neatly trimmed Van Dyck beard. In a video made at a right-to-die conference in Canada, his beard and attentive gaze reminded me of the face of Volkert Jansz, one of the black-hatted, black-robed officials of the Clothmaker's Guild, immortalized by Rembrandt's famed 1662 painting, *The Syndics*.

Admiraal is credited with more than seventy publications and has given more than three hundred lectures and countless interviews. He was the first physician to compile an authoritative guide to lethal drug dosages for Dutch doctors and pharmacists. The booklet, *Justifiable Euthanasia: A Manual for the Medical Profession*, was published by the NVVE in 1978 and was distributed to all Dutch physicians. It became a benchmark in the history of euthanasia and hastened death.

In 2003, Admiraal, Dr. Boudewijn Chabot, Canadian criminologist Russel Ogden, and several consultants co-authored *Guide to a Humane Self-Chosen Death*, an authoritative how-to manual that presents the practical steps involved in a suicide. The first edition, in Dutch, was published by the Wetenschappelijk Onderzoek Zorgvuldige Zelfdoding (WOZZ), a Dutch euthanasia think tank that Admiraal helped found in 2002.

Admiraal is adamant that dying patients should receive the best possible palliative care and pain management, provided by a team of dedicated nursing, medical, and spiritual caregivers. This team approach was developed at the St. Christopher's Hospice in London by Dame Cicely Saunders. Currently, a team of Dutch caregivers can work with patients in a hospital, a hospice, a nursing home, or in the patient's home. Admiraal noted, however, that after a seven-year study in a Rotterdam nursing home, "care in separate units had no advantages."[24] In other words, the dying could receive high quality end-of-life care whether in a hospital, in a hospice, or at home.

Despite the widely held belief that pain is what dying people fear most, researchers have found that end-of-life suffering has many components. In 1990, an extensive survey of Dutch physicians revealed that more than 90 percent of their terminally ill patients who requested physician aid-in-dying had serious or very serious physical suffering, and more than two-thirds had mental suffering. The most frequently reported forms of this suffering were general weakness or tiredness, dependency or helplessness, and degeneration or loss of dignity. Only 5 percent stated that pain alone was the reason for their request to be helped to die.[25] Admiraal discovered other considerations:

> It is important that many patients see their suffering as senseless, and they see no reason to continue to live in their own specific circumstances. But there is another factor, almost never mentioned. Many patients who have arrived at the point of total acceptance and acquiescence in their fate may no longer attach any value to their lives, relatives, or their world. They have reached a state of total detachment, something that

is especially difficult for relatives and caretakers to understand and accept. These patients long for an early, gentle death. They regard any hesitation from others in fulfilling their wish as un-justified and as a denial of their last wish. This longing to die is, in my opinion, also part of normal life. Some doctors may say that the above-mentioned reasons for requesting euthana-sia must be the result of depression and will prescribe anti-de-pressant drugs. These doctors, in my opinion, are unobservant and seem to be more preoccupied with their own concerns than with serving patients' needs.[26]

Admiraal is adamant that doctors should always put the needs of the patients above their own. "It is extremely difficult to termi-nate the life of another," he said. "Yet, moments of carrying out euthanasia have been the most decent and the most emotional mo-ments in my life as a doctor. These patients had become my personal friends during the long period of their terminal weeks.... Should I be asked, 'Do you think that it is right for a doctor to end the life of a patient, from a medical and ethical point of view?' I would counter with another question: 'Do you really think it is right to let a patient die in unbearable suffering?'"[27]

The legal framework for regulating euthanasia and assisted sui-cide in the Netherlands arose from the evolution of the collective will of the Dutch people and their physicians. The chief concept that protects physicians from legal repercussions is the "defense of necessity" concept. It arose from the need for a physician to commit a felony—euthanasia—to avoid a worse thing: extreme, unending, uncontrollable suffering. The earliest prosecutions arose when doc-tors faced a conflict between the duty to preserve life and the duty to relieve suffering at the risk of hastening death in the process. "

"Over some thirty years," wrote Professor Penney Lewis in her study of worldwide assisted dying practices, "the [Dutch] courts developed this duty-based defence of necessity in euthanasia cases, placing conditions on the defence, including an express and earnest request; unbearable and hopeless suffering; consultation; careful ter-mination of life; record-keeping; and reporting. These conditions became known as *requirements of due care* or *careful practice.*"[28]

One of the most challenging cases in the death-with-dignity de-bate surfaced when Dutch physician and psychiatrist Dr. Boudewijn

Chabot, a medical sociology researcher in end-of-life issues and options, agreed to help Hilly Bosscher, a fifty-year-old social worker. Chabot, a tall, intelligent, gentle man with blue eyes, a comforting smile, and a long, oval face topped by a full head of graying, medium-length hair, would learn a lot about Dutch euthanasia laws.

Born in 1941, Chabot was trained as a psychiatrist and psychotherapist at the Erasmus University in Rotterdam and at the Institute of Psychiatry and Maudsley Hospital in London. In 2007, he was awarded a Ph.D. in medical sociology at the University of Amsterdam.[29]

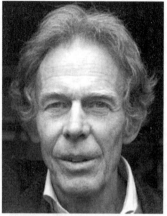

His first real contact with the realities of the right-to-die movement came in 1991. The NVVE had been trying unsuccessfully to find a psychiatrist who would consider a psychiatric patient's right to a hastened death. Chabot, who had eighteen years' experience in the fields of psychiatry and psychotherapy, volunteered to help. This led him to Hilly Bosscher.

Dr. Boudewijn Chabot

After spending thirty hours face-to-face with Bosscher over a period of two months, Chabot was convinced that she was profoundly and unalterably depressed and that her suffering was not amenable to psychotherapeutic treatment. She had suffered twenty-five years of beatings by her alcoholic husband before she divorced him. At the age of twenty, the elder of her two sons committed suicide. Five years later, her other son died of cancer. On the evening of his death, Bosscher attempted suicide via drug overdose and failed. Since then, she had only one desire: to end her own life in a dignified way with a physician's help and be buried between the graves of her two sons. She did not want to throw herself under a train because she remembered how distraught her train-conductor father was after removing the bloody remnants of a suicidal person from the tracks.

Bosscher had no appetite and a disturbed sleep, common symptoms of depression that occur in severe cases of mourning. However, none of Chabot's attempts at mourning therapy worked. Bosscher consistently refused anti-depressive medication. She showed no signs of psychosis or personality disorder.

With or without Chabot's help, she had resolved to kill herself. "Rope only offers a 70 percent chance of success, medication less than 50 percent," she told him. "I want to be certain this time that my next attempt at a dignified death will succeed."[30]

Chabot was intensely concerned. Neither he nor the NVVE had ever encountered such a tortured soul. Furthermore, if he facilitated Bosscher's self-deliverance, he could be charged with assisting a suicide, which was punishable with a jail sentence of up to three years and the loss of his medical license.

On the other hand, Bosscher did not want to live without her sons. She spent every waking moment wanting to die. Her only relief would be a dignified elective death.

Chabot asked four psychiatrists, a general practitioner, and a psychologist specializing in the treatment of psychological trauma to review her case. None of them met with Bosscher in person, but four of them (two psychiatrists, the general practitioner, and the psychologist) were convinced of her sincere and unalterable desire to die and had no realistic treatment options to offer. The fact that two psychiatrists insisted on mourning therapy and anti-depressants in a psychiatric ward, enforced by law if necessary, made Chabot's dilemma and ultimate decision even more complex.[31]

Bosscher asked Chabot for a series of prescriptions for pills which, if hoarded and taken collectively, would have killed her, with no one the wiser. "I do not want to burden you with the responsibility for my death and possibly legal consequences," she said.[32]

But Chabot was a principled man and believed that doctors should be accountable. When later asked why he did not offer the option of the pills, he replied, "What sort of psychiatrist would I be if I helped someone to die with a bundle of prescriptions, then washed my hands in innocence toward the outside world?"[33]

Convinced that it would be the best of a bad series of options, he went to Bosscher's little village and gave her a drink containing nine grams of barbiturate, which had been prepared by a pharmacist. In a note he wrote to accompany the fatal dose, he wrote, "I still hope you will flush this through the toilet."[34] She chose otherwise. With Bach playing softly in the background, and her closest friend at her side, Bosscher drank the mixture and quickly fell into a fatal sleep. Chabot then immediately reported the death to the local coroner and prepared to defend himself if charged with assisting a suicide.

The Dutch already had the world's most liberal policy on hastened death, but the Bosscher-Chabot case caused a worldwide sensation. Never before had a physician freely reported helping an otherwise healthy patient with extreme existential suffering commit suicide. The case also highlighted the difficulty of establishing whether a patient's free will had been influenced by depression.[35]

The local and appeals courts dismissed all charges against Chabot, but the Ministry of Justice made it a test case and took it to the Dutch Supreme Court. Defended by Eugene Sutorius, a longtime supporter of the right-to-die, Chabot stood trial in June 1994. The court made the principled decision that "suffering can be unbearable irrespective of its source," i. e., it is irrelevant whether the pain is physical or psychological. Chabot was found guilty. However, in view of the special circumstances of the case and the personality of the defendant, the court ruled that he would not be punished and would retain his medical license.

In 1995, Chabot was reprimanded by a medical disciplinary tribunal. Had he required one or more of his consulting doctors to evaluate Bosscher in person, the tribunal's case might have been dismissed because Chabot would have exhausted every avenue to try to deter her from committing suicide.

Chabot still stands by his decision, but to this day, he feels the pain of choosing to help end the life of a physically healthy woman because of her untreatable profound depression. "I do not know if I made the right choice," he said, "but I believe that I opted for the lesser of two evils."[36] As he told me in 2011:

> The court case of Mrs. Bosscher changed the course of my professional career. It started off a ten-year research project [1997-2007] to discover how patients can direct and be responsible for their own death with dignity without any punishable action by a physician. After reviewing 110 cases from a large sample of the Dutch population, I discovered and described in detail that stopping eating and drinking, with adequate palliative care, leads to a humane death in very ill or very old people.[37] But Mrs. Bosscher would have been too young for that. With the information in one of the recently published how-to-die books [including his own, *A Hastened Death by Self-Denial of Food and Drink*, 2008], she would have known how she could collect lethal medicines by herself.[38]

The Bosscher case set a major legal precedent. In Holland, a patient must no longer be terminally ill or suffering from unremitting physical pain in order to seek a physician-hastened death. Extreme and unrelievable existential pain had now been deemed a sufficient reason to warrant legal physician aid-in-dying. This result was hailed as a human rights victory by both the NVVE and the Royal Dutch Medical Association. It was also immediately decried by religious and secular opponents of the death-with-dignity concept as being proof that the morality of hastened death had made another huge slide down the moral slippery slope. The Dutch, they concluded, had just opened the gate for euthanasia-on-demand.

But even Chabot's strongest critics recognize that issues such as this one, which can be discussed *ad infinitum* in the abstract, are infinitely more difficult to deal with when a tortured, desperate, hopeless patient is sitting in a chair across from you. One person's ethical slippery slope, it appeared, was only the mirror image of another's concept of positive social change based on personal autonomy and the right of self-determination.

In 2007 and 2008, Chabot and Dr. Stanley A. Terman, an American physician, each expanded his views on personal end-of-life options through books describing how anyone could end his or her life through the voluntary stopping of eating and drinking (VSED), sometimes expressed as voluntary refusal of food and fluids (VRFF). The technique is recommended only for mentally competent patients who are terminally ill.

The procedure is outwardly simple. If a patient stops eating and drinking, he or she will die. This self-deliverance process falls within the right to refuse medical treatment. The most common form of VSED involves withdrawal of a feeding tube from a patient in a permanent vegetative state (as directed by the patient or his/her authorized proxy) or as directed by a competent and aware patient or his/her legal representative.

In practice, it is more complicated. Self-starvation at the end of a terminal medical decline can be extremely painful unless the discomforts can be alleviated with proper mouth care, thirst-reducing aids, pain relief for the underlying disease, or deep sedation. It generally takes seven to fourteen days before death occurs, so the patient has adequate time to stop the procedure if desired. A 2003 survey in Oregon concluded that hospice patients who voluntarily chose to refuse food and fluids are elderly, no longer find meaning in living, and usually die within two weeks after stopping food and fluids.[39]

Terman's 2007 book, *The Best Way to Say Goodbye*, is based on extensive research and on his own experiments with prolonged fasting. A medical advisor to the Hemlock Society's first Caring Friends volunteer training program, Terman earned a doctorate in biophysics from the Massachusetts Institute of Technology and a medical degree from the University of Iowa. He now heads Caring Advocates, a nonprofit counseling organization.

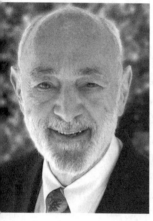

He believes that we are morally obligated to honor a patient's previously expressed wishes and to do everything possible to learn directly from the patient what he or she wants.[40] Terman emphasizes that VSED is extremely unlikely to be used by an irrational person because the process is relatively slow and requires expert supervision, whereas irrational acts are generally quick and impulsive. Another of his major themes is the need for creating strong advance directives, and he notes that most of the best-known right-to-die cases would not have evolved into enormously contentious and emotionally brutal court struggles if the patients had created an ironclad strategy to ensure that their advance directives would be carried out.

Dr. Stanley A. Terman

The extensive research reflected in Chabot's 2008 book, *A Hastened Death by Self-Denial of Food and Drink*, identified the circumstances and procedures that led to both bad and good deaths using VSED and provided critical information about how to achieve the latter. The key, Chabot found, was "to stimulate communication at the end of life between patients, their relatives, physicians, and nurses who might become involved with a hastened death by self-denial of food and drink."[41]

The acceptance of VSED within the medical and death-with-dignity communities was given a major boost when Compassion & Choices, America's largest right-to-die organization, announced a national information campaign, "Peace at Life's End, Anywhere," in August 2011. The program noted that VSED is legal in virtually all developed countries and is a peaceful process that causes patients minimal hunger or thirst when coordinated with hospice and palliative pain control measures. Compassion & Choices promotes this concept—as well as hospice or palliative care services in the home, withdrawal of life-prolonging treatment, and aggressive pain and/or symptom management, including palliative sedation—with a nationwide series of lectures and television interviews. The program was launched with a series of public talks and radio and television presentations.[42]

The next controversy arose in Holland in 1993 over the question of the termination of life of people who were not competent to make their own decisions. Ethically, the two most problematic groups involved are (1) seriously ill, disabled, or deformed fetuses and newborns and (2) older people who suffer from dementia.

In the first case, the *in utero* or newborn patient is known to have major disabilities or handicaps, suffers from inescapable pain, or has a combination of these. Examples include severely hydrocephalic infants and babies with severe cases of spina bifida. The patients are incapable of making decisions, so the parents and their physicians must do so. In some cases, the fetus might survive until birth, endure extreme pain, and die naturally soon after being born. Should such a child be euthanized in the womb or after birth? And if the child is euthanized, should the life-ending act be legal? In Holland, both scenarios are considered appropriate grounds for euthanasia if the parents and their physicians agree.

However, in the case of hydrocephalic infants, the degree of disability may vary enormously, and its course cannot be accurately predicted. Stephen Drake, a research analyst for Not Dead Yet, a highly vocal American disability rights group and outspoken opponents of euthanasia and assisted suicide, knows this from personal experience.

"I have hydrocephalus because of a brain injury at birth," he wrote. "I was born breech and the doctor used forceps. He told my parents that I probably would not live through the night and it would be better if I just died. Fortunately, my parents didn't take his advice."[43] Drake ultimately obtained a master's degree in special education from Syracuse University and entered their doctoral program. In 1997, he left academia and began his life as a disabilities activist.

The case that brought the issue of infant euthanasia to the headlines in the Netherlands was that of baby Rianne X, born in Alkmaar, Holland, in 1993. The baby had spina bifida, hydrocephalus, a spinal cord lesion, and brain damage. She seemed to be having severe pain that was difficult to treat. The parents did not want her to suffer and asked for termination of her life.

After Dr. Henk Prins, the attending gynecologist, consulted other specialists, who examined the baby, the parents' wishes were honored. Prins administered a lethal drug, and the child died in her mother's arms.[44] At his subsequent trial on charges of euthanasia, Prins said that ending baby Rianne's life had left him emotionally scarred, but he was in no doubt that his action had been correct.[45]

Prins offered necessity as his defense and was released without punishment. Judge Ben Posch said that Prins "had faced a difficult choice between two irreconcilable duties: preserving the child's life or ending her suffering." The court concluded that the defendant made a choice that—given the special circumstances of the case—could reasonably be considered justifiable.[46]

"Modern neonatology sometimes presents parents and caregivers with heart-rending situations," wrote Dr. Henk Jochemsen, Director of the Lindeboom Instituut's Center for Medical Ethics in Ede, the Netherlands. "What should the parents do? What should the doctors suggest? That is the conundrum."[47]

Because this scenario is repeated often in Holland—and worldwide—Dutch physicians and ethicists sought rational guidelines for helping make these difficult decisions for fetuses and infants. The result was the Groningen Protocol. Authored in 2004 by Eduard Verhagen, the medical director of the Department of Pediatrics at the University Medical Center Groningen, it was adopted for use in the Netherlands in 2005, and soon spread throughout the world.

To be eligible for termination of life under the protocol, an infant must meet the following five criteria:

1. The suffering must be so severe that the infant has no prospects for a future.
2. There is no possibility that the infant can be cured or relieved of his or her affliction with medication or surgery.
3. The parents must give their consent.
4. A second opinion must be provided by an independent doctor who has not been involved with the child's treatment.

5. The deliberate ending of life must be meticulously carried out with the emphasis on aftercare for the parents.[48]

The protocol has been labeled by some anti-euthanasia activists as a "Hitleresque style of eugenics, where people with disabilities are killed solely because of their handicaps."[49] Wesley J. Smith, an American author and a prominent spokesman for the religious right claimed, "[The protocol] is intended to legitimize eugenic infanticide and move it from a crime tolerated by the, oh, so tolerant Dutch, to outright legality. In other words, the last vestige of protection left in the Netherlands against infanticide—that is, the technical illegality of killing babies in the Netherlands—is to be stripped away, including the protection against the killing of disabled infants not dependent on intensive care for survival."[50]

Rationalists, on the other hand, view the protocol as a valid application of Occam's Razor: a method of reducing a complex problem to its basic elements. *And without some kind of rational guidelines,* ethicists ask, *how is a family to make a wise choice when faced with a decision that has horrible implications no matter what the outcome?*

In 2002, the Dutch legislature finally codified the parameters of the "defence of necessity," which releases physicians from legal liability if they provide euthanasia or assist in the suicide of a patient. The Termination of Life on Request and Assisted Suicide (Review Procedures) Act 2001 lists six criteria that must be met. This law, which governs hastened death in the Netherlands today, took effect on April 1, 2002.[51]

Often overlooked by those outside of Holland is the fact that the 2002 Dutch law has *not* legalized euthanasia or assisted suicide but, instead, sets strict rules specifying under what circumstances a doctor will not be prosecuted for either. The Dutch stipulate that *only* a physician, not a nurse or a general member of society, has the professional obligation to make these life-or-death decisions, and only they may use the "defense of necessity" argument. Non-physicians who are involved in euthanasia, assisted suicide, or mercy killings are still liable to prosecution for committing a crime.

The most recent major euthanasia-related development in the Netherlands is a movement to legalize voluntary euthanasia for anyone age seventy or over if they feel they have achieved completed lives and want to die before the onset of age-related illness, debility, or incapacity.

This concept of preemptive self-deliverance is often referred to as *completed life syndrome,* and the 2002 Australian case of Mademoiselle Lisette Nigot is often put forth as the perfect example of this concept.

In May 2010, a petition asking the Dutch parliament to debate whether all people over seventy have a right to self-deliverance gathered more than 117,000 signatures. The initiative, put forward by an activist group known as Out of Free Will, also hopes to decriminalize assisted suicide in the Netherlands by repealing Article 294 of the Criminal Code and permitting trained laypersons to facilitate the self-deliverances of qualifying persons.

The first formal organization to advocate the "completed life" concept came into being in 2009, when British euthanasia activist Dr. Michael Irwin founded the Society for Old Age Rational Suicide (SOARS). Enno Nuy, chairman of the Dutch euthanasia group Stichting De Einder, along with other right-to-die advocacy groups, including the NVVE, agree that "older individuals should be able to determine when they want to end their own lives, even if they are not suffering from serious illness. . . . Mostly it concerns people who are older, have no pleasant perspectives or expectations left, who have no friends or relatives, and who are facing Alzheimer's or dementia."[52] Dutch feminist Hedy d'Ancona, seventy-two, said the right to choose one's time of death is a "natural extension of her lifelong battle for emancipation."[53]

From the legal toleration of physician-hastened death that resulted from the 1973 Geertruida Postma ruling to the formalization of strict guidelines to regulate it in 2002, the Dutch euthanasia laws have been evolving under intense international scrutiny. The Dutch believe that their policies on euthanasia are the greatest hope for the future of personal autonomy. Their critics insist that the Dutch are sliding down an ethical slope that will inevitably harm financially, medically, and mentally challenged people. Others point out that according to the beliefs of the devout, Dutch end-of-life thinking directly refutes the concept that only God can create and end a life.

Refuting the latter belief, Else Borst-Eilers, the Dutch minister of health in 2002, a medical doctor and university professor, said, "Why would you think that this [voluntary euthanasia] is against God's will? I think that you are too formalistic in interpreting what people may or may not do according to God. People are allowed to extend life endlessly and manufacture all kinds of medicine. In any case it is difficult to believe in a God who does say: 'You may let a person die a week later,' but not: 'You may let him die a week sooner.' I just cannot understand that."[54]

Today, the Dutch system is viewed by most death-with-dignity advocates as a positive role model for providing and regulating hastened death. Nevertheless, the Dutch themselves note that their system is not necessarily exportable because it is based on a complex mixture of cultural characteristics not shared with other countries.

Dr. Aycke A.O. Smook, an oncologist and a past-president of the World Federation of Right-to-Die Societies, pointed out that the Dutch system is unique in several ways. "In the Dutch healthcare system, general practitioners, family doctors, and specialists know their patients and each other for a long time. As a result, a discussion of euthanasia is possible over a considerable period of time. Further, the health care system is accessible to everyone, both financially and otherwise, and guarantees unrestricted and palliative care, not only in hospitals but also at home and in nursing homes."[55]

"Autonomy in decision-making is a fundamental issue in our society," Smook said. "Fortunately, we have always had, and still have, extremists on the left and on the right sides, proponents and opponents of any subject. This forces us to carry on arguing with each other about difficult problems such as religion, abortion, and political issues, and about medical decisions concerning the end of life."[56]

"We have never tried to export our view of euthanasia," said Dr. Rob Jonquière, who served as CEO of the NVVE for ten years and is now the communications director for the World Federation of Right to Die Societies. He was born April 4, 1944, in Beverwijk, just northwest of Amsterdam during the German occupation of Holland, and his family moved several times for their safety. He grew up in Delft and then moved to Leiden. He graduated in medicine from Leiden University and has been a general practitioner since 1972. As a physician in a small town, he made euthanasia available to patients who qualified under Dutch law prior to assuming the leadership of the NVVE. He told me:

> I practiced general medicine, and my specialty was to treat the family. You had families on your list, so you knew them and you knew what was going on. One of the great advantages of

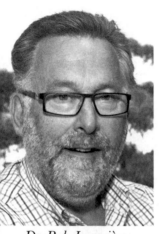

Dr. Rob Jonquière

the Dutch law is that all patients of one family are cared for by one GP. Not too long ago, you would see an old family doctor who, for example, birthed a child who was the grandchild of one of the first patients, so he knew the family history.[57] In 1975, I went with a group of colleagues in the U.K. I visited St. Christopher's Hospice and Dame Cecily Saunders and learned about good dying guidance.[58]

Jonquière gave me the key to understanding how controversial topics are dealt with in Holland. "The primary difference between the Netherlands and other countries," he told me, "is that in the Netherlands, not only do we practice euthanasia, but we also talk about it. Politicians, magistrates, doctors, public officials [and] everyone talks about it. It is not a secret."[59]

The Battleground States

The euthanasia debate requires us to confront the most basic of human concerns—the mortality of self and loved ones—and to balance the interest in preserving human life against the desire to die peacefully and with dignity.... This controversy may touch more people more profoundly than any other issue the court will face in the foreseeable future.
— Ninth Circuit Court Judge Stephen Reinhardt, 1996

The unquenchable thirst for legalizing death with dignity is most evident and persistent in the United States, where the debates and battles to establish a legal right to physician-assisted suicide can be traced back over a century. Brown University author and ethicist Jacob M. Appel documented extensive political debate over legislation (never passed) to legalize physician aid-in-dying in both Iowa and Ohio in 1906. His research discovered that both the supporters and opponents of euthanasia "generally agreed that the practice already occurred with frequency."[1]

The right-to-die debates peaked in the 1930s, when the Euthanasia Society of America was founded. The discussion waned in the face of almost universal optimism after World War II and then reignited in the 1960s and 1970s, inspired by the achievements of the civil rights movement. Right-to-die laws were proposed in Florida in 1967 and Idaho in 1969, but neither passed. Undaunted, the death-with-dignity movement was starting to build up at least a small head of steam.

The increased attention was fueled in 1978 by such popular and controversial books as Doris Portwood's *Commonsense Suicide: The Final Right*, and in the same year, Derek Humphry's immensely popular *Jean's Way*. On the stage, *Whose Life Is It, Anyway?*, a play about a young artist who becomes a quadriplegic, premiered in London in 1978 and gained international attention. In 1980, the syndicated

American newspaper advice column "Dear Abby" published a letter from a reader agonizing over a dying loved one, generating 30,000 requests for advance care directives from the Society for the Right to Die. That same year, the World Federation of Right to Die Societies was founded in London, and in California, Derek Humphry founded the Hemlock Society, which became the United States' largest right-to-die organization. By 1991, when *Final Exit* was published, the fight to establish the right to an elective death with dignity and without a physician's assistance had become a controversial national topic, and the movement's popularity began to grow.

The legal primer for creating future American right-to-die law laws was Humphry's *Lawful Exit*, published in 1993. In it, Humphry identified four possible ways that Americans could secure careful and legally protected physician aid-in-dying for the terminally ill.

1. By having state legislatures change the laws that forbid assisted suicide.

2. By having an appellate court, state supreme court, or the U.S. Supreme Court dismiss the conviction of a person for assisting a suicide.

3. By having guidelines for assistance in dying that are acceptable to both the medical profession and the law enforcement authorities.

4. By having a successful voters' initiative, which is democracy in its purest form. Currently, twenty-four states and the District of Columbia have this process. In these states, citizens who collect a predetermined minimum number of signatures on a petition within a specified time can place advisory questions, statutes, or constitutional amendments on a statewide ballot for voters to adopt or reject. If a majority of voters approve, the initiative becomes law after the procedures to administer the law are developed and put into place. In the United States, there is no initiative process at the national level.

The last two decades of the twentieth century were also the era when opposition from anti-euthanasia organizations, chiefly the National Right to Life Committee and its religious backers, the Roman Catholic Church and fundamentalist and evangelical Protestant churches, reached its peak. These groups had extensive experience in this kind of fight, having spent the previous two decades opposing the legalization of abortion. They portrayed the death-with-dignity battle as one between atheists, humanists, freedom of choice/personal autonomy advocates and conservative religious people, who believed that elective death contravened God's will.

The first major popular test of the nation's support for legalizing physician-hastened death came in 1986. Once again, Derek Humphry became a pioneer when he and the Hemlock Society drafted the California Humane and Dignified Death Act. "For those who believed in the right to choose to die and wished a physician to help them, the requirements [were] quite simple, a thoughtfully framed law that enables the patient to ask for death, and a willing physician to be able to provide the means, without fear of prosecution, persecution, or stigma," Humphry wrote.[2]

He first ventured into writing death-with-dignity laws in 1978, when the London *Evening Standard* asked him to write a charter for the legalization of voluntary euthanasia. The assignment arose from the enormous demand sparked by the publication of *Jean's Way*. Although a complete neophyte when it came to the legal ethics and legislation of euthanasia, he relied on his experience and instincts to fashion a charter that embraces substantially the same values and goals of current legislation.[3]

Starting in the first issues of *The Hemlock Quarterly* in 1980, Humphry made it clear that bringing about legislative change to allow physician aid-in-dying was a high priority. Because Hemlock was then in its infancy and lacked the financial and membership resources to launch any legal assault, his goal of achieving legislative change had to wait. "It wasn't until 1985 that we felt able to get to work on this, and we realized that there was no model law anywhere upon which to build," Humphry commented.[4]

Fortunately, they had his 1978 charter as a starting point. Humphry noted, "Every Saturday morning for many months in 1985, myself; Michael White and Robert Risley, two practicing attorneys in Los Angeles; and Curt Garbesi, a professor of law at Loyola Law School in Los Angeles, met to draft a law. It would specifically authorize direct euthanasia by a physician for 'individuals whose suffering at the end stage of life is so great that they wish to bring about their own death.'"[5]

The impetus for their action was the recent death of Risley's wife from cancer. Humphry wrote, "She did not ask him or a physician for help to die, but as he cared for her during the last days, Risley realized that, given her suffering, she might do so. His legal brain began to turn over the judicial consequences of assisting the death of another for humane reasons. A study of the cases and statutes showed that while it is not a crime to take one's own life, it is a crime to assist that action. Here's a legal ambiguity to start with: it is a crime to assist in doing something that is not a crime!"[6]

The group's hard work finally paid off. "[We] hammered out what we called the 'Humane and Dignified Death Act,' later renamed the Death With Dignity Act. Then we published the resulting prototype law in January 1986 as a supplement to *The Hemlock Quarterly*. So at last we had a draft law, the first in the United States, which set out what the right-to-die supporters wanted. And our lawyers urged Hemlock and our board of directors to start a citizens' initiative, which we attempted in 1988."[7]

Although Humphry and his lawyers had a good basic grounding in euthanasia law, they were unfamiliar with the mechanics and politics of successfully promoting a ballot initiative in a large and populous state such as California. State initiatives are extremely costly, and Hemlock could not muster the funds or the signature-gathering capabilities to defeat its medical and religious opponents. In a painful setback, Hemlock obtained less than half of the 372,000 signatures needed to get on the ballot.

"We were politically naïve," Humphry said. "None of us had any past political experience, whereas our opponents, notably the Catholics, had developed strong political ties and had a great deal of experience fighting off abortion rights laws since *Roe v. Wade* in 1973. They were much wealthier, and they were also better politically informed than we were as we started to do these things."[8] Intellectually, however, the attempt was highly successful in educating Californians about the pros and cons of physician aid-in-dying, and despite the failure at the ballot box, the Hemlock Society's membership doubled in the coming year.[9]

Ultimately, the California effort provided right-to-die supporters with a learning laboratory for the legislative change attempts that would soon follow. There were also two indelible lessons: "The religious right will not be changed. However word-perfect and abuse-free the *Death With Dignity Act* is, they will not be convinced. Let the members of the religious right die in their chosen fashion.

[Also, to negate its] stultifying attitudes, the medical profession must be offered a law which it feels comfortable with."[10]

To ameliorate hostility from doctors, the concept of direct euthanasia would have to be removed from any new proposed law and replaced with physician-assisted dying. A physician would write a prescription for a lethal dose of drugs, but the dying person would have to fill the prescription and administer the drugs. Having the patient ingest the lethal dose made it explicitly clear that he or she carried out the death, not the doctor.

The modern debate over state citizen initiatives originated in South Dakota in 1898, followed in 1902 by Oregon. There, almost ninety years later, the second major death-with-dignity rights campaign was the longest lasting, most expensive, and most brutal in American history. Eli D. Stutsman was the young Portland lawyer who, with Derek Humphry, had cofounded Hemlock of Oregon in 1987. Using the lessons learned in the defeat of the 1988 California initiative, he decided to initiate Oregon's first attempt at passing a bill that would enable terminally ill state residents to die with dignity. He drafted Oregon's Senate Bill 1141, which was introduced to the legislature in 1991 by Senator Frank Roberts, who was dying of cancer.

Despite sympathy for Senator Roberts, the bill went nowhere and died in committee in the Oregon legislature. "Of course it was instantly rejected, but it was a necessary step and got a good deal of attention," Humphry noted.[11] This rejection motivated Hemlock and its allies to found a political action committee, Oregon Right to Die, in 1993. The committee was better organized and wrote a more widely based bill dedicated to getting a law passed by a citizens' ballot initiative. This time the knowledge gained in California paid off handsomely, and they triumphed.

Applying their hard-won knowledge, the committee realized that the California effort had been massively underfunded. Half of the $210,000 Hemlock spent there had been used to hire people to gather ballot signatures, leaving only $105,000 for advertising and promotion. In Oregon, Humphry provided the campaign with Hemlock's 30,000-member mailing list. Hemlock and its supporters also raised $600,000 and spent it wisely on well-timed advertising and get-out-the-vote work.

With their newly honed skills, supporters of the initiative

achieved a voter turnout of 57 percent and countered their opponents' $1,500,000 budget. Oregon's Ballot Measure 16 of 1994 established the Oregon Death With Dignity Act, which was approved in the November 8, 1994, general election, with 51.3 percent of voters in favor and 48.7 percent against.

In 2010, at the World Federation of Right to Die Societies' nineteenth biennial congress, I learned about the basic components of the 1994 Death With Dignity Act from George Eighmey, who, for twelve years, was the executive director of Compassion in Dying and, after its merger, Compassion & Choices of Oregon. As he explained:

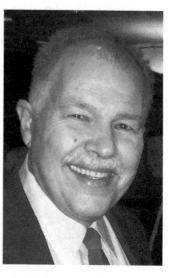

> Very briefly, it's a legal process. You have to have a terminal diagnosis; you have to be an adult; you have to be a citizen of the state of Oregon; you have to have two doctors who say that you're going to die within six months, and if either one of them questions your mental capacity, they can then insist upon a psychological

George Eighmey

> evaluation. You then have to make two oral requests, a minimum of 15 days apart, and then you then have to make a written request where your signature is witnessed by two people, one of whom can be a family member, but not both, and one of them can be a medical provider, but not both. This is to assure that it is an independent decision—that you weren't coerced into making the decision. Then, probably the most difficult part of the Oregon law, is that you have to self-administer medication. That means that nobody can pour it down your throat; nobody can inject you; nobody can pour it down your feeding tube. You must be physically able to end your life without an assistant. That means many people who meet all the other humane and secure qualifications fall through the gap. They don't qualify for death under the Oregon law because they are too sick to take the medicine.[12]

The victory notwithstanding, Measure 16 became the most controversial and contested bill in Oregon's history. After intense ongoing debate fueled by opponents seeking to amend or repeal the act, the state legislature returned it to the electorate for a second vote. Opponents of the measure argued that the original text lacked a mandatory counseling provision, a family notification provision, strong reporting requirements, and a strong residency requirement. The original authors argued that sending the measure back to voters was disrespectful because the citizens had already passed it via the initiative process, and the safeguards were adequate.

The challenge, named Ballot Measure 51, went before the voters on November 4, 1997. A solid 59.69 percent majority supported the right-to-die measure, up from the previous 51 percent. The vote unequivocally reaffirmed the will of the people, despite the fact that the opposition had pulled out all the financial stops to defeat the measure, raising four times more funds than the right-to-die supporters. The law finally took full effect on October 27, 1997. Although the state's legal issues had been conclusively dealt with, the law's opponents refused to give up. Politically inspired federal legal challenges were launched to negate the will of the people and fulfill conservative political agendas.

The next attempt to derail the law came in 1999, when both houses of the U.S. Congress passed the Pain Relief Promotion Act (PRPA), known as "The Hyde Act" after its cosponsor, Republican Senator Henry J. Hyde. "The act criminally punishes the use of controlled substances to cause—or assist in causing—a patient's death. The primary purposes of PRPA are to override the physician-assisted suicide law currently in effect in Oregon and prohibit other states from enacting similar laws," wrote doctors David Orentlicher and Arthur Caplan in *The Journal of the American Medical Association*.[13] At the beginning of the 2000 Congressional session, passage of the act seemed certain, but influential opponents, including the American Bar Association, the American Cancer Society, and the American Pain Foundation, came out against the legislation, and the act was allowed to die.[14]

Although Oregonians had twice voted upon and approved their death-with-dignity law, Republicans made a last-ditch attempt to derail it. On November 9, 2001, U.S. Attorney General John Ashcroft, with the explicit backing of President George W. Bush, issued an interpretive rule that physician-assisted suicide was not a legitimate medical purpose. Any physician who prescribed, dispensed, or administered federally controlled drugs for that purpose would be in violation of the federal Controlled Substances Act (CSA).

Eli Stutsman, who had drafted the first attempt at death-with-dignity legislation in Oregon, immediately jumped into the fray. He wrote about Ashcroft's unprecedented grab for power under the CSA, which had been enacted three decades earlier as part of the war on criminal trafficking in illegal drugs and drug diversion (the illegal use of legal drugs).

He pointed out the fabricated, flimsy political logic used to attempt to interfere with Oregon's law. "Neither drug trafficking nor drug diversion occurs under Oregon's Death With Dignity law, rather, the drugs are at all times lawfully possessed, prescribed, and dispensed by Oregon physicians and pharmacists in full compliance with the [federal] CSA." He continued, "[Ashcroft] does not argue that drug trafficking or diversion is taking place in Oregon. Rather, he simply disagrees with Oregon's determination that death with dignity is a legitimate medical practice under the narrow circumstances allowed in Oregon."[15]

The Ninth Circuit Court of Appeals summarily torpedoed Ashcroft's bald-faced partisan attack, stating that "the Attorney General lacked Congress' requisite authorization."[16]

The final vindication of the Oregon law came in October 2005, when the U.S. Supreme Court heard arguments in defense of the law in *Alberto R. Gonzalez, Attorney General, et al. v. State of Oregon, et al.* The federal prosecutor argued on behalf of the Bush administration, which challenged Oregon's right to regulate the practice of medicine when that practice entails prescribing federally controlled substances. On January 17, 2006, in a 6 to 3 decision written by Justice Anthony Kennedy, the court ruled that the federal government could not enforce the federal CSA against physicians who prescribed legal drugs in compliance with Oregon state law for the assisted suicide of the terminally ill. The Oregon Death With Dignity Law has been in force ever since.

When the law passed, hospitals, hospices, doctors, and nurses all had questions and concerns that needed to be resolved. Who would help the patients learn about the newly legalized right to hasten their deaths? When a state government has a new law, especially for a radically new concept such as death with dignity, there are often no trained internal experts to administer it. Consequently, the duty of educating the state government, physicians, and pharmacists fell to the backers of the new law. George Eighmey stepped forward.

He was the ideal candidate. A genial, frank, and forthright man, Eighmey had been both an attorney and a state legislator. In addition, he had extensive experience with death-with-dignity issues while serving as executive director of Compassion in Dying. When this organization merged with Compassion & Choices of Oregon, he served in the same capacity from September 1988 until his retirement in August 2010. "He was a very likeable and honest man," commented Derek Humphry. "He did a wonderful job stewarding the Oregon law, helping people work out the difficulties, finding doctors and pharmacists willing to cooperate, and being at the bedside of the dying if needed."[17]

In 2011, a study published in the *Journal of Palliative Care* compared the quality of life of dying patients who did and did not take advantage of the Oregon law. It found that according to the patients' families, patients who were given prescriptions to help them die (physician aid-in-dying) had more control over their symptoms and were more prepared for death than those who did not pursue physician aid-in-dying or, in some cases, those who requested but did not receive a legal prescription.[18]

Support also came from Ann Jackson, who was the director of the Oregon Hospice Association between 1988 and 2008, giving her extensive experience in the field before and after the passage of the law. She wrote, "The perspective of hospice workers is significant because (1) they visit patients and families frequently in the last weeks and months of life and (2) they are able to compare hospice patients who hasten death with hospice patients who do not. Their experience is important because 86 percent of persons who have used the Oregon Death With Dignity Act were enrolled in hospice.... Behind closed doors, hospice workers were frank in expressing their beliefs. One area where they were unanimous in agreement was that the Oregon [act] improved the quality of meaningful, important conversations about the end of life."[19]

When the Oregon bill was originally introduced, opponents described it as the "thin edge of the wedge": a tool for pro-euthanasia campaigners to get a foot in the legislative door, which would then lead down an inevitable "slippery slope" to horrible con-sequences never envisioned at the start. The transparency of Oregon's demonstrated results completely repudiated these contrived allegations.

In her 2005 article, "The Famous, or Infamous, Slippery Slope," philosopher Trudy Govier, the author of many books, including *Dilemmas of Trust* and *A Practical Study of Argument*, noted, "Many who allege slippery slopes have a recognizable theological perspective. They may use the slippery slope as cover for ideas that find their real source in religious teaching." She described the phenomenon itself as follows:

> It's alleged that legalizing assisted suicide will lead to legalizing murder, and for that reason we should not legalize assisted suicide. Or, it is feared, such legislation will lead to the de-valuing of the lives of the weak and handicapped, and ultimately to killing and a cult of death. This type of argument is referred to as *the slippery slope*, and is prominent in many discussions of assisted suicide. Slippery slope arguments go along the following lines: actions of a certain type may seem all right, but if we permit them, we will be led to permit further actions of related types, which are not all right; therefore, we shouldn't permit the first actions. Doing something that seems legitimate can lead us to do further, apparently similar, things that are not legitimate. Because we need to avoid the illegitimate actions, we should refrain from doing the apparently legitimate ones.[20]

Using the slippery slope argument, opponents claimed that Oregon's basic right-to-die bill would inevitably lead to incremental expansions of the law until death-on-demand for everyone became acceptable and legal. It might even lead to a Hitleresque mass murder of innocent people deemed to be physical or mentally inferior. The argument is fallacious because it assumes that a civilized society cannot be trusted to pass and regulate laws and build in safeguards to enable good things to happen without the process being inevitably perverted and society corrupted in the process.

Slippery slopers predicted that the law would victimize the nation's vulnerable classes: women, the poor, the disabled, the poorly educated, and ethnic minorities. In Oregon, and, more recently, in Washington State, reality has proven the slippery slope argument to be totally without foundation.

The official annual reports of Oregon's law covering the period

1998 through January 7, 2011, are extremely informative.[21] Because Oregon has one of the oldest and best-documented death-with-dignity laws in the United States, it and Holland are internationally viewed as primary sources of statistical information on the effects of legalizing physician aid-in-dying.

The statistics gathered and contained in the official Oregon annual reports show that the fears of the slippery slopers are totally unfounded. The following findings are from Oregon data on all 525 reported elective deaths under the law from 1998 through 2010.

- **Death by gender:** Slippery slope proponents alleged that women would be singled out and preyed upon. The reality: 53.7 percent of those who died under the law were men and 46.3 percent were women.
- **Death by age:** Opponents alleged that juveniles would find it easier to commit suicide because of the availability of the law. Only 6 of the 525 users (1.1 percent) fell in the 18- to 34-year age group, and all 6 met all of the standard end-of-life disease criteria. Because no one under eighteen was eligible to use the law, no juvenile was accepted or died under it.
- **Death by underlying cause:** Opponents maintained that people suffering from extreme but treatable depression might turn to the law to end their tortured lives, but those who were eligible to die under the law had to be terminally ill. People with transient or deep-seated emotional or psychological disorders, such as depression, were referred to appropriate specialists and were precluded from using the law.
- **Death by race:** Opponents alleged that racial minorities would be pressured into disproportionate use of death-with-dignity laws. However, in Oregon, 97.9 percent of those who died under the law were Caucasian.
- **Death by educational level:** Opponents were certain that the less-educated would be more likely to be persuaded to choose elective death than their better educated peers. However, in Oregon, 68.1 percent of those who elected hastened death had college degrees or some college education.
- **End-of-life care:** Slippery slope proponents said that the poor or disabled would be tempted (or forced) to commit suicide based on their lack of access to medical care. In Oregon, this

was not a significant factor. Nearly 89 percent of those who died under coverage of the law were enrolled in a hospice program.

- **Pain management:** It is frequently alleged that pain at the end of life is the greatest motivator to seek suicide, but Oregon's statistics show what researchers have known for decades. Pain is not usually the primary culprit. It ranked sixth in a list of seven major end-of-life concerns. Loss of autonomy (91.2 percent), being less able to engage in activities making life enjoyable (88.1 percent), loss of personal dignity (84.1 percent), and losing control of bodily functions (56.4 percent) rated far higher.[22]

Support for the official statistics provided by the state came from an independent study published in the *Journal of Medical Ethics* in 2007, which found that Oregon had "no evidence of heightened risk for the elderly, women, the uninsured, people with low educational status, the poor, the physically disabled or chronically ill, minors, people with psychiatric illnesses (including depression), or racial or ethnic minorities, compared with background populations."[23] Nothing of significance has changed between 2007 and the end of 2010.

Another fallacious idea promoted by the anti-euthanasia movement has also been disproven. In the months that preceded the enactment of the law, opponents railed that masses of dying people from other states would flock to Oregon to take advantage of the law, turning the state into a destination for suicide tourism. The argument was demonstrably irrational and deliberately misleading because the law specifically included a state residency requirement. No flood of dying refugees—not even one, to the best of anyone's knowledge—ever appeared on Oregon's doorstep. Unfortunately, that has not stopped opponents from endlessly repeating the baseless "straw man" claims.

All of the arguments for and against physician-assisted death would be repeated in Oregon's neighbor to the north, which became the next battleground. On a cool Seattle night in August 1993, Rev. Ralph Mero was pursuing his dangerous calling. Earlier in the day, as her mother looked on, Louise J.* had emptied the contents of forty Nembutal capsules into a small cereal bowl, hoping self-deliverance would provide relief from the pain of her terminal illness. Mero, a Unitarian minister for thirty years, a veteran end-of-life counselor, and the founder of Compassion in Dying in Seattle, had suggested that she mix the powder with something sweet to mask its notoriously bitter taste.

Louise chose a combination of ice cream and applesauce, mixed the pills into the concoction, and put it in the refrigerator. Only her fingerprints would be on the pill bottle and the bowl. "It would not do to implicate her new friend, Mero, or her mother, or her doctor, or the handful of others who knew about and helped her with her plan," wrote Lisa Belkin, a reporter for the *New York Times*.[24]

When Mero rang the doorbell of Louise's small apartment, her mother came to greet him. Inside, a medical assistant and a friend of Louise's were waiting. "After the initial greetings, Mero sat on the couch where Louise lay curled in her favorite flannel nightgown and thick woolen socks," wrote Belkin. "He took her hand in his, looked her in the eye, and told her she could change her mind, that no one would think less of her for it, that she could wait until another day."

"I'm ready now," she told him.

"Once you eat that, you're going to fall asleep very quickly," Mero said. "Don't you want to go lie on your bed before you start?"

"I've never really cared too much for my bedroom," Louise answered. "This room is where I want to die."

She lay back into the pillows and closed her eyes, as her mother stroked her hand. Her friend began to read a chapter from a fantasy novel Louise had not had time to finish. By the second page, Louise was snoring loudly. The friend continued to read quietly, not raising her voice above Louise's rattling slumber. She turned page after page, for nearly twenty minutes, until the chapter was over. Louise died a short time later.[25]

Louise had been sick for six years. The doctor who had diagnosed her terminal illness waited until she brought up the subject of suicide before discussing it. They talked of hospital care, hospice, and other options. Louise wanted none of them. She wanted an elective death while she was still lucid enough to make the decision. Her doctor agreed to prescribe the medication that would end her life. In addition, the physician contacted Compassion in Dying for general advice, which brought Reverend Mero into the picture. He agreed to comfort Louise when she chose to end her life.

Mero, by all accounts, is a cautious, deliberate man who is not necessarily joking when he says, "I was spontaneous. Once. When

I was nine years old." He speaks with the quiet understatement of someone who long ago wrestled with the shades of gray end emerged, as he describes it, "with no doubts whatsoever, absolutely none."[26]

His father's slow, difficult death, during which he threatened suicide, and his brother-in-law's deterioration in the final stages of AIDS led Mero to comment, "I was utterly horrified and outraged that lovely human beings should have to die in such a decimated state."[27]

A chance encounter at a 1988 conference sponsored by the Hemlock Society showed Mero a positive way to channel his outrage. With Derek Humphry's help, he started the first Hemlock chapter in Washington State and soon became an end-of-life counselor. With no legal way to help end the suffering of those seeking release from terminal pain and loss of autonomy, Mero was forced to become extremely innovative to help others without violating the state's existing anti-assisted-suicide law. His need for extreme caution forced him to turn down many suffering people because he knew that if he were arrested and convicted, he would lose his only opportunity to help others. "The temptation to make just one exception is overruled by the necessity of establishing responsible guidelines that society as a whole will accept," he said.[28]

In 1991, Mero became a proponent of Washington Initiative 119, pitting him and his aim of ending unnecessary end-of-life suffering against the well-organized religious opposition of the Washington Catholic Conference, the political arm of the three Roman Catholic bishops in the state, and by others with large bankrolls, who portrayed supporters of the initiative as "ghoulish doctors intent on murdering the poor and elderly."[29] The proposition would have allowed doctors to prescribe a lethal dose of medication and also to administer it if the terminally ill patient could not take it without help. Ultimately, the idea of physicians actively terminating lives was too much for many voters to accept. The proposition failed by a 46 to 54 percent vote.

Jack Kevorkian played a key part in sinking the effort. Word got out that he was planning two more deathings shortly before the vote. Mero said, "I called him and asked him if this was true, and whether he had considered that effect that might have on what we were trying to do. He was quite angry. He indicated that what he did was no one else's business and he really didn't care."[30]

Kevorkian carried out his threat. On October 23, little more than ten days before the Washington vote, he helped Marjorie Lee Wantz and Sherry Ann Miller die in Michigan, receiving his much-desired national attention. Mero and Humphry were outraged. "Those deaths took place in a cabin in the woods and provided a visual image for our opponents to use suggesting that doctor-assisted suicide was reckless and macabre."[31]

In April 1993, Mero and twelve colleagues—many of them ex-Hemlock members who had worked on the failed 1991 initiative with the Washington State Hemlock Society—formed Compassion in Dying, a nonprofit organization created to help terminally ill patients who choose rational suicide after medical therapy cannot help them any longer.[32] Compassion in Dying, though small, was a finely crafted, fully staffed organization. It had a nine-member board of directors and an advisory committee of five physicians, an attorney, a nurse, a psychologist, a minister (Mero), and a grief counselor. The advisory committee trained volunteers and provided input into policy decisions. As independent consultants, the physicians examined the patients to verify the terminal prognoses but were not asked to prescribe medicines or take over the patients' care.

Out of legal necessity, Compassion in Dying offered assistance only to people who were truly suffering in the last stages of terminal illness, were not suffering from depression or emotional illness, and could administer their own drugs, either orally or intravenously. As with the Hemlock Society's Caring Friends Program, Compassion was willing to provide a bedside presence at the time of death.[33] "We are being very clear that we are not promoting or encouraging suicide. We are only responding to the requests of people who are terminally ill and who have already made this decision," said Mero.[34]

"Americans are coming to realize that suicide is not always the tragic action of a mentally disturbed or emotionally distraught person," noted Barbara Dority, Compassion's president.[35]

Opponents of Compassion in Dying alleged that having lost the battle for Initiative 119, supporters were now moving to civil disobedience. Ken VanDerhoef, president of Human Life of Washington, a religious right-to-life group, commented, "You can't kill people no matter what you call yourself."[36]

The year 1994 ushered in a legal struggle to enact a death-with-dignity law in Washington State. In December, four physicians, three terminally ill patients, and Compassion in Dying brought suit in a district court seeking to modify the state's anti-assisted-suicide law. Over the next two years, the death-with-dignity advocates gained ground, only to lose it on appeal.

The tide of court support for liberalization of assisted suicide in Washington State, having risen in 1996, ebbed a year later. On June 26, 2007, the U.S. Supreme Court reversed the decisions of the Ninth and Second Circuit Courts of Appeals in *Washington v. Glucksberg* and *Vacco v. Quill* and upheld state statutes that barred assisted suicide. Justice William Rehnquist ended his opinion in the landmark case of *Washington v. Glucksberg* with the words, "Throughout the Nation, Americans are engaged in an earnest and profound debate about the morality, legality, and practicality of physician-assisted suicide. Our holding permits this debate to continue, as it should in a democratic society."[37] And continue it did.

In January 2008, Eli Stutsman, chief architect of Oregon's trailblazing Death With Dignity Act, helped to craft the Washington Death With Dignity Act. With a decade of experience behind them, the proponents rolled out their ballot proposal, Initiative 1000, on January 24, 2008, with rapid precision. The act was extremely similar to Oregon's, allowing physician aid-in-dying only for terminally ill state residents with six months or less to live.

Booth Gardner, an immensely popular man who had served as Washington's governor from 1985 until 1993, promptly filed the initiative with the secretary of state's office. A year after his retirement, Gardner had been diagnosed with Parkinson's disease and soon announced his support for assisted suicide. Ironically, he would not be eligible to die using the provisions of I-1000 because Parkinson's is not considered fatal, but Gardner strongly supported the initiative in his "last campaign" because he understood why other ill people would want the option.[38]

The get-out-the-vote effort was named "Yes on I-1000," and by June 2008, 3,600 volunteers were gathering signatures to get the initiative on the ballot. By July 2, Gardner turned in 320,000 signatures, far more than the 100,000 that were needed. The former governor also personally donated $470,000 to the campaign, becoming its largest contributor. "Yes on I-1000" ultimately brought in an astonishing $4.8 million, making it the first right-to-die campaign to collect more than its opponents.

As part of an urgent appeal sent out by the state's Catholic bishops, fundraising envelopes and anti-I-1000 information were distributed to the state's 290 local parishes, encouraging them to take up a collection for the Coalition Against Assisted Suicide. Despite their efforts, the opposition was only able to raise about $1.6 million.[39]

By the time the initiative got underway, Robb Miller was executive director of Compassion & Choices of Washington, which had merged with Compassion in Dying. To a skeptical reporter, he explained that I-1000 had a broad support base. "Democrats support this. Republicans support this. If you look at the Catholic Church, the laity are with us. It's the hierarchy that's opposing this."[40] Initiative 1000 won with a strong majority vote. On November 4, 2008, it was

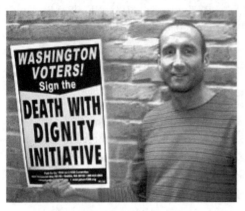

Robb Miller

approved with 57.82 percent in favor and 42.18 percent against. Thirty of the state's thirty-nine counties cast majority votes for the initiative.[41]

The law took effect on March 5, 2009. In 2010, the first full year of its use, lethal medication was dispensed to eighty-seven people. Prescriptions were written by sixty-eight different physicians. Medications were dispensed by forty different pharmacists. Of the eighty-seven participants in 2010, seventy-two died. Of these seventy-two, fifty-one took the fatal dose; fifteen died before taking the medicine; and six died with no indication of whether they took the medicine or not. [42]

Overall, the ages of the patients ranged from fifty-two to ninety-nine years. Seventy-eight percent had cancer; 10 percent had neuro-degenerative diseases, such as ALS; and 12 percent had heart disease or other illnesses. Eighty-eight percent were covered by public or private health insurance; 96 percent were white; and 62 percent had at least some college education. Of the patients who took the lethal dose, 90 percent died at home and 84 percent were enrolled in hospice care. There has been no evidence of any "slippery slope" pressure or discrimination.

Montana would be the next state to ponder the legality of death with dignity. Billings resident Robert Baxter was seventy-five, a clear-minded Marine veteran and outdoorsman who had retired from his career as long-haul truck driver. He had been dying from lymphocytic leukemia for twelve years when he stopped chemotherapy in 2007. "He was so skinny that he couldn't sit because his skin hurt," said his daughter, Roberta King of Missoula. "It pinched his skin together because there was no meat. It was that bad."[43]

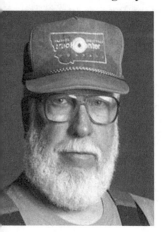

Robert Baxter

In 2007, Baxter filed a lawsuit to legally obtain assistance from a physician in dying. "It's always been a very important thing with me," said Baxter. "I watched people suffer so badly when they've died, and it goes on every day. You can just see it in their eyes: 'Why am I having to go through this terrible part of my life, when we can do it for animals? We put them out of their misery. I just feel that if we can do it for animals, we can do it for human beings.'"[44]

Robert Baxter, et al., v. State of Montana became the third round in the fight to legalize physician aid-in-dying. Arguments commenced before Helena District Court Judge Dorothy McCarter on October 10, 2008. The plaintiffs included Baxter, four physicians, and the death-with-dignity group Compassion & Choices. At issue was the question of whether the state's constitution guaranteed terminally ill patients a right to receive lethal prescription medication from their physicians.

The lead attorneys for the case, Compassion & Choices' veteran legal director Kathryn Tucker and renowned Montana litigator Mark S. Connell, sought a ruling that physician aid-in-dying was protected by the Montana constitution, which states that "the dignity of the human being is inviolable." They were supported by other human rights organizations and thirty-one Montana state legislators. They were opposed by the state's attorney general and by religious, ethical, and disability groups using the slippery slope argument as their chief weapon.

On December 31, 2008, Judge McCarter issued the landmark ruling that it is legal for a physician to prescribe a lethal dose of drugs to a competent, terminally ill Montanan who requests it, without being subject to arrest for violating Montana law. She said that she would not "deny the fundamental right of Montanans to die with dignity,"[45] adding, "We find nothing in Montana Supreme Court precedent or Montana statutes indicating that physician aid in dying is against public policy." Tragically, just hours after Judge McCarter made her ruling, Robert Baxter died naturally of leukemia. His family said he was unaware of the legal victory.

Montana Attorney General Mike McGrath immediately filed an appeal, asking the judge for a temporary injunction preventing assisted suicides from occurring until the Montana Supreme Court had ruled on the issue. Opponents of the ruling were shocked that the Montana Medical Association did not immediately take a stance or get involved in the case. In January 2009, Judge McCarter declined the appeal, meaning that physician-assisted suicides could proceed.

Kathryn Tucker triumphantly noted, "This ruling is consistent with a long line of cases recognizing that Montana's constitution protects the decision-making power of its citizens in the most intimate and personal areas of their lives. The court found that the decision of a dying patient whether to endure suffering or, instead, to cut such suffering short, is an intensely personal, private decision which must be reserved to the individual.... The court has found that it is the individual patients who should be entitled to make critical decisions for themselves and their families, and not the government."[46]

With the historic ruling, Judge McCarter added a third state where physician aid-in-dying is currently legal. The majority of Americans, who have consistently voted for a person's right to die when, where, and how he or she chooses, were jubilant that freedom of choice was being legally honored.

However, conservative blogger Wesley J. Smith, a prolific and articulate proponent of views matching the theology of the Catholic church, fundamentalist Protestants, and the ideology of the political right, dusted off the slippery slope argument once again. "Cases such as Baxter...among many others are really part of a slow motion *coup de culture*, a steady drive to topple the social order rooted in Judeo-Christian/humanistic moral philosophy and replace it with a dramatically different value system founded in utilitarianism, hedonism, and radical environmentalism. Once that process is complete, the courts will quickly make it clear that 'choice' has limits."[47]

Eventually, the case was appealed to the Montana Supreme Court, where the battle was settled once and for all. On December 31, 2009, the court upheld Judge McCarter's ruling, allowing physician aid-in-dying to proceed. No higher appeals were possible because the matter applied solely to the residents of Montana.

As they had in Washington, Compassion & Choices took the lead, informing Montana's physicians about the new law and its implications. By the end of March 2009, they had contacted all of the doctors, explaining how to comply with the new law. The group also emphasized its willingness to counsel physicians and their dying patients and provided referral cards to distribute to anyone who had questions about aid in dying, or who might benefit from Compassion & Choices' consulting service, which was free to anyone, whether or not they were members of the organization. Although physician aid-in-dying was now legal in Montana, finding doctors who were familiar with the new law and willing to hasten a dying person's death under its provisions was a challenge, as was finding pharmacists willing to fill the necessary prescriptions.

Despite Judge McCarter's original ruling, no physicians immediately stepped forward to issue lethal prescriptions to those who were eligible. Janet Murdock, sixty-seven, who had terminal ovarian cancer, was one of the first to ask a member of Montana's medical community to help her die. "I was so hopeful when the court recognized my right to die with dignity. I have suffered so much that I have considered throwing myself into a snow bank to die of hypothermia. Does Montana's medical community care more about anti-choice extremists who may disapprove, or about people like me who may suffer, and be left to an unbearably painful end of life?"[48] Murdock, who was under hospice care, died of her disease two months after futilely seeking help.

In 2011, in a last-ditch attempt to derail Montana's death-with-dignity ruling, Montana Senator Greg Hinkle introduced Senate Bill 116, the Elder Abuse Prevention Act, to overturn the *Baxter v. Montana* decision. The bill was strongly supported by Alex

Schadenberg, the Canadian leader of the Euthanasia Prevention Coalition, one of the most politically active and vocal recyclers of the discredited slippery slope theory. Schadenberg insisted, "Legally assisted suicide is a recipe for elder abuse because it empowers heirs and others to pressure and abuse older people to cut short their lives."[49] In Oregon, where assisted suicide is legal, the official statistics refute Schadenberg's claim.

Bill 116 was soundly defeated by a majority of state senators of both parties, who voted 35 to 15 in favor of maintaining the Montana Supreme Court's Baxter ruling. The senate vote left the responsibility to develop the standard of care for aid in dying where it should be: in the hands of Montana's medical community.

Because there is no actual law to *regulate* physician aid-in-dying in Montana, there is no mandatory statistical reporting of physician-hastened deaths, resulting in a total void of information. "There is no way to track how many people have ended their lives this way, but a spokesperson for Compassion & Choices has said that 'more than one patient' died with the aid of a physician since the [Montana] Supreme Court decision, but declined to say how many, where, when, or which doctors participated."[50]

Emboldened by the successes in Oregon, Washington, and Montana, Compassion & Choices announced that the organization would embark on a state-by-state drive to legalize physician aid-in-dying throughout the United States. Its plan was to offer legal expertise, headed by Director of Legal Affairs Kathryn Tucker; leadership coalition-building expertise, led by president Barbara Coombs Lee; and a substantial financial base—a $7 million annual income, most of which comes from bequests, including a $10 million donation ($2 million each year for five years—the largest sum ever given to an American choice-in-dying organization) by liberal philanthropist George Soros.

Currently, the magnitude and acceleration of the death-with-dignity movement's initiatives are enormous when compared with the tiny first step taken in 1985, when Derek Humphry and three colleagues created what would become the first draft of all U.S. ballot initiatives and the laws that followed.

Amazing things are happening with increasing frequency in the United States as the momentum for legalizing the right to die with dignity increases. Progressive laws are being enacted; unreasonably punitive laws are being revised or revoked; and other statutes thought to condemn assisted suicide are found to be baseless. Following is the status of some current activities in states other than Oregon, Washington, and Montana.

In California, Governor Arnold Schwarzenegger signed the California Right to Know End-of-Life Options Act in 2008. Now, when a patient diagnosed with a terminal illness asks a physician, "What are my choices?" the doctor must answer the question. Knowledge empowers patients and gives them comfort.

New York State passed the Palliative Care Information Act in 2010. This act requires physicians and nurse practitioners to offer terminally ill patients information and counseling concerning palliative care and end-of-life options.

Residents of Vermont, "The Green Mountain State," are currently considering Bill H.274, which would allow physician aid-in-dying. Patient Choices Vermont reports that as of February 2011, 64 percent of Vermont residents supported the bill.

In Connecticut, "The Nutmeg State," where I was born, two doctors asked the courts in 2010 to declare that the forty-year-old state law on assisting a suicide does not necessarily prohibit "aid in dying...a recognized term of medical art, which may, in the professional judgment of a physician, be a medically and ethically appropriate course of treatment.[51]" The petition was dismissed on June 8, 2010, without allowing the physicians to present their evidence. Supporters included Compassion & Choices' Kathryn Tucker, who stated that an appeal was considered but has not yet been acted upon. The case was opposed by the disability rights group Not Dead Yet.

After massive research by Tucker and other legal experts, it was discovered that Hawaii was the first state—in 1909—to pass a death-with-dignity act, originally enacted to help people with leprosy. Robert Orfali, one of ten members of a panel convened to explore the subject "Is Physician-Assisted Dying Already Legal in Hawaii?" wants to work with Compassion & Choices to help physicians establish a system of safeguards similar to those in Oregon.

On February 6, 2012, as a result of a case involving the Final Exit Network, the Georgia Supeme Court unanimously declared the state's 1994 anti-assisted suicide law null and void because it violated the First Amendment by denying freedom of speech. In response to the court's decision, Georgia legislators are expected to pass a new law making the physical act of assisting a suicide a felony punishable by a prison sentence of one to ten years. However, the drafters of the new legislation wanted to make sure that no one would be charged with a crime for giving detailed instructions on how to commit suicide or by attending the death, provided there was no physical assistance in the suicide. They specifically have said that counseling will not be challenged.

And the beat goes on. In another dozen states, carefully researched challenges to existing anti-assisted-suicide legislation and physician aid-in-dying laws continue. Whether or not every effort is successful, each will give dying patients a little more hope that they will not be forced to endure needless, unwanted suffering at the end of their lives, and each will re-energize the death-with-dignity movement to continue the fight to establish death with dignity as an inalienable civil right.

Countries south of the U. S. border are also experiencing an awakening of interest in the right to die with dignity—and changing laws. This right is consistently gaining ground in some unexpected places all around the world—especially those areas where the Catholic Church dominates the local culture.

Esta Es Mi Voluntad

Euthanasia is not a choice between life and death, but the choice
between two different ways of dying.
— Jacques Pohier, French Catholic theologian[1]

D r. Gustavo Alfonso Quintana does not fit the stereotype of a
lawbreaker. The robust, sixty-six-year-old Bogotá, Colombia, physician, survivor of two heart attacks and a serious
car crash, and father of four children, is warm-hearted and quick to
laugh. A bald, deeply tanned man with an easy smile, he looks more
like a successful plantation manager and horseman than a family
doctor, especially when he wears his favorite walnut-colored leather
vest. But from 1981 to 1997, in violation of the existing Colombian
law, he helped more than forty terminally ill patients end their tortured lives at their request through direct euthanasia.

The oldest of seven children, Quintana was born in Tuluá (Valle
del Cauca) in 1946. He enjoyed competitive swimming in high school
and later entered a Jesuit seminary to become a priest. "The education I received from the Jesuits enabled me to become a freethinker,"
he told me in an interview held in Cali, where my wife and I were
visiting relatives in her native city. "They always told me about having the right to have doubts; to question anything, even the doctrines of my own church."[2]

He remained in the seminary for four-and-a-half years, but he
ended his studies two months after receiving his priest's robes. Es-
chewing ordination, he turned to medicine. He earned his degree in
general medicine from the medical school of the National University in Bogotá, specialized in gynecology, and later earned a diploma
in gerontology. He now practices medicine from a modest office in
Bogotá.

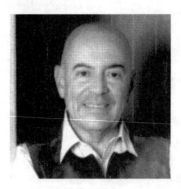

*Dr. Gustavo Alfonso
Quintana*

Quintana was forced to confront his own life-and-death issues in 1981. On the way home from a medical conference one night, his small car hit a deer, and he was knocked unconscious when his head slammed against the interior of the car's roof. When he regained consciousness in the hospital, he had no feeling in his feet, legs, or arms. He feared he had a spinal cord injury and might become a quadriplegic. A vigorous man who loved scuba diving and water-skiing, he could not conceive of being confined to a bed and a wheelchair for the rest of his life. He told one of his medical professors that if he had any incapacitating injuries, he would prefer to die.

"It was the first time that I had faced my own death," he told me. Fortunately, X-rays showed that he had spinal-cord contusions that would only temporarily cause numbness in his arms and legs. "Being very near death gave me a different perspective on every minute of my life," he said.[3] It was a pivotal point in his medical career. He had learned an extremely important concept: not to jump to conclusions about voluntarily ending a life. He vowed to help do so only after assuring himself that all other ways of making a patient's life endurable had been exhausted, and only after the patient's wish to die was not only clear but authentic, independent, and repeated.

> The first time I administered euthanasia was in 1981, eight months after my car accident. The patient, Teresa,* was a fifty-seven-year-old woman with a brain tumor. I knew the family well. She had the tumor removed, but three years later, it reappeared. She could not move anymore. She became bedridden and eventually fell into a coma. The cancer had spread rapidly and ravaged her entire body. As time passed, she became more and more like a fetus, curled up and not able to move or communicate. After three years of agony and emaciation, she had lost forty kilos (88 pounds) and wasted away to 28 kilos (62 pounds)—just bones wrapped in skin. I saw that many people were coming to see her out of morbid curiosity, not from love and affection.

With the exception of a home healthcare nurse, Teresa's daughter had been her only caregiver, and she consulted me what to do about her mother's condition. I told her that I believed Teresa had lost all the dignity in her life. She had already been unconscious for several months. I told her daughter that maybe it would be the right decision to end Teresa's life through euthanasia. She thought it over for a good amount of time.

After Teresa had the first brain operation, she told her doctor that if some time in the future she could not make any decision about herself, she did not want to stay in a bed without any capacity of being conscious. She expressed that two times, and I was told of her wishes by her daughter. None of her wishes had been written down. At that time—the early 1980s—living wills and advance directives were not common.

Her daughter agreed to the euthanasia. Teresa's death took place in her home on a day when the nurse took her day off. Her daughter held her hand and stroked her hair. I gave her the injections. It all happened in about two minutes. I think it was very easy for her breathing and heartbeat to stop because of the great deterioration she had already experienced.[4]

Quintana believes that people have the right to die well and to choose when and where to die. As for his personal philosophy, he explained that he is "obsessed with life, not death," and above all, he agrees with the idea that "people who cannot lead a fulfilling life are entitled to choose a dignified death."[5]

Of his own existence, he said, "I would buy fifty more years of life if someone would sell it to me. But I love life with quality so much that if the time comes when I no longer have any good quality of life, I will choose my own euthanasia. This is, of course, a very personal question. Each person has the right to decide how they die."[6]

In 1999, Quintana became the first Colombian physician to state publicly that he had administered euthanasia to terminally ill patients who requested it.[7] He continues to do so to this day.[8] He does not rush to judgment or fulfill every request to die. Prior to euthanizing a patient who wants to die, he asks himself, "If I were that person, would I want to end my life? If I find that the answer is yes, then I would be willing to proceed to induce death."[9] If the patient is incapable of making the choice personally, Quintana consults with the closest family members and asks if the patient expressed the wish not to be kept alive after all hope for recovery had been lost. He then reviews the patient's medical records and consults his own heart. "Helping [someone die] is never easy, but I do it with respect and affection for my patients."[10]

Quintana does not regard death as sad, preferring the term "culmination of life," and he hopes to help change society's attitude toward it. He charges patients only for the material he uses. Although he accepts donations, he is not interested in making money from the procedure.[11]

Colombian interest in the emerging field of bioethics and the right to die dates as far back as 1954, when Dr. Fernando Sánchez-Torres became a frequent contributor to *El Tiempo*, one of Bogotá's

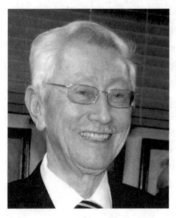

largest newspapers. In 1985, he chaired a select group of professionals from various departments at the National University in Bogotá, and the group formed the Colombian Institute of Bioethical Studies.

Dr. Jaime A. Escobar-Triana of Bogotá is one of Colombia's most respected physicians and educators. A prolific scholarly author, he is known as one of the pioneers of bioethics studies in Colombia and led the creation of the first Colombian Ph.D. program in bioethics at the Universidad El

Dr. Jaime A. Escobar-Triana   Bosque, Bogotá.

He holds a pragmatic view of euthanasia. "These concerns [about euthanasia] have been with me for many of my professional years as a surgeon, as a director of an ICU, and especially the use of technologies that can prolong a patient's agony, prolonging the process of dying and affecting the patient's dignity. We doctors have always been afraid of talking about euthanasia, but today, a person has the autonomy to decide about his life and death. If life is no longer worthy for them, then the situation warrants euthanasia if a person of sound mind requests it. If the doctor agrees, it will be a mutually friendly and private agreement between the doctor and the patient."[12]

Although he lives in a country where the Catholic religion is dominant, Dr. Escobar-Triana respects total freedom of belief—and non-belief: "For some people there is not another life after this one, and the only opportunity to live is in this life. No one has the right to impose their religious views on people who don't agree with them. That is against human dignity." In his book, *Death as a Final Exercise in the Right to a Dignified Life*, he stated that if life is to be lived with dignity, and death is a part of living, one must have the right to die with dignity.[13]

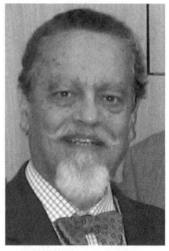

In the 1970s, when the search for a firm definition of death was a major research topic, neurosurgeon Dr. Juan Mendoza-Vega's article, "Brain Death: Considerations in Colombia," became a seminal position paper on the subject, as did his article on the gross inequality between medical services provided to the upper and lower classes of Colombian society.[14]

Mendoza-Vega's first encounter with the ultimate death-with-dignity option arose when his brother was diagnosed with an inoperable cancerous abdominal tumor. His brother's fate was sealed. Imminent death

Dr. Juan Mendoza-Vega

was unavoidable, and the accompanying pain would be excruciating. The only option was terminal sedation. Mendoza-Vega described the prognosis to his brother, his sister-in-law, and their children. All of them agreed to the use of terminal sedation. His brother's physician then started an intravenous morphine drip to render him unconscious. The flow was increased until his brother's heart stopped. He died painlessly.[15] Dr. Mendoza-Vega has remained a prominent leader in the international death-with-dignity movement ever since. Most recently, he was elected to serve as the director of the World Federation of Right to Die Societies from 2008 to 2010.

Both Mendoza-Vega and Sánchez-Torres took the basic concepts of bioethics out of the classroom into the popular media.[16] It was also in the late 1970s that both medical schools in Bogotá began holding seminars on the rights of ill persons, especially the right to a dignified death. That concept was introduced by Dr. Escobar-Triana, then the director of the intensive care unit at Bogotá's San Juan de Dios Hospital.[17]

One of the most influential people in the evolution of the right-to-die movement in Colombia was Beatriz Kopp de Gómez. A Bogotá native, she studied ballet in Paris. A highly respected, socially promi-nent, practicing Catholic, she majored in Oriental Studies at the Universi-dad de Los Angeles in Bo-gotá. In 1947, she founded Bogotá's National Ballet Academy and served as its director for many years.

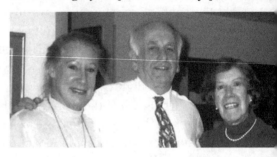

Kopp de Gómez, the mother of four children, was both a consummate

Clemencia Uribe, Derek Humphry, and Beatriz Kopp de Gómez

liberal and a talented diplomat. When she heard that Bogotá's Catholic archbishop feared that the Ballet Academy dancers might appear scantily clad on stage, she invited him to her home for tea. There, she assured him that the young women would be wearing full-length tights and dresses with high necklines. Her diplomatic skills would serve her well in the future, when she took on causes more radical than the design of ballet costumes.

In addition to being a patron of the arts, Kopp de Gómez was a driving force for positive social change. While living in New York in the 1970s, she was active in the Society for the Right to Die and served on the board of Concern for Dying. In addition, she was a board member for the Family Planning Center of Colombia and was an executive member of the International Planned Parenthood Foundation.

Through her trips abroad, she learned of European organiza-tions that advocated euthanasia for those who no longer wanted to suffer when the pain of incipient death was too great to bear and could not be alleviated. In 1979, she became the founder and pres-ident of Soledad Humanitaria, later renamed the Fundación Pro Derecho a Morir Dignamente (The Foundation for the Right to Die with Dignity [DMD]), in Bogotá. It was the first death-with-dignity group in Central or South America.

Under her leadership, DMD joined forces with the progressive elements of the Colombian medical profession and started taking the message of death with dignity to medical schools, nursing associations, palliative care facilities, and public groups and promoting discussions about the right to die in the media. As a result, public awareness of end-of-life options rose progressively, and the subject was more likely to be discussed in Colombia than in any other Latin American country.

Kopp de Gómez led DMD into the international spotlight when she attended the founding meeting of the World Federation of Right to Die Societies in Oxford, England, in 1980. Her organization was a founding member of the federation and remains active. Early in its history, DMD originated an aggressive awareness program, *Esta Es Mi Voluntad* (This is My Choice), to promote and distribute living wills. It also established a national living will registry for more than 250,000 people who filled out this form.

Her intellectual and diplomatic talents earned enormous respect from Colombia's ruling political elite. On August 20, 1999, Kopp de Gómez was presented with a special medal struck in her name by Colombia's Congress for her long service in the cause of a dignified death in Colombia. Dr. Virgilio Galvis, the minister of health, presented it to her at a ceremony in Bogotá.

Five years later, her leadership, tenacity, and tact earned her the first biennial Marilynne Seguin Award, presented at the international congress of the World Federation of Right to Die Societies in Tokyo for the person who had contributed the most to the death-with-dignity cause worldwide. She donated the accompanying $2,000 USD prize to the DMD.

On August 15, 2006, two years after this honor, she died peacefully at her home in Bogotá at the age of eighty-four. At the time of her death, DMD had more than 10,000 members. Despite her strong views on the right to die, which were diametrically opposed to those of her church, Kopp de Gómez was accorded a Catholic funeral.

Under its current executive director, Dr. Carmenza Ochoa de Castro, DMD has raised its already high media profile and increased its work to educate scholars, physicians, and other caregivers about end-of-life options. It now has over 27,000 members, most of whom are in Bogotá, with the rest in regional chapters in Ibagué, Manizales, Pereira, Armenia, and Cali. The DMD now has a larger membership than all other right-to-die groups in Central and South America combined.

In 1997, José Euripides Parra Parra, a Bogotá lawyer and a

strong opponent of euthanasia, brought a case before Colombia's Constitutional Court, the highest in that country, to right a perceived wrong. At that time, Article 326 (now 106) of Colombia's Criminal Code stated, "He who kills another person out of compassion, to put an end to intense suffering caused by physical injuries or grave or incurable illness, will be punished with imprisonment of six months to three years."

Parra argued that Article 326 gave lesser penalties to those who assisted in mercy killings than to those who committed murder.[18] In his eyes, the law failed to protect those who lacked the ability to defend themselves against exploitation by others who sought their deaths (false "mercy killings") because mercy killers were given a much lighter penalty than murderers. Parra sought to have Article 326 declared unconstitutional.

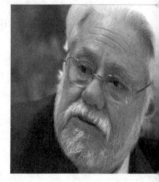

In a landmark ruling on May 20, 1997, both pro- and anti-euthanasia supporters—and Parra especially—were shocked by the court's decision. In a 6 to 3 vote, Chief Justice Carlos Emilio Gaviría Díaz, who wrote the majority opinion, stated that a terminally ill person of sound mind had the right to end his or her own suffering. Further, the

Carlos Emilio Gaviría Día

court ruled, that since he or she would have to have expert medical advice to properly determine the extent and likely outcome of his or her medical problems, the patient was also entitled to have a physician's assistance in ending his or her life if that was needed to end the suffering. That being the case, the physician could not logically or legally be punished for providing either the information or the actual assistance in helping a terminally ill person die. The result was the decriminalization of the assisted suicide law in Colombia, shielding a doctor acting in good faith from any criminal liability for having assisted a suicide.[19]

The ruling established that physician aid-in-dying was legal in Colombia, and specified who would qualify for it: "Patients who in fact are suffering from a terminal disease or injury certified in their medical records by two specialist physicians, experiencing intense, ongoing pain, which cannot be alleviated by modern medical science, and with no hope for a cure or relief."[20]

In early June 1997, Eduardo Cifuentes Muñoz, the outgoing vice president of the Constitutional Court, stated that the ruling would have to be reconsidered because it contravened Article 11 of the national constitution on the inviolability of the right to life.[21] But on June 13, 1997, the court confirmed its original decision by a vote of 7 to 2. Colombia had become, and remains today, the sole Catholic nation and the sole developing country where active euthanasia is legal, practiced openly, and unregulated.

One of the pivotal points of the ruling was based on whether or not life, as defined by Colombian constitutional law, needed to be respected and legally protected as a sacred gift from God. If so, life would need to be fully protected until death occurred naturally, despite the specific situation of an individual. If not, life could be regarded as a value of extreme importance but its voluntary ending would be a secular, personal matter. Since the Constitution of 1991 defines Colombia as a secular state, it followed logically that the constitutional interpretation of life needed to be viewed from a secular perspective.[22]

Following its ruling, the court strongly advised the Colombian national legislature to enact a law to provide appropriate safeguards and reporting procedures for all acts of euthanasia or assisted suicide, as was the case in Switzerland. But to enact such a law would validate a medical action that was anathema to many Catholic legislators, about half of their constituents, and the Vatican.

In 1999, attempts were made to regulate physician aid-in-dying. After Chief Justice Carlos Gaviría Díaz stepped down from the court and became a senator, he personally introduced such bills in 2004 and 2005. All of these bills failed to pass.

In March 2007, Senator Armando Benedetti, with the backing of Diego Palacio Betancourt, the minister of social protection, held a public hearing on the idea of regulating euthanasia, but proposed legislation was never voted on. In September 2008, a congressional commission approved a preliminary draft of new legislation, including a provision to preclude suicide tourism by specifying that anyone seeking to use the act would have to have been a resident of Colombia for at least one year. Eventually, Benedetti acknowledged that there was no chance of getting the necessary majority of votes in the legislature to pass such a bill, and he withdrew his motion.

Currently, in Colombia, physician-hastened death has been decriminalized, but there is no required reporting system. The matter remains solely a private decision between doctor and patient. For that reason, the annual number of physician-hastened deaths in Colombia is unknown. Since the 1997 decriminalization, doctors who aid a death or perform euthanasia on competent patients are protected from prosecution. Since that time, no Colombian physician, including Dr. Quintana and several others who have openly admitted to practicing euthanasia for appropriate patients, has ever been sued by a family member or been questioned by any police or medical authority about the hastened deaths.

In Venezuela in 2001, the first proposal to allow active euthanasia set off a rousing debate when it appeared in the publication of a draft of a law under review by the health subcommittee of the Presidential Commission for Social Security. The ministry of health defended it; the Catholic Church condemned it; and the proposal was not approved.[23]

On March 6, 2006, with the support and assistance of DMD in neighboring Colombia, the Asociación Venezolana Derecho a Morir con Dignidad (AV-DMD) was launched in Venezuela to promote personal autonomy and self-determination at the end of life. Its president, Professor Rafael Aguiar-Guevara, became interested in euthanasia and its legal implications in 2002 at the Congress of the World Association for Medical Law in Maastricht, Holland. He visited the headquarters of the Dutch right-to-die society NVVE and spoke at length with its CEO, Dr. Rob Jonquière, about the challenges the Dutch experienced during the evolution of their euthanasia laws. Aguiar-Guevara's visit to the Netherlands prompted intense research that resulted in his 2003 work, *Euthanasia: Myths and Realities*, the first right-to-die book published in Venezuela.

In 2004, Venezuela's Supreme Tribunal of Justice proposed to the National Assembly a new legal amendment that would decriminalize euthanasia in certain circumstances. This new law would indemnify physicians from deaths resulting from the "law of double effect" or from direct euthanasia, as long as these acts were taken with the consent of a mentally capable patient. If the patient was unable to personally communicate his or her wishes, the doctor could proceed if the person had a valid living will. But the amendment lay dormant until 2010, when a revision of the national criminal code proposed to legalize physician aid-in-dying for the terminally ill.

The new draft stated that all individuals have the right "to die with dignity, to request their attending physician to perform an appropriate procedure or for related advice, as long as the person is in the final stages of life or presents with a serious, chronic illness that causes suffering."[24]

Again, the proposal met stiff opposition. Alberto Arteaga Sánchez, a former dean of the faculty of political and juridical sciences of the Central University of Venezuela and a devout Catholic, questioned the bill's constitutionality using the "sanctity of life" argument. "Life must be respected from the moment of conception until death, and it is not a disposable right," he said.[25]

Any proposed Venezuelan euthanasia law faces predictable opposition by the Catholic Church. Professor Aguiar-Guevara noted, "Traditional and orthodox doctrinaires, jurists, politicians, and healthcare professionals, under the authoritarian influence of the Catholic doctrine, have done their best to obstruct the access of the community to fulfill their rights of free speech and discussion of this special topic. Even the press refused to write on the subject and, according to information that I have had from several journalists, the orders came from editorial management and media owners; so that it has been the private sector itself, and not the government, who [violated] the right to free speech and information."[26]

Nevertheless, the revised law has the backing of Venezuela's Minister of Health, Gilberto Rodriguez Ochoa, who considers it "a humane act to allow people to die with dignity when they are in a terminal state or suffer a chronic, painful, and irreversible illness."[27] Another major source of support came from a poll conducted by Venezuela's largest private communication company—before the poll was shut down for unknown reasons. The poll showed that approximately 80 percent of the population favored euthanasia.[28] The fate of the bill, however, is in the hands of the Venezuelan National Assembly and President Hugo Chávez, not the voters.[29]

In 1996, an Argentinean study of 407 young doctors who had been in practice for ten years or less showed a diverse range of opinions on end-of-life choices. Seventy percent of respondents supported the withdrawal of life-sustaining care when requested by competent patients and more than 50 percent of those who supported it had already withdrawn such care. Ninety-seven respondents (24 percent) supported physician-assisted suicide. Surprisingly, almost two-thirds supported active euthanasia in terminally ill patients who were unable to request or consent to it, and 40 percent of the respondents had already practiced this. More than half of the doctors had withdrawn life-sustaining treatments or practiced active euthanasia or both. Given the unusual variants in the answers, the authors of the report noted, "This subject has rarely been explored, and official data is lacking. We consider that there is an urgent need to open the debate in our community."[30]

Argentineans are debating the most ethical paths for the most primal decision people face: when and how to die. In 2011, the case of a two-year-old girl in a permanent vegetative state drew attention to the issue of euthanasia in Argentina, where it is now a crime. "Camilla [has been] in a vegetative state since she was born," said her mother. "She doesn't cry; she doesn't blink; she doesn't swallow; she doesn't move."[31] Camilla's parents want their daughter to have a dignified death. In response, the Argentine Senate and the legislature in Buenos Aires began hearings on whether to legalize euthanasia.

In 2007, a professionally conducted poll of 5,700 Brazilian adults found that 57 percent of respondents opposed allowing the intentional death of someone who suffers from an incurable disease. However, a 2009 study of Brazilian doctors and caregivers concluded that the definition of euthanasia was unknown by one-third of the physicians and most of the laypeople involved.[32]

The law in Mexico differentiates between active and passive euthanasia. In 2008 and 2009, in Mexico City and in the states of Aguascalientes and Michoacán, laws were enacted to allow the terminally ill, or close relatives, if the patient is unconscious, to refuse further medical treatment that may extend life (passive euthanasia). For a hastened death to be legal, the patient generally must have granted permission via an advance medical directive certified by a notary public.

At the federal level in Mexico, the Party of the Democratic Revolution and the Institutional Revolutionary Party have introduced bills to decriminalize euthanasia, but a federal law concerning euthanasia has been emphatically opposed by the Catholic Church. As a result, as of December 2010, eighteen of thirty-one Mexican states have revised their constitutions under pressure from the church to protect the right to life from the moment of conception until natural death.[33]

But throughout the world, the definition of a "natural death" has yet to be decided. A century ago, natural death was triggered by hundreds of conditions and diseases that now are routinely cured by modern medicine. And a generation from now, the list of "lethal conditions" will be even shorter. Indeed, the concept of what constitutes a natural death is simply an arbitrary line drawn in the sand based on current knowledge and technology.

According to a poll conducted in February 2008, 59 percent of Mexicans think doctors should have the legal right to end the life of a person suffering from an incurable illness upon a request by the patient and his or her relatives.[34]

In Mexico, the veterinary drug Nembutal (the world's most sought-after euthanasia drug) is available without prescription from numerous veterinary pharmacies, making Mexico the prime destination for terminally ill elderly foreigners. Although many Nembutal sources in Mexican towns just over the American border have dried up because of extreme demand (which triggered a government crackdown), veterinary pharmacies in more remote areas still sell Nembutal under local trade names without a prescription for the modest price of $25 to $45 per bottle, which contains six grams of the drug. Two bottles would provide a lethal human dose. Oddly enough, the massive demand for the drug by foreigners has had little or no effect on the use of Nembutal for self-deliverance by Mexicans themselves.

In other instances in Central and South America, Panama is dealing with the pressure to legalize euthanasia and physician aid-in-dying by stepping up the promotion of palliative care. In 2006, the first Paraguayan Congress on Palliative Care took place in Asunción to develop a "moral alternative to euthanasia."[35]

In Latin America and everywhere else, the entire debate about the right to die revolves around two different and irreconcilable theories. On one hand is the sanctity of life argument, which claims that only God can create a life, and, therefore, only God can decide when that life should end. A terminally ill person does not get to vote on the quality or timing of his or her death. On the other hand is the personal autonomy argument, which holds that only the person who is enduring an unavoidably painful or debilitating medical condition should have the right to decide when to ask for assistance to end the pain through physician-hastened death.

One striking difference between North America/Europe and Latin America is the almost total lack of knowledge about non-medical methods of self-deliverance in Latin America. The use and advantages of the helium method, which NuTech invented and field tested, are virtually unknown to Latin American right-to-die groups and their medical advisors. Nembutal is also seldom used for self-deliverance, despite the fact that, unlike in the United States, Canada, and Europe, where it is rigidly banned, it is readily available from most veterinary pharmacies throughout Latin America.

No studies have been done to determine why the helium and Nembutal systems of self-deliverance have not gained the popularity that they have in North America and Europe. One strong reason is that, in Latin America, the physician is more of a patriarchal authority figure commanding greater respect. In addition, traditionally educated Latin American physicians are not exposed to NuTech-style options during their medical training.

Another major reason for the paucity of self-deliverance information in Latin America is the dearth of Spanish-language publications that describe the procedures. Derek Humphry's *Final Exit* (*El Ultimo Recurso* [*The Ultimate Recourse*] in the 1992 Spanish language edition) is the only how-to manual that is readily available throughout Latin America, usually through Amazon.com. On the other hand, Amazon.com is not as widely used in Latin America as it is in North America and Europe.

The legal status of physician aid-in-dying is constantly evolving throughout Latin America. The chief deterrents are the pervasive influence of the Catholic Church and the relatively low per capita income of the majority of the citizens. The low availability of funding for even basic medical care in many developing nations is also a huge challenge. As a result, advanced concepts such as palliative care and death with dignity end up at the bottom of the list of concerns for lawmakers and caregivers.

But the next generation of Colombian physicians will have more sensitivity to patient autonomy than the previous one. In 2011, Andrés Castellana,* a third-year medical student in Colombia, reflected on what he and his classmates were being taught about the right to die. "We had our first medical ethics course in our second year," he said. "We learned the basic requirements of practicing ethical medicine, such as 'First, do no harm,' and 'the welfare of the patient comes first.'"

Although his teachers did not go into any great detail at that time, they left him with the belief that when all hope of recovery has passed, a hastened death might be allowable if specifically requested by the patient. "It depends a lot on the religious values of the doctor," Castellana said. "The doctors who are strict Catholics or Jehovah's Witnesses think voluntary euthanasia or physician-assisted death is unethical or a crime, and they would never be involved in it. But those who do not have strong religious beliefs or put the desires of their patients first think that it is an option if it is the request of the patient."[36]

Progressive thinkers throughout Latin America actively campaign for better healthcare, a better understanding of the options at each stage of the dying process, better palliative care, and the right to physician aid-in-dying. Given the clearly evident trends, countries throughout Central and South America are definitely moving toward greater acceptance of the death-with-dignity concept. It will take years, however, for these countries to accept something as radical as the brainchild of Switzerland's Ludwig Minelli.

– 14 –

One-way Tickets to Zürich

My main problem is that troubled people from all over the world are denied assisted suicide in their own countries and are so desperate they have to come here.

— Ludwig A. Minelli, founder of Dignitas

I may look all right, but I'm not. I know that people say that I look well, but I'm not. My condition has deteriorated an awful lot, particularly my speech. I hate talking on the phone now and, really, I don't like talking much at all," said Dr. Anne Turner to BBC interviewer Fergus Walsh in January 2006. The retired family planning physician, a resident of Bath, England, was about to turn sixty-six. She had cheated the Grim Reaper once already after being diagnosed with breast cancer and undergoing a mastectomy.[1]

But now she was three years into a rapidly progressive case of supranuclear palsy, a rare and incurable degenerative disease that causes gradual loss of brain cells, leading to loss of control of movement, especially walking, balancing, swallowing, speaking, and moving the eyes.

Turner continued, "I don't have a good quality of life now. . . . While I still can go to Switzerland, I'm going to go. In a month's time or two, I might not be able to."

At the time of the BBC interview, Turner spoke with a heavy slur and could walk only with a cane. She knew firsthand what a lingering, degenerative disease with certain death would be like. In 2002, she had retired from her medical practice to care for her wheelchair-bound husband, Jack, also a physician, as he died slowly from Multiple System Atrophy. Both she and Jack had earlier been forced to sit helplessly by as his brother wasted away and died from ALS, known in Britain as motor neurone disease. And she did not want to end up like British actor, Dudley Moore, also a victim of progressive supranuclear palsy, who could not walk, talk, or even blink at the end of his life.

Anne Turner clearly wanted to die peacefully when she chose, not from another of her bone-breaking bad falls or from choking to death while attached to feeding tubes. In October 2005, she attempted suicide by drug overdose but failed. Shortly thereafter, she joined Dignitas, a nonprofit organization in Zürich that assists elective death.

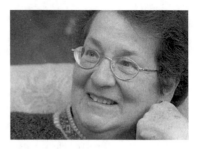

Dr. Anne Turner

Turner felt that her fellow doctors in England should be able to help people die, but she knew it was a felony offense if they did. She contacted BBC television to document her situation and to publicize the lack of compassion in Britain's vindictive law against assisting a suicide. She was angry that because she wanted to die while still capable and coherent, she had to fly to a foreign country in order to do so. That meant dying earlier than necessary abroad, while she could travel, instead of living a still-rewarding life somewhat longer and dying among friends and family in England. She was far from alone. As of December 31,2011, 882 Britons were part of Dignitas' 6,000 active members and more than 180 Britons had made the one-way trip to Zürich.[2]

Dr. Turner's case was far more clear-cut than some of those that Dignitas has handled. Her death was near, and the lethality of her condition was unquestionable. After she paid the Dignitas initiation fee, she forwarded full copies of all her medical records to them. They and outside physicians review the complete documentation of a member's medical condition. If it meets their acceptance standards—and less than half do—then Dignitas gives the member a "provisional green light," which authorizes him or her to travel to the headquarters office building in Forch, a Zürich suburb. If Turner had waited much longer, the window of opportunity for her to die of her own free will would have passed because she would have lost the ability to swallow pills or liquids. At that point, Dignitas could not have legally helped her because Swiss law would have deemed that an act of homicide rather than an assisted suicide.

The morning of January 24, 2006—a day short of Turner's sixty-seventh birthday—was predictably grey and freezing cold. After breakfast, Turner; her son, Edward; and daughter, Sophie; along with two BBC newsmen, took a taxi to the Dignitas office to consult the physician. Turner's other daughter, Jessica, who could not bear to watch her mother die, stayed at the hotel.

After an hour-and-fifteen-minute consultation, Turner was formally approved for her "accompaniment," the Dignitas term for an assisted suicide. She and her children were driven to the Dignitas apartment, which was then in a working-class residential block of Gertrudstrasse in Zürich. There, they were met by two trained Dignitas volunteers, or escorts, who offered them tea and coffee and helped Turner fill out the required legal documents. When her escort asked her if she wanted to proceed, she said, "Yes, of course." Then, she was given a glass containing a mild-tasting anti-emetic to ensure that the lethal dose she would take later would not be vomited up.

The half-hour that followed was consumed with remembrances and tearful last good-byes. When Turner signified that she was ready to die, the video camera at the end of her bed was turned on. As it rolled, the escort asked again, "Are you certain you want to proceed?"

Turner again answered "yes" and drank a small glass of Nembutal. A few minutes later, with her two children by her side, she fell asleep. Within a half hour, she was dead. Afterward, her son Edward explained, "She was ready to go and that makes it all the easier for us. We will respect her choice and . . . are very thankful that her suffering is over."

Although active euthanasia—a doctor directly helping someone to die—is illegal in Switzerland, that country has the world's longest standing law that permits assisted suicide. In 1918, the Swiss Federal Council stated that suicide assistance should not be punished if it was benevolently motivated. In the process of adopting a federal criminal code that year, the council proposed that suicide should not be a crime and that "aiding and abetting suicide can themselves be an act of friendship."[3]

It has long been part of Swiss mentality that simple suicide should not be an offense, and this became law in 1942. However, Article 115 of the Swiss Penal Code says that a person who aids or abets another person in suicide for selfish motives will be imprisoned for up to five years. Assisting a suicide is legal as long as the assistance is provided solely for altruistic reasons.

Dr. Jérôme Sobel, president of Exit-ADMD Suisse Romande, a 15,000-member right-to-die group for French-speaking Swiss, explained that a political debate in the Swiss National Council on December 11, 2001, confirmed this interpretation of the law and legitimized the actions of associations that defend the right to die with dignity.

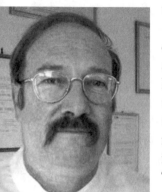

Dr. Jérôme Sobel

On November 3, 2006, the Swiss Federal (Supreme) Court at Lausanne ruled that a person's decision as to when, where, and how to end his or her life is part of the right to self-determination protected by Article 8(1) of the European Convention on Human Rights (ECHR), as long as the person is capable of free will and can act upon it.[4] The same court ruled that this right belongs also to mentally ill persons, on the condition that in those cases, a physician may write a prescription for a lethal medicine only if a psychiatrist has conducted an in-depth review of the patient's condition to determine whether or not he or she has the capacity of free will. Patients whose suicidal impulses are simply the product of depression and not the result of a carefully made rational decision are excluded.

In Switzerland, anyone may carry out an assisted suicide, although if a controlled substance, such as Nembutal, is required, the provider must be a physician licensed to prescribe it. As a result, doctors review and approve cases and then write prescriptions for the lethal drugs. The patient must take it by his or her own hand, usually under the supervision of a staff member of one of the four Swiss assisted-suicide groups.

The lack of legal aid in dying in their own countries drives people to Switzerland. Swiss law makes no distinction about residency. "The Netherlands, Belgium, and Luxembourg do not have a residency requirement, but their solution to prevent suicide tourism is to require the patient to have a good doctor-patient relationship," said Dr. Rob Jonquière. Almost every other locality in the world that has legalized physician-hastened death or assisted suicide has strict residency requirements. The other exception is Colombia, where the constitutional court decriminalized euthanasia and assisted suicide in 1997 without mentioning a residency requirement.

Anyone may come to Switzerland to die, as long as they meet

the legal qualifications. At first, Swiss assisted aid-in-dying organizations catered only to their own citizens. That changed in 1999, when Dignitas, a nonprofit organization created and led by attorney Ludwig Minelli, began to permit citizens of other countries to use its facility—and immediately became a lightning rod for controversy.

Minelli has a simple explanation for opening his doors to outsiders: fairness. "I said to myself, *what is the difference between a woman with breast cancer with metastasis in the German city of Konstanz, and the Swiss city of Kreuzlingen, neighbour city of Konstanz? Only the distance of half a kilometer. Should this difference be the reason to say yes to the person who lives in Switzerland and no to the one who lives in Germany?* Therefore, I have decided we will accept members in our association from outside of Switzerland."[5]

Today, anyone, anywhere who meets its eligibility requirements is welcome to join Dignitas. Between its founding in 1998 and December 31, 2011, 182 members from the United Kingdom, 25 from the United States, 15 from Canada, and a total of 1,076 people from more than 32 other countries chose to voluntarily end their lives at the Dignitas clinic, turning Minelli's native Zürich into the undisputed world capital of legal assisted suicide.[6] The total of British citizens will soon top two hundred. Minelli views this as a great human rights achievement. Some Swiss officials do not.

Andreas Brunner, general prosecutor for the canton of Zürich, said, "Suicide is not something Switzerland wants to be known for. This kind of tourism isn't the proper thing for Zürich."[7]

Dr. Margrit Leuthold, a member of the Swiss Advisory Commission on Biomedical Ethics, holds a different perspective. "We really hope to raise awareness among the countries who send us the most patients: Germany and Great Britain….It's a call to these countries not just to export the problem."[8]

In addition to Dignitas, there are three other right-to-die groups in Switzerland. Exit Deutsche Schweiz, headed by Saskia Frei, serves the German-speaking region. Founded in April 1982, it is headquartered in Zürich. In its first five years, it grew to 20,000 members. Now, with about 55,000 members, it is the largest of its kind in Switzerland, a nation of only 7.8 million people.[9] In 1984, it published the first German-language manual for voluntary death, *Humanes Sterben in Würde unter Selbstverantwortung (Humane Dying with Dignity and Self-Responsibility)*. The eighteen-page booklet, updated in 1993, gave specific lethal doses for various drugs and was only sold to people who had been members for at least three months.

In the early 1990s, the association broadened its services to include drafting living wills and distributing do-it-yourself instructions for voluntary death. About 1995, it began to openly assist suicides of Swiss members. It assists with about one hundred twenty voluntary deaths of Swiss citizens per year, generally using Nembutal.

Its sister group, Exit Association pour le Droit de Mourir dans la Dignité (Exit-ADMD), based in Geneva, serves the French-speaking residents of Switzerland. Its leader is Dr. Jérôme Sobel.

Ex International (formerly Exit International, which has no affiliation with Philip Nitschke's Exit International in Australia) was formed in 1997 and is based in Bern. It was founded by Dr. Rolf Sigg, former managing director of Exit Deutsche Schweiz. As of 2007, the group was also willing to provide assisted suicide for foreigners who come to Switzerland.[10] Sigg claims to have helped more than three hundred people die.[11]

I first met Ludwig Minelli at the 2008 World Federation of Right to Die Societies' conference in Paris. He impressed me as a typical well-educated European professional man: well-mannered, conservatively stylish, multilingual, and unostentatious. Timid he is not. Over lunch, he chuckled as he told me a story about being invited by Vatican Radio to describe what he does and why he does it. He declined the interview, stating that religious dogma and wars have led to the deaths of millions of innocent people. Moreover, he said, a peaceful death at Dignitas was always a free-will personal choice, but being burned at the stake for being a witch or being killed for being an infidel was not. Needless to say, Minelli, although he once considered studying for the priesthood, is an atheist.

The eldest of four children of a house painter, Ludwig Amadeus Minelli was born on December 5, 1932, in Zürich and grew up in Küsnacht, a village on the shore of Lake Zürich. Despite thinning hair, glasses, and hearing aids in both ears, he walks and speaks with the vitality and enthusiasm of a man twenty years younger. His clear blue eyes are attentive, and his skin has a rosy glow, which Swiss winters virtually guarantee. His thoughtful demeanor evolves from a mind that is focused and attentive. Like many well-educated men, his tastes in music and literature are classical, and his speech is precise and articulate. Among his heroes he names Sir Thomas

More, a sixteenth-century English lawyer, humanist, statesman, and author,
and Sir Winston Churchill.

Minelli began his career as a free-
lance journalist. In 1964, he became
the first Swiss correspondent for the
prestigious German news weekly, *Der
Spiegel.* By 1973, he became aware of the
European Convention on Human Rights,
an electrifying moment that sharpened
his latent interests in law. He began to
work as a citizen advocate for Swiss citizens after the Swiss ratified the ECHR in
1974. Three years later, after having filed

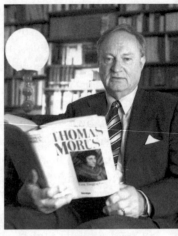

Ludwig Minelli

applications for Swiss citizens at the ECHR at Strasbourg, he started
his law studies at the University of Zürich, eventually receiving a
master of law degree in 1981.

His empathy for the dying began in 1966, when he saw his beloved grandmother die a lingering, painful death from kidney failure.
When the doctor visited her, she would ask him, "Couldn't you give
me something so that it would go a little bit quicker?" She was evidently unable to take a lethal dose unaided, as the physician replied,
"I'm not allowed to, but I will do nothing to make it go slower."[12]

In 1992, Minelli—a close friend of Manfred Kuhn, then vice
president of Exit Deutsche Schweiz—was asked to join the group as
legal advisor and to help its director, Rev. Dr. Rolf Sigg, re-establish
peace within the organization. The majority of Exit's board wanted
to dismiss Sigg and no longer wanted to discuss matters with the
rest of the board. Minelli was asked by both factions to chair Exit's
Tenth General Assembly at Bern. This assembly dismissed the majority of the board, elected replacements, and ended Exit's internal
turmoil.[13]

On May 17, 1998, the day after dealing with another Exit power
struggle, Minelli left the group and created Dignitas. "I designed
the statutes of Dignitas to create an association which would defend
the right to die in a peaceful manner and without power struggles,"
Minelli wrote.[14] He neatly solved the problem of internal management dissension when he created Dignitas' organizational structure.
There are only two active members of its general assembly, which is

the only authority empowered to make decisions and to alter its statutes. One is the secretary-general, currently Minelli. On any issue, if the other member disagrees with him, the two must seek a compromise in order to find a unanimous solution. In case of a serious discord, the secretary-general is entitled to overrule the other member of the general assembly. Hence, Minelli's rules are Dignitas' rules.[15]

Any mentally competent person over the age of eighteen can join Dignitas, whether they want to seek a hastened death immediately or want to have an "end-of-life insurance policy." People usually want to join because their lives are unbearable, but on average, Dignitas approves only a small proportion of the applications for an assisted suicide that it receives.[16] Dignitas' consulting physicians routinely turn down questionable cases after a thorough examination, and Minelli himself sometime carries out personal counseling when a member seems to be making an ill-considered choice to end his or her life. This often leads the member to seek medical or psychiatric help before making any irrevocable decisions.[17]

"An assisted suicide with Dignitas will never be an action of an insane person because . . . we can help only if this person has the capacity of discernment in the view of their own death," Minelli said.[18]

In December 2005, Dignitas refused to help former Qantas Airline pilot Graeme Wylie, seventy-one, who had advanced Alzheimer's disease. Dignitas said the information provided on Mr. Wylie's behalf did not provide clear evidence of his ability to rationally consent to assisted death.[19]

Minelli believes that death with dignity at the time and place of one's own choosing is a fundamental human right, which he defends vociferously and with unflagging tenacity. As a result, he has created the most controversial assisted-suicide organization in the world. A confrontational, high-profile international figure, Minelli is under continuous scrutiny and attack by his opponents.

His philosophy of total personal autonomy clashes head on with ancient traditions invented and enforced by church and state. "Suicide is a marvelous solution for a situation which you can't alter," he commented. That phrase is very often quoted by the media, but they do not quote the rest. Minelli finds that people who have chosen voluntary death often have not had the opportunity to talk openly about it—or to explore the alternatives. "So we will first [help them] find out whether something other than death might solve the problem."[20]

The Swiss suicide law breaks the age-old patriarchal lock once held exclusively by religions and governments. Supported by a large and growing percentage of people in the Western world, the "Swiss option" unnerves conservatives and traditionalists and gives hope to those faced with end-of-life scenarios that have no other happy ending.

All four of the Swiss assisted suicide groups will accept clients suffering from three general classes of disorders.

1. **The terminally ill.** The least controversial cases resemble those of Dr. Turner, who was terminally ill and would have died within a few months, no matter what kind of care she received.

2. **Degenerative, severely painful, or debilitating conditions that are not necessarily terminal.** These cases include people who are enduring extraordinarily painful lives, although their conditions are not defined as terminal, and they could survive more than six months. Included are those with degenerative diseases, such as Parkinson's disease, muscular dystrophy, or paralytic conditions from genetic defects or traumatic injuries. These conditions may bring on complications that degrade the quality of life but are not necessarily fatal. These sufferers usually seek voluntary death because of a combination of uncontrollable pain and loss of autonomy.

3. **Progressive, lethal dementia.** The third, and most controversial, cases consist of those people suffering from progressive lethal dementia, such as Alzheimer's disease. In the earliest stages, the patients are lucid and in control of their intellectual faculties, leaving them competent to make legally binding end-of-life decisions. As the disease progresses, it is harder for a doctor or psychiatrist to say with certainty that such patients are in sufficient control of their intellectual ability and have sufficient capacity to make a sound decision. It is legal in Switzerland for these people to receive assistance in dying, as long as their capacity for rational thought is still beyond any doubt.

However, Dignitas has taken a stand beyond that of the other, similar groups. In 2002, it caused an uproar when it announced that it had helped several mentally ill—but not legally insane—people end their lives. Some degree of depression is frequently part of the reason that people want to die, but often the depression can be treated.

"Someone suffering from depression may not be capable of making a rational decision," said Thomas Schläpfer, a psychiatrist at Bern University Hospital. "Suicidal impulse is not uncommon in people with severe mental disorders, and they see Dignitas as an easy, clean way out. It is morally and ethically wrong to help them die."[21]

Minelli disagrees, arguing that those with mental problems have periods when they are fully competent to make a decision to die. "There are cases of longtime chronic mental disorders that defy treatment. And many of these people have long periods of lucidity when they are capable of deciding for themselves. As a human rights lawyer I am persuaded that the right to make an end-of-life decision belongs to every person who has the capacity of discernment."[22]

Then there is the profound conundrum of adult death pacts, such as those between a husband and a wife, both rational, where one is severely ill and the other is not. These pacts have been immortalized (and often romanticized) in legend and literature for centuries. News that Sir Edward Downes, eighty-five, the world-renowned conductor *emeritus* of the BBC Philharmonic, and his wife, Lady Joan Downes, seventy-four, an accomplished dancer and choreographer, chose to die together at Dignitas on July 10, 2009, ignited an international controversy. She had terminal liver and pancreatic cancer. He, although virtually blind and increasingly deaf, was not terminally ill. Their son and daughter stated, "After fifty-four happy years together, they decided to end their own lives rather than continue to struggle with serious health problems."[23]

The couple held hands for their final moments before lying down on separate beds to drink Nembutal. Dignitas was criticized for allowing Sir Edward to end his life, but he had stated that he would be bereft without his wife and would soon be completely blind and deaf, unable to enjoy the music he had created. For the couple, the choice was crystal clear. And who had the authority to tell them that their decision was unacceptable?

Certainly not Ludwig Minelli. He also thinks that the choice to stop living belongs equally to the elderly, who may have typical old-age health problems, perhaps compounded by having no surviving family or friends. Once again pushing the envelope of acceptable reasons to choose elective death, he told the BBC News, "I think this capacity to make an end-of-life decision should also apply to a healthy person, so the British discussion about terminally ill persons is completely obsolete.... If these people have lost all interest in life, Minelli says, "Why should we say no [to hastened death]?"[24]

These are cases of those who suffer solely from existential angst: the settled decision that life no longer has meaning and there is no longer a reason to prolong it. This has sometimes been called "tired-of-life-syndrome." Minelli believes that Dignitas should provide an assisted suicide for such people. "I am opposed to the idea of paternalism. We do not make decisions for other people."[25] The Dutch would agree.

The core concept of the death-with-dignity movement, namely, personal autonomy vs. patriarchal authority, provokes the same levels of passion—and sometimes the threat of fanatic violence—as the ongoing abortion debate in the United States. Dignitas is not immune to such threats.

Despite the predictable protests of some Catholics, conservative Christians, and disability rights activists, the response of the viewers was overwhelmingly positive when *A Short Stay in Switzerland,* a serious dramatic recreation of Dr. Anne Turner's case, was broadcast by the BBC in January 2009. But Gillian Gerhardi, a fifty-year-old British mother of two suffering from cerebral palsy and advanced multiple sclerosis, was angry that Turner had taken "the Swiss option" far too soon.

She felt that the phrase "dying with dignity" was terribly misleading. "A dignified death is one where the person has fought for life and has not taken the easy way out," said the stoic, resolute woman. "I understand people are frightened of having a bad death full of suffering. But where did we get this idea that we are due a so-called dignified death?"[26]

She told a journalist that she had a plan. "I thought to myself that . . . the only way to make my point was to book myself into their death flat, and then blow myself and Dignitas founder, Ludwig Minelli, sky high," she said, adding with a wistful laugh, "I would become the first anti-suicide suicide bomber." Gerhardi concluded, "By killing herself, [Turner] was saying that life as a disabled person is not worth living."[27] Had her plot succeeded, Gerhardi would have stopped Ludwig Minelli and Dignitas once and for all.

Dignitas faced other challenges as it grew. Because most of the members traveling to Dignitas are in very poor health, the administrative office needed to be close to a major, handicapped-friendly international airport. Therefore, the organization's official head-quarters is in Forch, a suburb of Zürich about twelve miles (twenty kilometers) from the airport.

Dignitas' first assisted suicides in 1998 were Swiss members, and the deaths generally took place in the members' homes. After the organization decided to accept foreign members, it needed a fa-cility for its clients. Of necessity, the facility changed locations a number of times. From early on, the neighbors of Dignitas' vari-ous apartments touched off the dreaded "not in my backyard" re-sponse. No one wanted to live or work near or in a building where elderly people continually hobbled in on crutches or in wheelchairs, followed two or three hours later by the arrival of a police car, a coroner's car, and finally, a hearse to remove a plain wooden coffin. They could see only the trappings of death, not the profound peace that came with making a rational decision for self-deliverance.

From December 1, 2005, until August 31, 2007, Dignitas had an apartment in a residential building on Gertrudstrasse, Zürich, where Dr. Anne Turner died. But they were forced to move out after tenants grumbled that empty coffins were piling up.[28] "It doesn't belong in an apartment building," said Pius Schwendimann, who lived downstairs from Dignitas. "Every time a coffin is carried down, it's creepy."[29]

Then came "the nomadic period," from September 2007 until February 2008, during which Dignitas could not find an apartment that would accommodate its needs. Members would not stop dying just because Minelli did not have the perfect place to help them. This forced him into emergency response mode.

Dignitas had been evicted from its most recent apartment after only one month, so twenty members received their lethal doses in their hotel rooms, much to the displeasure of the hotel managers. At one point, Minelli gave up his own living room for two deaths. Dignitas carried out the assisted suicides of two German members in cars parked in scenic public parking areas with a view of woods and meadows.[30] When the media got hold of that story, they played it as a lurid feature for months.

From February 2008 until June 2009, Dignitas rented an apart-ment in a drab, grey, five-story office building at Ifangstrasse 12, in Schwerzenbach, near Zürich. The location had a dubious distinction. Prostitution is legal in Switzerland, and the apartment was locat-ed just doors away from The Globe, Switzerland's busiest brothel.

A spokesman for the Schwerzenbach town council lamented, "We didn't want the country's biggest sex club and largest death factory side-by-side on our doorstep." Ultimately, Dignitas was evicted from the building after complaints from other tenants.[31]

Minelli secured a loan for a building in Wetzikon, another Zürich suburb, but lost it because of complaints from neighbors. He turned to his loyal members for help, and the problem was solved. In July 2009, he announced that 276 members from 60 countries had loaned him CHF 885,000 ($809,000 USD) for the project, with Minelli personally putting up the balance for the $1 million-plus (USD) cost. This enabled Dignitas to occupy premises from which they could never again be evicted, for Minelli owns it and Dignitas is the tenant. He has subsequently repaid all the loans.

The "Blue Oasis" is an esthetically dignified facility. Minelli is proud of the tasteful, soothing design of the two-story building and

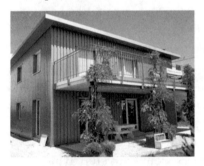

its site. It is located at Barzloostrasse 8 in Pfäffikon, a rural industrial suburb of Zürich. Flowering trees and tall grasses visually separate the blue edifice from a road, nearby buildings, and a soccer field. A pond flecked with lily pads and stocked with goldfish, surrounded by slate flagstones and gravel walks, provides a Zen-like peacefulness. Inside, hardwood floors, white walls, large windows, and original paintings of Swiss and Norwegian landscapes give the interior a light, bright, appearance.

The Blue Oasis

Two pleasantly appointed accompaniment rooms are available for members who come to die. The larger of the two includes chairs, a table, and a big, L-shaped, white couch for visitors and is decorated with plants. The bed where the member will die is covered with a rose-and-yellow duvet and faces a window overlooking the garden. This room is used for members with family or friends who have traveled to be with them during their final minutes. A somewhat smaller room is similarly decorated. As a Swiss resident noted, the location was not stolen from *The Sound of Music* film set—a modern machine factory lies just behind its back door—but it was the best that could be achieved, given the complex social and logistical necessities involved.

After the Dignitas member has passed the evaluation process in Forch, escorts drive the person to the Blue Oasis, or the journey from the hotel is made by taxi or in the car of friends. The member enters through the glass front door and goes to a small room containing five padded wooden chairs, which surround a circular table covered by a yellow throw. Atop it are a candle, a bowl of Swiss chocolates, and a box of facial tissues. There, a Dignitas escort carefully explains the client's Voluntary Death Declaration form, a lengthy legal document that provides all the official information required by Swiss law and exonerates Dignitas from all legal liabilities.

After the form is signed, the escort specifically asks if the member wants to call off the procedure or wants to proceed. Few people change their minds by that point. Next, the member is given a small glass of an anti-emetic. While waiting for it to take effect, the member has time to say good-bye to family and friends.

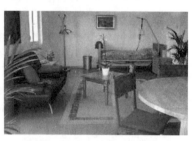

An accompaniment room

Meanwhile, the Dignitas escort dissolves fifteen grams (about one rounded tablespoon) of powdered Nembutal in a small glass of water. Dignitas tells the patient in advance about the well-known bitter taste of the drug. As Minelli told me, "The bitterness is our last test in order to know whether or not the person *really* wants to die."[32]

There was a hiatus in the use of Nembutal in January 2008, when the medical director of the canton of Zürich declared that he would no longer tolerate physicians writing a prescription for Nembutal after only one consultation, and he would prosecute such physicians for unprofessional conduct if they continued to do so.[33] Minelli recoiled against this rule because of the added difficulty it would pose for foreign members and because he believed the measure was directed solely against Dignitas. He decided to use the helium self-deliverance method with four patients, after discussing the procedure with them and gaining their consent. Since no drug prescriptions would be required, the process of dying at Dignitas would be totally demedicalized, and the new rule would become irrelevant.

Problems arose, however, when Dignitas, for aesthetic reasons, chose not to use a standard plastic exit bag because they thought the sight of it might upset family members. Instead, they used much smaller plastic medical partial face masks, which, if not precisely adjusted, can fit badly because of the variation in face shapes. A poor fit can allow air to leak in and lower the concentration of the inhaled helium, which is exactly what happened. The lower concentration increased the time until unconsciousness and death and exposed the staff to an unnerving sight—involuntary spasmodic muscle contractions and random eye movements that often occur with the helium system while the person is unconscious and insensible.

A detailed examination of videotapes of the four deaths led a panel of North American experts on helium self-deliverance to conclude that the Dignitas members experienced no pain as they died, but the time to unconsciousness and death was longer than normal, probably due to the ill-fitting face masks. After these four cases—all effective and painless for the members but anxiety-laden and emotionally disturbing for the escorts—Dignitas ceased using the helium method and reverted to its standard dose of Nembutal.[34]

When the member signifies that the time to die has arrived, the escort turns on a video camera to record the member's actions when consuming the Nembutal. The escort asks for a final time if the member wishes to proceed and then films the member and at least one other witness to show that taking the lethal dose was entirely voluntary and unassisted. Most physically able members drink the small glass of Nembutal through a straw quickly, relaxed and composed in the face of death, knowing that they will no longer have to bear any further suffering.[35]

Under Swiss law, every unusual death must be reported to, and examined by, the police to determine if a crime was committed. After each assisted suicide at Dignitas, a staff member calls 117, the police emergency number, to report the death. A police detective, a police officer, a prosecutor, and a public medical officer generally arrive within an hour. After they review the video, interview the witnesses, and are satisfied that the death occurred legally, the witnesses are free to leave. Swiss law has been complied with, and the body is released to whomever the member has directed: the crematorium or a funeral director, if the member has made provisions to have his or her body embalmed and returned home.

The majority of members who come to Dignitas request to be cremated after death, with the ashes placed in urns either for transportation back to the member's home or as a temporary storage container until the cremains are scattered, as directed by the member's written orders. Some ask that their ashes be spread in the fields or mountains of Switzerland, and some choose interment in Lake Zürich.

Bruce Falconer of *The Atlantic* reported that Minelli stored urns until he had enough to fill the trunk of his car. He then drove at night to a quiet spot on the lake and sent the urns to the bottom. The burial of urns and their sterile contents in the lake was not a health hazard, but in 2009, Minelli received an official warning from Zürich's water authority that disposing of human cremains in the lake without a permit was a violation of law.

One day in April 2010, while divers were searching for a sun-shade they had lost from their powerboat, they found sixty-seven red-clay cremation urns. All but one bore the embossed rampant lion logo of Zürich's Krematorium Nordheim—the largest in the city—which Dignitas and numerous local mortuary and funeral facilities use. Police later found evidence that the Küsnacht shore, where the urns were found, had been used for many years by local people to bury urns at the request of deceased relatives. As part of the investigation, Minelli was questioned, but the case against him was dropped for lack of evidence.[36] The urns have since been reburied in Küsnacht Cemetery.[37]

An assisted suicide through Dignitas is not cheap. As of December 2008, the listed expenses (in USD with conversion rates as of June 2010) were as follows:[38]

- Initial membership fee: (Swiss francs: CHF) 200 = $180
- Annual membership fee: CHF 80 = $72
- Preparation contribution: CHF 3,000 = $2,700
- Doctor's consultation in Switzerland: CHF 500 = $450
- Completion of the assisted suicide: CHF 3,000 = $2,700
- Administration: CHF 1,500 = $1,350
- Funeral director and cremation: CHF 2,000 = $1,800
- Total: CHF 10,280 = $9,252

These costs are only for fees paid to or through Dignitas. They do not include fees associated with obtaining certified copies of the necessary medical records and documents. In addition, there is the cost of transportation, food, and lodging for the member and traveling companions to and within Switzerland and the cost of transporting traveling companions back home from Switzerland. Dignitas offers reduced fees for pensioners and those in poor financial circumstances, but the reduction must be approved in advance. "This provision is not at all rare," said Minelli, "but of course, it must be financed by those who pay the full fees."[39]

Minelli's daughter, Michèle, stung by accusations that her father is making huge profits from death, noted that she and her sister will have no inheritance when her father dies because everything has been spent on his assisted suicide campaigning work. Minelli himself points to the large debt he has incurred, rather than a large income.

In response to allegations about poor conditions at the apartments and mistreatment of members, Dignitas sends out forms asking the surviving relatives about their experiences with the organization. The responses are overwhelmingly positive. Edward Turner, Dr. Anne Turner's son, praised Dignitas as "superb." He stated, "We are full of admiration for the way they have helped my mother through this very difficult time."[40] Shortly thereafter, Edward Turner became a prominent and outspoken public advocate, as well as a trustee, for the British right-to-die group Dignity in Dying.

In November 2009, when the Manchester *Guardian* wrote an extended feature story about Dignitas, it generated 127 reader comments. Along with the usual pro-and-con knee-jerk reactions, one thoughtful one caught my eye. "Chrystaline" (her online persona) wrote:

> This article gives me hope. When I was twelve my mother told me she wished she had killed herself while she was still able to do so. She had MS, and could no longer move of her own accord. She was fed through a tube in her stomach and had gym socks on her hands to keep herself from tearing her own skin apart from the constant uncontrollable tremors. She lost the ability to speak the following year. It was two more years before she finally died. She had to live on many years past what she should have, in constant pain that no drug could treat, in a convalescent home at the age of 45, with a medical staff dedicated to *preventing her death*. Until you've seen that happen to someone you love, you have no business condemning this man [Minelli] or his work. If you have seen it... you probably wish there were more like him.[41]

Those who work at Dignitas would agree with her. As of 2011, the staff consisted of five men and nine women, a mixture of professionals, college students, and retirees, who work part-time. Most staff members come to Dignitas through friends and family. Minelli's chief assistant is Silvan Luley, a tall, affable, forty-year-old master of law graduate. At the 2010 World Federation of Right to Die Societies' congress in Melbourne, Australia, Luley told me that his mother, Erika, was one of Dignitas' first employees, and she worked there as an accompaniment escort. According to Luley, others had come as members to end their lives but wound up working for Dignitas instead. "Minelli always tries to motivate people to make more of their lives. That's why I work for him, his human approach," he commented."[42]

Despite the fact that Dignitas is a small, nonprofit organization run by one man with a small staff of part-time employees and a total membership of only about 6,000, it has sent high-magnitude legal shockwaves throughout the world, especially in Britain. There, the legal system struggles with potential assisted suicide cases that still threaten friends and family with up to fourteen years in prison, even though the death does not take place on British soil.

Switzerland, however, remains firm in its humanitarian convictions. In 2011, a small group of Swiss citizens who oppose the legality of assisted suicide and the right for foreigners to travel to Switzerland to take advantage of the law brought both subjects to a vote. Of more than 278,000 ballots cast in the referendum, the initiative to ban assisted suicide was rejected by 85 percent of the voters and the initiative to outlaw it for foreigners was rejected by 78 percent.[43]

–15–

The Disunited Kingdom

Society gives us pious advice and help on how to bring a baby into this world. Why do we not provide equal guidance and assistance about how we can safely leave this earthly life?
— Dr. Michael Irwin

No place in the world faces greater turmoil over the right to die with dignity than Great Britain. The challenges there have deep roots, for England is home to the world's oldest right-to-die organization. An article in the *British Medical Journal* on November 2, 1935, announced the organization of the Voluntary Euthanasia Legalisation Society (VELS, later VES, then Exit, and now Dignity in Dying) advocating "the legalisation of voluntary euthanasia, that is, painless death for persons desiring it who are suffering from an incurable, fatal, and painful disease."[1]

Dr. Charles Killick Millard, of Leicester, the visionary pioneering author of "Euthanasia: A Plea for the Legalisation of Voluntary Euthanasia under Certain Conditions," was the driving force behind this movement. He was a free-thinking libertarian, a political radical, and a Unitarian who cared little for the Christian moral embargo on taking one's own life. A thorough iconoclast, he and a number of other intellectuals of his era also believed in the now-discredited philosophy of eugenics, which sought to improve the genetic composition of a population.

The long list of VELS founding members and sponsors included physicians and surgeons; clergymen; prominent writers, including Havelock Ellis, Virginia Woolf, H.G. Wells, and Aldous Huxley; and many other British notables. Even with this socially prestigious membership list, the formation of this noble-minded group was a brave act.

At about the same time, a scandal-to-be was already brewing

within its ranks, although it would not become public until fifty years later. Bertrand, Lord Dawson of Penn, a VELS founding member and also His Majesty's personal physician, had become a national celebrity by saving King George V from death by respiratory arrest in 1928. On the evening of January 20, 1936, however, King George was in more dire distress. In the final stage of cardio-respiratory failure, he was already comatose and close to death. To ensure that the monarch's imminent and unavoidable demise would be announced in the London *Times* and other prestigious morning newspapers rather than in the "less appropriate evening journals," Dawson gave the monarch a lethal dose of morphine and cocaine.[2]

Prior to doing so, at 9:25 p.m., he issued a bulletin alerting the *Times* "that the king's life was moving peacefully towards its close" and advising the editor to hold the presses for a forthcoming announcement. The king died by Dawson's lethal injection about 11:00 p.m. It was not a mercy killing, for the king was already comfortably sedated, but a convenience killing. Lord Dawson died in 1945 with his secret intact. It was not made public until 1986, when his private diary entry containing the exact details was published.[3] It is exactly this kind of secret end-of-life activities that the death-with-dignity movement wants to end by passing transparent, safe-guarded laws governing physician aid-in-dying and assisted suicide and by decriminalizing the distribution of authoritative guides to self-deliverance.

Britain has never been a welcoming place for people who want to end their lives prematurely or peacefully. In medieval times, ordinary citizens were considered to be the property of the sovereign. Suicide was viewed as depriving the crown of its property without permission. "The property belonging to the person who committed suicide was confiscated by the crown as a substitute for the taxes and labor which the deceased would have rendered had he still been alive."[4] The body of a person who ended his own life was often drawn and quartered, with the head mounted on a wooden stake in a public place. It was forbidden to bury the body on church grounds, a ban still enforced by some Catholic and other denominations. In more modern times, those who attempted suicide and failed were presumed to be mentally ill and were often involuntarily committed to psychiatric institutions for arbitrary and indefinite periods.

However, most of the turmoil about voluntary euthanasia in

modern Britain revolves around a fifty-year-old law. At the time it was enacted, the Suicide Act 1961 was a considered a major social advancement. The previous law considered attempted suicide, actual suicide, and assisting a suicide all to be crimes.

The 1961 act decriminalized attempted suicide and suicide so that those who failed in the attempt would no longer be prosecuted and could seek mental or medical help without stigma. Assisting a suicide, however, remained a crime. Section 2(1) of the act currently states, "A person who aids, abets, counsels or procures the suicide of another, or attempt by another to commit suicide shall be liable on conviction on indictment to imprisonment for a term not exceeding fourteen years." This posed a bizarre and unique legal concept: someone could be convicted and imprisoned for assisting in the commission of a non-crime. There is no other instance in law where an accessory can be criminally liable when the principal does not commit a crime.

Ever since the 1961 law took effect, the British people have been fighting to obtain the legal right to die with dignity. By 1970, more than 50 percent of Britons supported physician aid-in-dying, and as of January 2010, that support stood at 71 percent.[5] However, four bills introduced in Parliament to amend or replace the law have failed, for the simple reason that the politicians are too timid to endorse this (or many other) controversial subjects. As a result, the public cart continues to drag the balky legislative horse.

Now, right-to-die cases are front-page news in British papers almost weekly. News stories and court cases have educated the public about the grotesque problems posed by the 1961 law, and opposition to it has steadily risen as a result of the public debate. Although the law has yet to be amended or repealed, its foundation is cracking, and unrelenting public opposition demands that it be liberalized.

Outright censorship—and the dark shadow of prosecution for aiding and abetting a suicide—has long put a virtual stranglehold on the publication of right-to-die materials in the United Kingdom and most of its former colonies until fairly recent times.

The 1974 publication of Dr. George B. Mair's *Confessions of a Surgeon* shocked and mesmerized the British people. With great candor, Mair disclosed that he and his colleagues routinely helped hopeless, suffering patients accelerate their deaths with barbiturate overdoses, frequently with the legendary "Brompton Cocktail."

Developed in the Royal Brompton Hospital in London in the first quarter of the twentieth century, this potent mixture consisted of morphine or heroin, cocaine, and sometimes Thorazine (to counteract nausea) dissolved in ethyl alcohol, commonly in the form of gin. Mair's book shined a spotlight on the two-tier deathbed caste system: if one could afford a sympathetic private physician, a discreet, peaceful death was frequently available. But for the majority of the dying, that luxury was rarely an option, and terminal misery went unabated.

In 1978, Derek Humphry's emotionally powerful book, *Jean's Way*, which told of his pact to help his wife end her pain-filled, cancer-riddled life, became an immediate best-seller in Britain—and quickly led the police to Humphry's door. However, the book told of Humphry's devotion to his wife, and her unquestionable will to die, in such a way that it was unlikely that any jury would convict him, and no charges ever followed.

In 1979, the VES voted to publish a guide to self-deliverance, and membership quadrupled. But publication was derailed by severe legal actions, including the arrest of VES president Nicholas Reed and a formal legal inquiry into the lawfulness of publishing the book itself.

In 1981, Reed was convicted and sentenced to two-and-a-half years in prison for aiding and abetting a suicide. His colleague, seventy-year-old Mark Lyons, who had helped numerous people in unending pain commit suicide by providing pills and alcohol, was given a two-year suspended sentence.[6] The pair was apprehended after a coroner's autopsy of the body of a multiple sclerosis sufferer revealed that she had died from a barbiturate overdose accompanied by alcohol—a classic form of self-deliverance in the 1980s and still used in a slightly modified form today.

On the heels of the Reed-Lyons case, Britain's Attorney General held a hearing to determine whether publishing the VES members' booklet, *A Guide to Self-Deliverance*, constituted aiding and abetting a suicide and was, therefore, a criminal offense. Although sufficient grounds for prosecution were not found, the fear of future criminal prosecution convinced the VES to scuttle the booklet.[7]

Despite the hostile political climate in Britain, international acceptance of the right to die with dignity took a major leap forward there in September 1980. In Oxford, England, twenty voluntary euthanasia societies banded together to form the World Federation of Right to Die Societies. British Exit (previously and later renamed the VES) hosted the meeting. Professor Gerald Larue, an American and president of the newly launched Hemlock Society, was named to the federation's board of directors, and Derek Humphry was named executive director. That first meeting in Oxford initiated a fierce debate over a critical subject that remains unresolved: should right-to-die groups focus on finding methods of achieving peaceful death and on teaching their members how to use them, or should they focus solely on promoting changes to outdated and repressive anti-euthanasia laws?

A bitter, turbulent argument took place at Oxford over this subject. Writer and television personality, Sir Ludovic Kennedy, whom Exit had asked to speak on "Why I Believe in Voluntary Euthanasia," made headlines when he criticized booklets on self-deliverance being produced in England and Scotland. He stated unequivocally that he did not agree with the 1970s do-it-yourself methods, such as a barbiturate overdose and a plastic bag, but argued for physicians to be able to provide, upon written request, euthanasia for rational people who were terminally ill. This issue—perfecting and promoting effective do-it-yourself methods vs. working endlessly for legislative change—plagues the death-with-dignity movement to this day.

Dr. Colin Brewer, one of the authors of VES' controversial and ill-fated booklet, *A Guide to Self-Deliverance*, noted that until the laws on assisted suicide were changed, and doctors were willing to help, terminally ill people who wanted to end their lives usually had no alternative but to use one of the well-known, commonly available (but often gruesome, painful, and frequently unsuccessful) methods, such as jumping from heights, shooting or hanging themselves, or drinking corrosive household chemicals.[8] Even though the formation of the World Federation of Right to Die Societies had drawn international attention to the repressive conditions in Britain, all attempts to force revisions to the Suicide Act 1961 still failed.

In 2001, however, political storm clouds began to brew over the home of Diane Pretty, an English mother of two. Two years earlier, she had been diagnosed with motor neurone disease (MND), known in the United States as ALS, a degenerative, fatal condition, which gradually made her completely dependent on her family for her care. Pretty wanted Brian, her husband of twenty-three years, to be able to legally help her die when her life became unbearable and she could no longer act for herself.[9] Brian had agreed to this, but he told the BBC, "There is no way we are going to go against the law. So we will go to court. We shall fight in court and we will appeal if we lose because I want her to have her final wish."[10]

Brian Pretty wrote to then Prime Minister Tony Blair, pleading with him to change the law. When that failed, his wife asked the Director of Public Prosecution (DPP) for assurance that her husband would not be charged if he helped her end her life.[11] The DPP expressed his sympathy, acknowledging that Pretty and her family were experiencing "terrible suffering," but upheld the law and refused to grant Brian Petty immunity from prosecution.[12]

In August 2001, Diane Pretty, described by her admirers as a "tough lady," demanded the right to appeal the DPP's decision in the courts, claiming that his ruling violated her human rights. She argued that being required to go on living in the advanced stages of her disease was subjecting her to ill treatment contrary to Britain's 1998 Human Rights Act, which states that "no-one shall be subjected to torture or inhuman or degrading treatment or punishment."[13]

Pretty's lawyers argued that the DPP's decision discriminated against the disabled because an able-bodied person could easily end his or her own life with dignity and without help. Two months later, three High Court judges rejected Pretty's appeal, concluding that Britain was "not ready to sanction the idea of assisted suicide."[14]

In an unprecedented move, Pretty filed an emergency appeal to the European Court of Human Rights. She traveled twelve hours in an ambulance to Strasbourg, France, to attend the hearing on her case. On April 29, 2002, the court rejected her appeal. Five days later, deteriorating rapidly, she developed a chest infection and the accompanying breathing difficulties and was admitted to Pasque Hospice, Luton, near her home. Under heavy sedation, she died on November 19, 2002, in the way she had always feared most: a slow and painful death by choking and asphyxiation. In stark contrast, Dr. Ryszard Bietzk, the head of medical services at the hospice where Pretty was cared for and died, characterized her death as "perfectly normal, natural and peaceful."[15] After her death, her husband presented Prime Minister Tony Blair with a petition signed by fifty thousand people that called for legalization of voluntary euthanasia and assisted suicide.[16]

Pretty's case attracted enormous media coverage and generated tremendous sympathy for her cause. George Levvy, head of the Motor Neurone Disease Association (MNDA) in England, said, "Diane showed great courage and determination, both in her battle against motor neurone disease and in her campaign through the courts."[17]

Members of the MNDA were divided over the debate. Many supported Pretty's application, but some would have been horrified by any change in the law.[18] Rachel Hurst, director of Disability Awareness in Action, said it would be "very wrong for justice to say in certain circumstances people can die. It would be a slippery slope and many people who did not want to die could be affected."[19]

Unlike the general public, most of the British medical establishment was immensely relieved that the courts had decided against legalizing assisted suicide. Dr. Michael Wilks, chair of the British Medical Association's committee on medical ethics, said, "The European Court of Human Rights has made the right decision."[20] But major breaks were already evident in their ranks, and some British physicians boldly supported Pretty's case.

Just months before Pretty's death, doctors Len and Lesley Doyal published "Why active euthanasia and physician assisted suicide should be legalised" in the *British Medical Journal*. They made the point that the Strasbourg ruling, while consistent with legal precedent, was morally wrong and that the law should be changed. "In the face of so much moral right," they asked, "where is the wrong?"[21]

The event that triggered a blaze of demand for legal reform in the United Kingdom happened in 2003, when British citizens, unable to achieve a peaceful death in their own country, started traveling to the Dignitas facility in Zürich to end their lives. Reginald Crew was the first. On Monday morning, January 20, 2003, Crew, seventy-four, flew from Liverpool with his wife, Winifred, and a daughter to Zürich to die. The retired auto and dock worker had been dying for four years from MND, and he had had enough. "I'd never say I was tired of life, but I'm tired of the life I'm in and I know I am never going to be cured.... I couldn't live another six or seven months like this. I'm gradually going out of my mind because this is not living."[22]

Crew wanted to make his death in Switzerland a public statement about Britain's antiquated 1961 law. To do so, he invited a British television crew from ITV-1's *Tonight with Trevor McDonald* to be with him. After Crew's arrival in Zürich, a Swiss physician confirmed that his condition was terminal and his death was imminent.

At the Dignitas apartment, with his wife at his side, Crew drank a small glass containing fifteen grams of Nembutal dissolved in water. He fell asleep within a few minutes and died without pain about twenty minutes later.

Winifred described her husband's death as "dignified," noting, "Although I am a Roman Catholic, like many others in my position, when Reg said he wanted medical assistance to die, to avoid a long and painful death, I felt this was the right thing to do.... He loved England. He always said it was the best country in the world and he should have been able to end his days there in peace like he did here."[23]

Back in England, she and the television crew, who had been passive observers, were interrogated by police. After Winifred endured a long, nervous wait, authorities notified her that there was insufficient evidence that she had violated the law and that there was no public interest in prosecuting her. This landmark decision set the precedent for every subsequent British death at Dignitas. To this day, no friend or family member who attended an assisted suicide there has ever been prosecuted. It seems clear that the DPP has no interest in taking a case to court, for if the defendants were acquitted, the Suicide Act 1961 could be found to be a violation of the right to self-determination.

Outraged by this flouting of the law, Colin Hart, a member of the British pro-life group Alert and director of the Christian Institute, a conservative Anglican organization, told the BBC, "I would think that it is unreasonable to choose death over life."[24] Numerous viewers were quick to note that Hart might have taken a more pragmatic view if he had been the person doing the dying, not Reg Crew.

The news that Dignitas was available as an end-of-life option brought a flood of membership applications from Britons. By 2004, only a year after Crew's death, more than nine hundred had joined—the single largest group of non-Swiss members after the Germans.

Because Swiss law and practice recognized both terminal illness and intolerable pain and suffering as valid reasons to receive a legal assisted suicide, other people began to take the plane to Zürich. Just three months after Crew died, Robert and Jennifer Stokes of Bedfordshire, England, also chose "the Swiss option." Mr. Stokes, fifty-nine, suffered from epilepsy, and his wife, fifty-three, had diabetes and severe back pain, none of which were considered to be terminal conditions. Nevertheless, the Stokes died in Zürich on April 1, 2003, the first British couple to do so.

Encouraged by the authorities' decision not to prosecute Winifred Crew, the VES asked the DPP to clarify the policy in the "aiding and abetting" section of the Suicide Act 1961 as it related to assisting suicides of Britons on foreign soil where it was legal. A month after the deaths of Robert and Jennifer Stokes, Lord Charles Falconer, Minister of State for the Home Office, sent the following—and strikingly candid—reply:

> As you know, section 2(1) of the Suicide Act 1961 makes it an offence in this country to aid, abet, counsel or procure somebody to commit suicide. Provided that the aiding, abetting etc takes place in this country, we believe (though the point is untested by the courts) that the offence under section 2(1) is committed even where the suicide occurs abroad. However, aiding, abetting etc, of suicide abroad is a matter for the authorities in whose jurisdiction the suicide occurs. It is therefore for the Swiss authorities to determine whether any offence has been committed under Swiss law (whether in the Stokes' or any other case). We are of course concerned that UK citizens, whether terminally ill or not, may be helped to die in countries where this is legal in certain circumstances. But this is a matter of law *in the country concerned* and not one in which the [British] Government should intervene.[25]

In 2003, as the list of Britons traveling to die in Zürich grew longer, Baron Joel Joffe introduced the "Assisted Dying for the Terminally Ill Bill" in the House of Lords to legalize physician-hastened death in England and Wales. A native of South Africa, Joffe worked as a human rights lawyer, representing Nelson Mandela in the 1960s, and with the international charitable organization Oxfam.

The bill, drafted by Deborah Annetts, chief executive of the VES, was designed to enable a competent adult who is suffering unbearably as a result of a terminal or serious and progressive physical illness to receive medical help to die at his or her own considered and persistent request and to provide pain relief medication for such people. The bill lacked enough support to reach the House of Commons, leaving the Suicide Act 1961 intact.[26] In 2006, Joffe reintroduced the bill, but it again failed to get past the House of Lords.

After numerous attempts to persuade Parliament to amend the law, a group of euthanasia activists decided to force the issue. On February 28, 2007, Raymond Cutkelvin and four supporters, including Dr. Michael Irwin, boarded a plane for the one-hour flight from London to Zürich. Two days later, all but one returned. Cutkelvin, fifty-eight, a former British post office clerk, had been diagnosed with inoperable pancreatic cancer. Alan Rees, his civil partner of twenty-eight years, held Cutkelvin's hand as he drank a lethal dose of barbiturates and quickly fell into his final sleep. "My only regret is that we had to travel to Switzerland," Rees said. "We should have been able to do this in our own country."[27]

Because the suicide took place abroad, it might have been tacitly ignored by the authorities had it not been for the bravery of Rees and Irwin. Two years afterward, in 2009, when the "Swiss option" was everyday news, the two men sent Director of Public Prosecution Keir Starmer ironclad proof that they had directly aided and abetted Cutkelvin's suicide in violation of the Suicide Act 1961. The evidence included signed, detailed descriptions of their plans for the trip and copies of their airplane tickets and of the checks used to pay for them. They then demanded to be prosecuted for their crime, to force the Crown to acknowledge that the law was impossible to enforce. With great reluctance the police opened an investigation.

Irwin told a London newspaper, "I expect to be charged and want to be charged…. I want to highlight the two-tier system where 'assisted suicide' is only available to those who can afford it. That, to me, is a form of hypocrisy."[28]

Pro-life groups also wanted Irwin to be charged—and convicted. Nuala Scarisbrick, spokeswoman for the group Life said, "We are opposed to any form of 'assisted suicide.' The law must be enforced, particularly if someone has admitted breaking it. This is not a matter of vengeance but of principle—our laws need to be respected."[29] Or, in other words, a fifty-year-old law is itself inherently more important than the wishes of the majority of the citizens who want it repealed.

For Irwin, a veteran international activist, it was just one more tilt at bureaucratic legal windmills. For Rees, it was a ghastly emo-

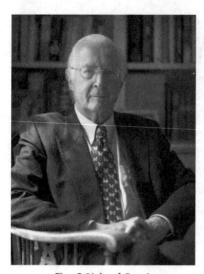

Dr. Michael Irwin

tional nightmare while the DPP left them swinging in the breeze of legal indecision for nearly a year after charging both with being parties to aiding and abetting a suicide. All charges against them were ultimately dropped, as the DPP ruled that prosecution was not in the public interest.

Michael Irwin was no stranger to legal wrangling or the fight for human dignity. Born in London in 1931, he was trained as a physician at St. Bartholomew's Hospital Medical College, London, and earned a master's degree in public health from Columbia University in New York City. Beginning in 1957, he held numerous top-level international medical positions for the United Nations, culminating in service as their medical director. He went on to play the same role at the World Bank, from which he resigned in 1990.

Free of officialdom, and having seen, as most doctors do, numerous examples of unnecessarily ghastly deaths, he turned his skills to promoting death with dignity. A parliamentary candidate in 1999, he campaigned for the implementation of living wills. He served as president of the World Federation of Right to Die Societies and was chair of the VES. In 2003, he retired from active practice as a physician.

A vigorous, intelligent, and impeccably dressed professional man, the eighty-one-year-old euthanasia activist looks more like the lord of a baronial estate (which he is not) than a reformist firebrand (which he is). Irwin and many other Dignitas members and supporters deliberately use well-publicized civil disobedience to fight for the death-with-dignity cause.

A controversial act of mercy cost Irwin the chair of the VES. In 2003, he traveled to the Isle of Man to bring an overdose of sleeping pills to his friend Patrick Kneen, seventy-four, who was terminally ill with prostate cancer. When Irwin arrived, he found Kneen too ill to swallow. Kneen died naturally while receiving care from his own physician. Nevertheless, a police interrogation of Irwin and Kneen's wife followed, revealing their intent to help Kneen die. Irwin gave the Manx police a detailed diary of his involvement in planning to assist his friend's suicide. Oddly, Mrs. Kneen was charged for conspiracy to aid and abet a suicide, but Irwin was not. Months later, all charges were quietly dropped. It was yet another unprosecutable case.[30]

After the Isle of Man incident came to the attention of the British General Medical Council, Irwin was struck off the medical register, revoking his physician's license.[31] Irwin shrugged off the reprimand. He was already retired, and he considered many of his medical colleagues hypocrites for not publicly endorsing legalized physician-assisted suicide, which many of them already practiced unobtrusively and *sub rosa*.

Irwin's controversial actions did not sit well with the VES either. Irwin had been affiliated with the venerable group since 1993, ultimately rising to be its chairman and chief spokesman. At a board meeting in 2004, he was stripped of his position as chairman because of his blatant activism, which clashed with the society's stated goal of supporting only legislative change.

The opposing board members, as well as VES' chief executive, Deborah Annetts, eventually forced Irwin completely off the board. Annetts made it clear that the group's leadership should be seen as working within the law to promote legal reform and should not condone mercy killings or exit-guide activities.

No longer constrained by his position in the VES, Irwin and a small group of like-minded colleagues founded The Last Choice (TLC). This organization provided information, logistical assistance, financial aid, and, if needed, a traveling companion for terminally ill British citizens who wanted to go to Dignitas. Because of the risk of prosecution, Irwin was the group's only identified member. By 2005, TLC had collected £5,000 in pledges and had opened a bank account outside of Britain to hold the funds. However, by 2010, TLC had been absorbed by the Scottish group Friends at the End (FATE), with which Irwin had long been closely associated.[32]

When a friend chose suicide at the age of ninety, Irwin asked himself, *Why shouldn't there be more attention given to this category of people by the right-to-die movement?* Noting that the elderly had a more imminent stake in making their final choices, Irwin commissioned a national polling organization to ask British adults whether elderly, competent individuals who suffer from a variety of health problems should be legally allowed to receive physician-assisted suicide.

When the results came in, more than 67 percent of respondents agreed.[33] With this show of support, Irwin and eleven colleagues founded the Society for Old Age Rational Suicide (SOARS) in 2009 to promote the right of people who had "completed lives" or had accumulated sufficient medical problems to legally seek assisted self-deliverance.[34] Although the group does not solicit membership, Irwin reported over five hundred supporters in its first year.

As do many other physicians, Irwin has a "twinning" agreement with a fellow doctor to help him achieve a peaceful passing should a "bad death" stare him in the face at the end of his life. If his "twin" were struck first, Irwin would do the same. He speaks openly of his arrangement, as it helps him demonstrate how the medical community will provide compassionate care for its own members while denying the same to those outside its ranks.

Confrontational activism in the style of Michael Irwin was probably the last thing on mind of thirty-one-year-old Debbie Purdy in 1995.[35] She was on a roll. The attractive, outgoing Englishwoman had an exciting career as a world-traveling independent writer.

"I was getting paid to indulge my greatest passions: diving in Malaysia, white-water rafting in Indonesia, water-skiing in Thailand. I couldn't have been happier," she wrote.[36] At the end of January, she got an assignment to write about a Cuban band that had just arrived in Singapore. Its leader, Omar Puente, also thirty-one, was a gifted musician who had studied classical music. But popular Cuban rhythms were in his blood, and when he went off to tour the world, that is what he played.

Charmed by his warmth, Purdy was smitten. Puente felt the same way. Having noticed some weariness in her feet after dancing with him in Singapore, she saw a doctor upon her return to England. The results were terrifying. A lumbar puncture and an MRI showed that she had primary progressive multiple sclerosis. The prognosis was not good. She would suffer from progressive loss of muscle control with a strong likelihood of a premature death. Nevertheless, she returned to Singapore and Omar.

In 1997, with her health and mobility both in decline, the couple moved back to Purdy's home in England, where they married in 1998. By then, she was confined to a wheelchair and needed assistance getting in and out of bed. The energetic, ambitious writer knew her life would end in spiraling misery. She decided that when her condition became worse than her ability to cope with it, she would go to Dignitas.

"I love my life, but I have always been a fiercely independent woman," she wrote, "and I want to have choice about how and when I die. Should living become unbearable to me, I want to be able to ask for and receive help to die with dignity. British law does not allow this. . . so my options are to attempt suicide myself, and risk making matters worse, or to travel to Switzerland to have an assisted death."[37]

She did not want to wait until she required her husband's help to travel and expose him to possible arrest for assisting a suicide. Applying British law to a country over which England had no legal jurisdiction was, to say the least, confusing. If Purdy and her husband departed England and arrived in France, they would immediately be ruled by French law. When they drove over the border to Switzerland, they would then be bound by the Swiss legal code, which permits assisted suicides. Upon returning home, though, their actions might be subject to all of the penalties of British law.

Referring to the British assisted suicide law, one legal commentator stated that if this perverse interpretation of the law were applied, "This would say, 'We own you! Wherever you go, you're ours! You can never escape!' That's the sort of attitude the old Soviet Union used to have towards its unfortunate subjects."[38]

Fearing for her husband's legal future, Purdy demanded that the DPP rule in advance on the likelihood that he would be prosecuted if he accompanied her. She won a hearing on October 2, 2008, before Britain's High Court of Justice. In a case reminiscent of Diane Pretty's, Purdy and her counsel argued that the DPP was infringing on her human rights by failing to clarify how the Suicide Act 1961 is enforced. At the end of July 2009, Purdy's long fight was rewarded with a court ruling that the current lack of clarity was a violation of the right to a private and family life. The DPP, Keir Starmer, was ordered to issue clear guidance on when prosecutions could be brought in assisted suicide cases.

Caught between the standing law and the flood of people risking prosecution when they helped someone die, Starmer released

his proposed "Interim Policy for Prosecutors in Respect of Cases of Assisted
Suicide" for purposes of public discussion in September 2009. The debate period was set at 120 days and produced
an enormous outpouring of response.
One of the brightest and most dedicated
public servants in the British legal system, Starmer clearly wanted to achieve
the best possible outcome for his nation.

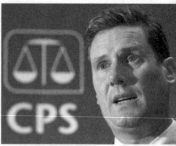

*Keir Starmer, Director of
Public Prosecutions*

Commenting in *The Telegraph,* journalist Mary Riddell wrote,
"Over the next few weeks, Keir Starmer will take up the challenge
that the Parliament dare not face and write the rulebook on assisted
suicide. King Solomon might have balked at producing interim guidance on such a thorny issue."[39]

On February 25, 2010, Starmer released the new rules for the
Crown Prosecuting Service to use when deciding to prosecute those
accused of assisting a suicide. These rules closely paralleled the
standard for assessing criminal liability for assisting a suicide under
Swiss law: lack of malicious motive. The revised guidelines "make it
clear that there is a distinction between compassionate acts to assist
someone to end their own life [which are unlikely to be prosecuted],
and malicious encouragement or assistance of suicide [which likely
will be prosecuted]," said Sarah Wootton, chief executive of Dignity in Dying, the new name for the VES. She hailed the guidelines
as a victory for common sense and compassion.[40]

On April 16, 2011, Debbie Purdy revealed that Starmer's clarification of the law led her to defer the decision to go to Dignitas until her condition worsened considerably because her husband could
then accompany her to Switzerland without fear of prosecution. If
she had not pursued this clarification, she would have ended her life
two years earlier, when she was still physically able to make the trip
unaccompanied.[41] For Purdy, the clarification brought a dramatically
positive change. In September 2010, she noted, "I was preparing to
lose and was in the middle of organising to go to Dignitas. Winning
was like being given permission to be alive."[42]

The DPP's guidelines did not change Britain's Suicide Act 1961.
Those suspected of violating it will continue to be interrogated by
the police, as will those who accompany friends or family members

to Dignitas. The guidelines clarify only how the evidence against such people will be evaluated. But the likelihood of being prosecuted is much lower now because people will be judged chiefly on their motives, not simply their presence at a death. So far, no one interrogated after helping someone end his or her life in Switzerland has been charged with breaking the law.

The ongoing struggle for death with dignity in Britain has attracted some high-profile figures. In early 2010, internationally acclaimed British author Sir Terry Pratchett made a radical proposal that drew the attention of his countrymen. He suggested that tribunals of British coroners should decide who could voluntarily end his or her life by assisted suicide without legal penalties.

"There needs to be, for the safety of all concerned, some kind of gentle tribunal, to make certain that requests for assisted death are *bona fide* and not perhaps due to gentle persuasion," he said.[43] He then volunteered to be the first person to have his case reviewed.

His immensely popular science fiction/fantasy novels, particularly the *Discworld* series, which satirizes modern life, along with his white beard, wide-brimmed black hat and black leather coat made Pratchett a literary icon. Long a supporter of the right to die, Pratchett was diagnosed with Alzheimer's disease in 2007 and wanted to be able to end his life when he no longer considered it meaningful, saying, "[I] do not believe in a duty to suffer the worst ravages of terminal illness."[44]

Naturally, the right-to-life faction violently disagreed. Disability activist Clair Lewis was appalled by Pratchett's idea. "In the UK this week, affluent writers like Terry Pratchett and Martin Amis are swamping the press with calls for death clinics (again!) for those with nothing else to worry about except their impairments," she blogged, "while those of us in poverty, and lacking the services and resources we need, know that should assisted suicide become legal here, people will end up being killed because of things which could be fixed."[45]

But not all members of the death-with-dignity movement saw Pratchett's proposal as a step in the right direction. They noted that instead of broadening the scope of personal autonomy, it would create yet another layer of paternalistic bureaucracy with the power to grant, delay, or deny what euthanasia advocates saw as a civil right, not a political privilege.

Perhaps the most dramatic example of taking charge of one's own death in Britain came from John Hicklenton, a brilliant, world-famous illustrator of intense graphic novels. He was best-known for visceral characters such as Judge Dredd and Nemesis the Warlock in the cult British comic series *2000 AD*. Stricken with multiple sclerosis, Hicklenton watched his ability to control his body steadily decline and knew that his creative days were numbered.

His final work, *100 Months*, was a magnificent mosaic that interpreted his own path to death. According to *The London Telegraph*, he finished *100 Months* just one day before his trip to Dignitas on March 19, 2010. Instead of meekly accepting the withering away of his life, he wrote the final page of his story with the same intensity that filled his characters. His friend and colleague, Pat Mills, the founder of the *2000 AD* series, said that Hicklenton's attitude toward his death reflected his attitude toward every other challenge. He stared his killer in the face and said, "MS, you have a week to live. You've met someone you shouldn't have fucked with!"[46]

More than two hundred people have made the one-way journey, usually accompanied by friends or loved ones. They come forward nearly every week, giving interviews about their plans to protest the indignity of what they are being forced to do, piling one impossible-to-prosecute case on top of another in the lap of Britain's agonized DPP.

Dignitas founder Ludwig Minelli blamed the increase in British "suicide tourism" in Switzerland solely on the British government. "The question for politicians in Britain today is this: Why do you force your citizens, people in the most terrible circumstances, who are determined to end their suffering in a way of their own choosing to leave your country and travel to Switzerland in order to exercise their free will? Where is the humanity in this policy?" he asked.[47]

Minelli's perspective was validated yet again in October 2011, when new Royal College of Nursing guidelines instructed British nurses that they could go to prison for talking to patients about assisted dying. The gag order was seen by many as paternalistic prima facie evidence that the British medical establishment believes elderly people are incapable of rationally considering and acting logically on the life-and-death issues that they are personally confronting.

"They will be warned they face prosecution if they are found to have discussed any aspect of euthanasia with a patient who goes on to commit suicide," wrote Sophie Borland in the *Mail Online*. "The new Royal College of Nursing guidelines will remind staff that it is illegal to offer information about assisted dying—including contact details for Dignitas in Switzerland—in case it is seen as 'encouragement.' The RCN produced the guidelines after nurses came forward to say they had been asked for advice from patients and relatives about assisted suicide."[48]

But in the same month that timid British medical officials were telling their nurses to treat their rational adult patients as if they were incompetent children, groups of retirees fortunate enough not to be under their thumbs were demanding exactly the information that the physicians were working hard to suppress. Older Citizens Advocacy York, a retirees' lobby group in the ancient city of York, called for a "free and frank debate" as the Australian right-to-die campaigner Philip Nitschke was arriving there for a planned Exit International lecture and workshop on November 18, 2011. Protests promised by Catholics failed to materialize outside St Mark's Unitarian Church in Edinburgh, where the lecture-workshop was held for about thirty people. This indicated an incremental shift in public opinion in England, where a number of Nitschke's presentations had formerly been blocked.

While England struggled with end-of-life issues, the Scots brought their own independent perspective to the discussion. A young rebel and a spirited, pioneering grandmother led the way.

– 16 –

Those Feisty Scots

People who promote legislative change are working to help future generations. People who are involved with self-deliverance are trying to help people here and now.
— Christopher Docker, Director, Exit (Scotland)

To put it mildly, the Scots are a highly independent lot, quick to bristle in the face of outside authority. They have a long tradition of refusing to be ruled by others, especially their powerful English neighbors to the south, and are determined to chart their own course. Frustrated by the inability of the British voluntary euthanasia society (then called British Exit) to produce a practical self-deliverance manual for terminally ill people, Scottish members separated to form Scottish Exit. Their specific goal: to publish reliable self-deliverance guidance.[1]

In their autumn 1981 newsletter, they published a paper by noted investigative journalist and death penalty opponent Sir Ludovic Kennedy, "Why I Want to Choose My Moment of Death." It advocated that every adult sign a legally binding advance medical directive specifying what medical practices the person wanted—or wanted to ban—if he or she became terminally ill or was in "great pain and/or distress." He also advocated that "in every hospital there should be kept under lock and key a supply of lethal pills, and when a patient feels that he can no longer stand the pain and misery of being kept alive, he should have the right to call for one of these."[2]

On October 23, 1981, Scottish Exit's *How to Die With Dignity*, the world's first manual for rational suicide, was launched. It was written by Dr. George B. Mair, a retired surgeon horrified at the pain and suffering he had witnessed in his practice. His radical and eagerly anticipated guide was available only to those who had been Exit members for three months or more to help avoid impulsive, irrational suicides.[3] As did his previous book, *Confessions of a Surgeon*, in which he described cases where he provided assisted suicide to terminally ill patients, Mair's new publication severely rattled British public opinion.

By 1992, younger blood was running in Scottish Exit's veins. Christopher "Chris" Docker, then thirty-nine—just a baby in an organization whose members had a median age of seventy plus—

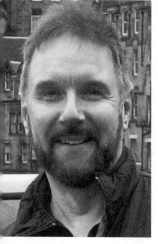

was becoming progressively more active. A native of Birmingham, England, Docker adopted Scotland as his home in his teens.

The nonconformist streak that led him to become involved in human rights and civil liberties issues started at the age of fifteen. Having read the barbarous history of the Christian church and compared it with the gentler ideologies of creeds such as Buddhism, the precocious young man wrote to his Anglican vicar and resigned from his religion.[4]

He began to make his mark in the field of voluntary euthanasia as assistant editor of the Exit newsletter. In 1992, during the Ninth Biennial Congress of the World Federation of Right to Die Societies, held in Kyoto, he made a fortuitous connection. The research-oriented Docker met Cheryl Smith, then the staff attorney for the Hemlock Society.

Christopher "Chris" Docker

He asked her whether anyone had ever methodically collated evidence about the efficiency of self-deliverance drugs. Docker, who would soon earn a master's degree in philosophy with a specialization in law and ethics in medicine, wrote, "We were distributing Derek Humphry's *Final Exit* to our members, as well as *How to Die With Dignity*, yet there seemed to be little or no agreement within the scientific community about what drugs and what dosages could be relied on to cause death."[5]

Two years later, he and Smith instigated an unpaid, nonprofit research collective known as the International Drugs Consensus Working Party to help identify, sort, and evaluate a huge mass of evidence about the relative lethality of various drugs.

"After about eighteen months' work, we got near a final draft," Docker told me.[6] "We even did some practical experiments with Dr.

Colin Brewer—who probably was the first to think of compiling a suicide guide—with a plastic bag over his head, asking us to watch for blue fingertips, which is the sign of anoxia."[7]

In 1993, the result of the collaboration was the first edition of *Departing Drugs*, a seventy-eight-page booklet that became a valuable reference for the right-to-die community and was published in English, German, Spanish, and Dutch. As a safeguard, it was available only to those who could prove that they had been a member of a right-to-die group for at least three months. *Departing Drugs* was followed in 1995 by a collection of Docker's articles published in *Beyond Final Exit* by John Hofsess' Last Rights Publications.

In 2007, Docker crystallized his thoughts into a book, *Five Last Acts*, which was expanded upon in 2010. A review in the World Federation of Right to Die Societies' newsletter described it as "what may be the most comprehensive guide to self-deliverance techniques available." It focused on the five self-deliverance methods Docker believed to be most useful:

1. The helium and exit bag system, developed by NuTech in 1999
2. A sleeping pill overdose combined with a plastic bag, an older, but still viable, technique
3. Drug overdoses alone, with special attention to a combination of chloroquine and a strong sedative, such as Nembutal
4. Voluntary refusal of food and fluids (also known as stopping eating and drinking or voluntary death by dehydration), under controlled medical supervision and palliative pain control
5. Ligature compression, i.e., self-compression of the carotid arteries and jugular vein to stop blood flow to and from the brain.

In addition to creating publications to help suffering people end their lives peacefully, Docker used the power of a new medium to reach those who needed this guidance. In 1995, he took his organization to the internet, providing what would become a vast reference resource for information on voluntary euthanasia, living wills, and voluntary refusal of food and fluids.

Like John Hofsess' DeathNET (now offline), which was launched the same year, the Scottish site got massive media attention, most of which was sensationalistic. The *London Times* produced a cartoon of a computer with "Game Over" and the heading, "Deathly Hush Falls on the Internet." Others ran headlines such as "Scottish Group Spreads Euthanasia on the Internet."[8]

As Docker noted, "This [was] the fastest response the Society [had] ever seen on such a scale. Within three hours of circulating a press release on a bank holiday we had achieved four media interviews. Death on the 'Net' [was] obviously of interest to a lot of people."[9]

Since 2004, Docker has run hands-on workshops for Scottish Exit members in Scotland and England, teaching them legal ways to make or acquire the means for self-deliverance. This is a clear dividing line between Exit and its current English counterpart, Dignity in Dying. In Scotland, it is not an offense to assist a suicide, but in some cases, a person might be charged with homicide.

"Exit's primary focus is providing self-deliverance information," Docker told me. "We publish a newsletter and do workshops. The [London-based] society is much better equipped to handle politics, but they don't handle self-deliverance information."[10]

That was a diplomatic understatement. Dignity in Dying considers promoters of do-it-yourself, self-deliverance techniques to be poison in the well; a major obstacle to achieving reform of the antiquated British anti-assisted-suicide laws. Docker's comments summed up the right-to-die world's primal internal policy split: legislative change vs. do-it-yourself deathing education.

"We need both," Docker continued. "They [Dignity in Dying] are focusing on what they're good at: legislative reform. We're focusing on what we're good at: educating people how to help themselves right now. There's no conflict of interest. People who promote legislative change are working to help future generations. People who are involved with teaching self-deliverance techniques are trying to help people here and now."[11]

However, there is one thing that Scottish Exit and British voluntary euthanasia groups agree upon: their disdain for the well-publicized, controversial, "safe suicide" workshops that Australia's Philip Nitschke runs in England, Ireland, and Scotland. To the British, Irish, and Scots, Nitschke is a foreign poacher, making trouble for them on their own turf—and then leaving. In England, Jo Cartwright from Dignity in Dying exclaimed, "What he is doing is irresponsible and unlawful and we had hoped that he would be deported. We now want the various police forces to stop the meetings from happening!"[12]

To avoid being banned in Britain, as was Nitschke, Docker em-

ploys the pragmatic strategy espoused by Canadian euthanasia activist John Hofsess. He believes that right-to-die activists who skirt
the edge of the law should fly under the radar, giving them a better
chance to reach and help the people they seek to serve, rather than
scream the message from the housetops and draw return fire from
opposing groups and law enforcement agencies.

Instead of providing right-to-die advice to individuals in person
or on the telephone, which might be construed as aiding and abetting a suicide, Docker runs how-to seminars. He makes it clear that
he will tell attendees the best means that anyone can use to end his
or her life, but he will not make recommendations or engage in any
personal counseling.

"If you tell me, 'Chris, I'm going to end it all tonight, can you just
run through the method with me again?' and I do so, I'm probably
committing a crime," Docker said. "And if I go to prison, then I
won't be able to help anybody. I can either be a sounding board for
you at the end of life, or I can provide you with information. But if
I only provide you the information, it's without the knowledge that
you're about to use it for suicide."[13]

Docker's cautious approach was not enough for some Scottish Exit members. Fundamental differences of opinion over goals,
methods, management, and finances resulted in the birth of a second Scottish right-to-die organization, Friends at the End (FATE),
in 2000.

Dr. Elizabeth "Libby" Wilson, a death-with-dignity advocate
from Glasgow who refuses to be muzzled, was one of those who
did not agree with quiet, under-the-radar methods. Wilson publi-
cally confronts social injustices head-on and has for more than fifty
years. While she was still an Exit member, Wilson's chapter in Glasgow established a program similar to the Hemlock Society's Caring
Friends group. It offered person-specific advice on self-deliverance,
which was a legal concern for Exit and later for FATE. But for Wilson, her personal counseling involvement in the right-to-die movement was a logical progression from her role as a pioneer family
planning physician in the slums of Glasgow in the 1970s and 1980s.

Born Elizabeth Bell Nicoll in 1926 in South London, she attended a boarding school staffed largely by Quakers, whose ethics
and compassion she greatly admired. "I think if I had any religious
belief I would identify most closely with their doctrines," she wrote.

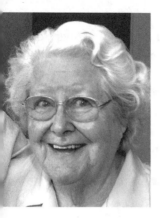

Dr. Elizabeth "Libby" Wilson

"They have intellectualized religion and discarded most of the irrational dogma I find so repugnant."[14]

Her parents were both Church of Scotland missionaries, serving first in Chamba, a small hill state in the foothills of the Himalayas in India, and then in Nyasaland, Portuguese East Africa.[15] From her mother, in particular, she saw what it was to stand strong in her beliefs and hold a passionate commitment to helping others.

Before the end of World War II, Libby entered medical school at King's College, London. There, she earned a degree in medicine and surgery and fell in love with Graham Wilson, an ex-Royal Air Force medical officer. They married two weeks after she received her degree. Her entire medical career was spent at the cutting edge of medical ethics. In 1954, she earned a certificate in family planning and began work in the Sheffield branch of the Family Planning Association. This office was run by a group of highly committed Nonconformist and Quaker ladies ready and willing to defy the political correctness and religious orthodoxy of the time by championing the cause of birth control, especially for overburdened poor women. Later, Wilson worked with local policewomen, training them how to deal with the special health needs of rape victims and prostitutes.

The storm over female empowerment raged in the 1960s, when the birth control pill came on the market, allowing women to effectively control their own reproductive options for the first time. The opposition from the Catholic Church was ferocious.

When Wilson and a colleague created a clinic in Sheffield for the unmarried, "There was a big headline in the *Sheffield Telegraph,* 'Bishop condemns sex clinic.' Absolutely brilliant! We had all the free publicity we were quite unable to have gotten in any other way."[16] And the Sheffield postman knew where he should deliver mail addressed to 'The Den of Iniquity. Ecclesall Road.'"[17]

When her husband died of cancer in 1977, Wilson made a major change. At the age of sixty-four, when many women would be taking up gardening and focusing on their grandchildren, she left Scotland to spend a year as a volunteer physician in poverty-stricken, war-torn Sierra Leone.[18] There she saw a whole new level of suffering, particularly among children. Often deprived of even the most basic medical supplies, and surviving serious threats from the warring factions, she returned home in 1991, acutely aware of the enormous number of those for whom no medical help would ever be available.

"I have no illusions about 'doing good,'" she wrote. "I learnt as much about life and humanity as I had taught about conception…. One can only do the work in front of one on a day-to-day basis, as each patient deserves one's whole attention and skill."[19]

Throughout her career, Wilson believed it was imperative for patients to know all their options. When she retired from medical practice, it seemed logical to campaign for those who wanted a choice at the end of life. Recruited by Scottish Exit, she transferred her caring skills from medicine to death-with-dignity advocacy. She helped to organize the Glasgow and West of Scotland chapter of Scottish Exit and published a regular newsletter.[20]

Wilson knew her opposition: "Well-organized, well-funded, and from exactly the same people I was opposed by in my earlier life. Mostly people who have strong religious beliefs. I respect people with strong religious beliefs. They're entitled to have them, but I don't see why their religious beliefs should override mine…. [They] produce a lot of specious arguments about slippery slopes and vulnerable people and all sorts of things, which actually has very little validity in fact."[21]

After she parted company with Docker's Scottish Exit organization in February 1999, Wilson continued her end-of-life counseling without skipping a beat. Her newly apostate group temporarily adopted the name Phoenix but formally changed it to Friends at the End (FATE) in November 2000.[22] Started from scratch with about twenty-five members, FATE currently has more than five hundred, with equal numbers in England and Scotland.[23]

In August 2005, FATE faced an important test. May Murphy decided to end her life at the Dignitas facility in Switzerland. The seventy-five-year-old widow from Glasgow was suffering from the end stages of multiple system atrophy. She was the first Scot that FATE helped to die using "the Swiss option."

To avoid an effective prosecutorial legal challenge, FATE organized a group of elderly helpers, each with a separate role, so that prosecutors would have to identify, collect, and try an entire herd of golden-agers for the alleged crime. It was the same mass-civil-diso-bedience defense strategy used earlier by other death-with-dignity activists, such as Philip Nitschke.

"One person. . .got money out of the bank for [Murphy]," Wil-son said. "Another got the airline tickets at the airport, and some-body else went to the Registry Office in Edinburgh to get her birth certificate and marriage certificate and all the papers the Swiss au-thorities demand. Michael Irwin [a member of FATE's board] came up from England. . . . [He] flew off with her to Zürich, and I took her wheelchair back to her house."[24]

Soon afterward, FATE developed a working relationship with Dignitas. In an announcement that made front-page headlines, FATE declared that it had produced a booklet outlining the costs and step-by-step procedures necessary to obtain aid in dying at the Dignitas facility.[25]

Written and edited by Wilson and her colleague, Nan Maitland, and published in February 2007, the *UK Guide to Dignitas* was avail-able only to FATE members. The content made it clear that Dignitas was not a death-on-demand service or a walk-in deathing center. The Swiss required extensive pre-screening of medical records and two face-to-face meetings with doctors in Switzerland to determine if the candidate (who had to be a member of Dignitas) was eligible to receive an assisted suicide there.

When FATE advertised the *UK Guide to Dignitas*, its most vo-ciferous opponents—the Catholic Church, the Church of Scotland, and right-to-life campaigners—were outraged. Julia Millington, po-litical director of the ProLife Alliance, was indignant, "We would be very concerned about the move to promote the services of Digni-tas....We feel that it would be appropriate for police to investigate the activities of FATE."[26]

That never happened. Wilson and her colleagues ignored the pro-tests. Other books about assisted suicide had already been published in Scotland since 1981, starting with Dr. Mair's revolutionary *How to Die With Dignity*. Hence, *The UK Guide to Dignitas* broke no new ground at all. It has never been challenged by Scottish prosecutors, a testament to the fact that its information is entirely legal and that the demand for accurate information about end-of-life issues can no longer be stopped by calls for state censorship by religious zealots.

Wilson's compassion, and the price that altruistic people some-times have to pay, came to international attention in 2009 in the form of Caroline "Cari" Loder. A former lecturer at London University's Institute of Education, she was a prominent multiple sclerosis researcher. In 1994, she discovered a new treatment for multiple sclerosis that came to be known as "The Cari Loder Regime." While it was cruelly ironic that the disease she studied for so many years finally came to claim her own life, Loder's intimate professional knowledge of the illness and its progression put her in the best possible place to evaluate her own end-of-life options rationally.

Research on the internet directed her to FATE, and she contacted Libby Wilson. Although she had already chosen the fast-acting helium self-deliverance system to end her life, Loder wanted advice on some critical steps. Like everyone with a degenerative disease, Loder knew that she had only a narrow window of opportunity to end her life on her own terms. She had to act soon so that she could turn the knob on the helium canister using her own hands, without exposing anyone else to possible prosecution.

Always independent, Loder lived alone despite her disabilities and was determined not to go into residential care.[27] "She knew her condition was worsening and she told me she wanted to do this sooner rather than later. I asked her if she was utterly sure," Wilson said. Loder immediately replied, "Yes, absolutely."[28]

After asking a neighbor to walk her dog, Loder died at her home in Surrey on June 8, 2009, to the sound of Frank Sinatra's "I Did It My Way" and wearing a T-shirt with the poignant message, "Live life to the full."[29] She had used the helium system. When the police searched her home, they found Wilson's email address on Loder's computer, making Wilson a suspect in a potential assisted suicide.

Wilson was legally required to travel the four hundred miles from her home in Glasgow to Surrey to be interrogated about her involvement with Loder's death. She was well prepared for police questioning, having learned from other right-to-die activists what to expect.

On September 28, 2009, when the holding-cell door slammed shut on Libby Wilson, the cheerful, eighty-three-year-old, white-haired, retired Scottish physician was calm and relaxed.

"My granddaughter, Elizabeth, who thought she might be interested in joining the police, asked if she could come down and watch me get arrested," she beamed after her release on bail that afternoon.[30] When she arrived at the police station, the cherubic-looking mother of six and grandmother of eighteen was arrested and put in the holding cell. Next, she was fingerprinted, photographed, searched, and had DNA samples taken by the Major Crime Investigating Team. They also confiscated her shoelaces, in case she was inclined to try to take her own life with them.

To pass the time in the bare, whitewashed jail cell, she brought along a thick book of crossword puzzles. "I wasn't even allowed to use my own pen," she chuckled. "I had to borrow theirs."[31]

After six hours of interrogation by detectives, most of which was consumed by equipment problems and red tape, she was released on bail on suspicion of aiding and abetting a suicide, with instructions to return on November 18.

Wilson was the first person to be arrested after English Director of Public Prosecution (DPP) Keir Starmer released guidelines outlining how he would decide who would and would not be prosecuted in such cases. Two others, including a male neighbor of Loder's and a friend from West London, had already been taken into custody on suspicion of helping Loder die and were also charged and released pending possible trial.

Loder had ordered the helium tank as part of a standard party balloon kit via the internet, along with the plastic hood designed specifically for a helium self-deliverance. She also bought the latest edition of *Final Exit*, which explained the helium exit procedure in detail.[32] She left a detailed written statement explaining that she had ended her own life, hoping to forestall a police investigation of her friends.[33]

"I provided information," said Wilson. "That's it. And, under the European Convention on Human Rights, individuals who want to commit a legal act are entitled to have all the information possible to enable them to perform it efficiently."[34]

Based on their new guidelines, the Crown Prosecution Service ultimately dropped all charges against Wilson and Loder's two other accused friends. The DPP's spokesman noted, "Ms. Loder had plainly intended to commit suicide, and there is no evidence that the advice given contributed significantly to the outcome. It has been concluded [that] a prosecution of [Wilson] is not required in the public interest."[35]

When asked if she thought the battle for legalized assisted suicide could be won, Wilson replied, "Eventually, but not till after I'm dead because politicians are lily-livered skunks. They haven't got the courage of their convictions. . . .[They] are afraid of the religious vote....The great majority of them won't stick their necks out."[36]

Margo MacDonald was a striking exception to this rule. According to her colleague, Tom Brown, "Margo has attained the status of national treasure. Politics apart, in our frequently disappointing Scottish Parliament, if a voice can be raised for straightforward commonsense and an unflinching ability to face the hard facts, it is usually Margo's."[37]

MacDonald first won election as member of the Scottish Parliament (MSP) in 1973 and served two terms. During the 1980s, she had a successful career as a dynamic presenter of Scottish radio and television programs. In 1999, she returned to Parliament as a representative for the Lothians District as an Independent and was still representing her district as this book went to press. She has a personal stake in Wilson's cause.

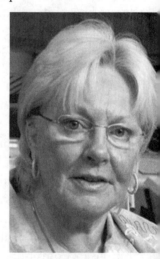

The vivacious sixty-eight-year-old stared in amazed bewilderment as she watched the video playing on her computer. In order to prepare a bill to legalize physician-hastened death in Scotland, MacDonald was researching death-with-dignity concepts and had come across the internationally famous YouTube sensation, "Do It Yourself with Betty."[38] Produced by Philip Nitschke's Exit International, the video shows Betty Peters, a smiling, chirpy great-grandmother and former registered nurse educator, giving a

Margo MacDonald, MSF

detailed demonstration on how to create a homemade helium exit bag from readily available materials. It was YouTube's most viewed video on voluntary euthanasia in 2007 and made the almost-octogenarian Betty an unlikely poster child for the death-with-dignity movement. The video quickly went viral.

"I'd never seen anything this bizarre in my life, I think," MacDonald laughed. MacDonald is slowly dying from Parkinson's disease. With a little more research, she learned that professionally made exit bags could be purchased for $60 online and ordered one.

"Until I saw the exit bag, I think I still had a valid academic approach to this; perhaps theoretical," she said.[39] Holding the exit bag in her hands made the fact of self-deliverance quite clear. Those who are physically able can choose when, where, and how their deaths will occur. But those who do not have the physical ability can use other means of elective dying, such as closely monitored voluntarily refusal of eating and drinking.

In March 2008, MacDonald stood before her fellow MSPs at the Parliament Building in Edinburgh's Holyrood District and delivered a short speech in favor of the new End of Life Assistance Bill. The bill, which she had authored, would legalize euthanasia and assisted suicide in Scotland.

"I think it's very healthy for all of us to consider the value of our life. I think it's just as healthy . . . . that you should concern yourself with your contribution to the general society throughout your life, that is, right until the moment of death."[40] Speaking from the podium in a firm voice, with both arms shaking noticeably from her disease, MacDonald continued:

> As you know, I have a degenerative condition, and I would like to have the right to determine by how much my capacity to fulfill my social function, my familial function, my personal function, is going to be truncated. And I would like the ability to make that decision. I don't want to burden any doctor; I don't want to burden any friend or family member. I want to find a way that I can make a decision to end my life in case I am unlucky enough to have the worst form of Parkinson's at the end of life.
>
> You will have noticed from letters I have received that the medical practitioners here admit that in every case, palliative care is not necessarily as effective as everyone would want it to be, and I'm mindful of that.... I am mindful of what the doctors say and how difficult it is for them. However, I have read the personal testimony of doctors and have seen doctors who have admitted in court to assisting a suicide. They are no less doctors in my estimation. And can I congratulate Jeremy [Purvis, MSP] for [having brought this bill] to Parliament as

quickly as he could. There are many, many people who have a lot less time than I have.[41]

She was the second MSP to undertake firsthand research on assisted dying. The first had been Jeremy Purvis, whose attempt to have the issue debated had fallen at the first legislative hurdle in 2005. Purvis was not alone. Similar bills had failed, even though, for more than two decades, the majority of Scots have frequently and unambiguously stated that they want access to voluntary euthanasia and assisted suicide for the terminally ill and those in extreme, uncontrollable pain.

MacDonald's bill faced rough sledding. According to James Park, an American existential philosopher and strong proponent of such safeguards in physician-hastened-death laws, it lacked adequate safeguards. A Scottish colleague concurred. "One problem they [politicians] have is that each time they put forth a bill, they think they are inventing the wheel," commented Chris Docker. "In spite of the fact that [Scottish] Exit spent a considerable sum enabling Glasgow University to research and propose good legislation, the politicians only ask [the death-with-dignity movement's] opinion *after* they have written the draft. By that time it is too late to suggest the type of legislation that would stand a better chance of getting through, as it contains superior safeguards."[42]

In addition, the bill had already fallen victim to behind-the-scenes political skullduggery. Opposition MSPs who managed the parliamentary diary ordered that it be considered by a special ad hoc committee, rather than by the health committee, where it belonged. MacDonald was furious.

Another familiar hurdle was the highly organized opposition from the Catholic Church (which comprises only 16 percent of the Scottish population) and conservative Protestants, despite the fact that the majority of Scottish citizens are unchurched. The Reverend John Cameron, a leading Church of Scotland (Protestant) minister—in defiance of the official position of his denomination—praised the concept of voluntary assisted suicide and physician-hastened death. "At present, we force citizens facing terrible deaths to fly out prematurely to Switzerland since they must be sufficiently fit to travel. As a society, we are refusing to face this matter head-on and are offloading our ethical dilemma to another country. This is surely morally unacceptable."[43]

In April 2010, a few months before the final vote on MacDonald's bill, an international professional polling firm posed the following question to 1,001 adult Scots: "The Scottish Parliament is considering the End of Life Assistance (Scotland) Bill, which would allow people with intolerable terminal illnesses to be assisted if they wish to end their own life. Do you agree that this option should be available to people in Scotland?" The result: 77 percent of those who responded supported the legislation; 12 percent opposed it; and the remaining 11 percent were unsure.[44]

The decisive parliamentary vote on MacDonald's bill took place on December 1, 2010. It failed to pass, with sixteen votes supporting it, eighty-five against, and two abstentions. With wry humor, Christopher Docker wrote, "With a landslide parliamentary vote against assisted suicide—and a landslide public opinion poll in favour—one has to ask if any members of the Scottish Parliament actually support the Scottish people?"

George Anderson, representing the senior citizens' group, Militant Retired, found a unique way to vent his disgust with the public's inability to penetrate the personal prejudices and political intransigence of their elected representatives. He challenged the Scottish Parliament to authorize a public referendum. Colorfully and succinctly, he posed the question to be discussed: "Why are terminally ill people being forced into exile in the same way as lepers in medieval times?"[45]

The response was a thundering silence from Holyrood.

In April 2011, despite the recent poll showing 77 percent support in Scotland for physician aid-in-dying, a spokesman for the Catholic Church nevertheless made a completely false, baseless, and totally predictable knee-jerk response. "The fact that the Scottish Parliament last year rejected the Assisted Suicide Bill was widely accepted as representing the settled will of the Scottish people and it's difficult to imagine that public opinion could have shifted in such a short period of time. The vote showed Scottish public opinion is not in favour of euthanasia."[46] Indeed, the twelve-month-old poll showed exactly the opposite.

Undaunted by the unsubstantiated claims, MacDonald stated her plan to reintroduce the bill in 2011. "Because the Swiss have open minds and big hearts, politicians here are dodging the dilemma posed by the small number of people for whom palliative care and drug therapy do not afford the peaceful death which all of us seek."[47]

Undeterred by Scotland's legislative stubbornness, Nan Maitland, Libby Wilson's close friend and collaborator on the *UK Guide to Dignitas*, took her own advice and ended her life in the Swiss fa-

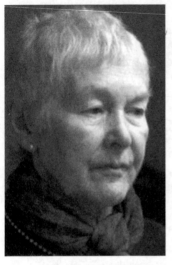

cility on March 1, 2011. She had cofounded the Society for Old Age Rational Suicide (SOARS) with British euthanasia advocate Dr. Michael Irwin and was also a member of Wilson's FATE. A mother of three and a retired occupational therapist, Maitland was passionate about helping the elderly retain their independence for as long as possible. She provided advice from her home in Chelsea. She was not terminally ill but had crippling arthritis and did not want to face further deterioration.

Nan Maitland

In the company of Dr. Irwin and Liz Nichols, another friend and FATE member, Maitland enjoyed a convivial three-hour meal at a five-star hotel in Zürich. The next day, she and her companions made the short trip to the Dignitas facility in Pfäffikon. There, with her friends beside her, she drank a lethal dose of Nembutal and quickly died. In her final note, she wrote, "For some time, my life has consisted of more pain than pleasure and, over the next months and years the pain will be more and the pleasure less. I have a great feeling of relief that I will have no further need to struggle through each day in dread of what further horrors may lie in wait. For many years, I have feared the long period of decline, sometimes called *'prolonged dwindling,'* that so many people unfortunately experience before they die. Please be happy for me.... I have had a wonderful life and the good fortune to die at a time of my choosing."[48]

Dr. Michael Irwin said, "There are many elderly individuals who get to the last years of their natural lives and have to seriously consider whether departing this existence will be much more attractive than struggling on."[49]

Sue Brayne, director and moderator of MyHealthtalk.org., wrote:

[Maitland] planned her death, to my mind, purposefully, courageously, and without drama. In the note that she left behind, she made it clear that she had no wish to enter a prolonged period of painful decline before death that many elderly experience. It really is time that we as a society learned to respect *quality* of life more than life at any cost. For me, Nan Maitland's selfless action of ending her life with such composure is a lesson to us all. It's a travesty that she wasn't allowed to die in her own home, in her own bed, surrounded by those she loved, at the time of her own choosing. Rather, she had to get on an airplane and fly to a foreign country to take a lethal dose in a location that meant nothing to her. Shame on us all.[50]

Support for Maitland's beliefs came both from the professionally conducted Scottish poll and from one commissioned by SOARS in the United Kingdom in 2011. There, two-thirds of those who responded agreed that elderly people who suffer from serious (but not necessarily life-threatening) illnesses should have the right to physician aid-in-dying.

The number of assisted suicides at Dignitas by members from the United Kingdom continues to rise every month. The English and Scottish publics have decided that their anti-assisted-suicide laws are now dysfunctional and obsolete. But the British law is the model for virtually identical versions in Canada, Ireland, Northern Ireland, Australia, and New Zealand. If the British law, now creaking and groaning under the strain, finally crumbles, it will force other countries to reconsider their own.

A Rising Tide Lifts
All Ships

All truth passes through three stages. First, it is ridiculed. Second, it is violently opposed. Third, it is accepted as being self-evident.
—Arthur Schopenhauer

Throughout the world, people now have access to a wide variety of end-of-life choices, many of which did not exist two decades ago. Right-to-die societies worldwide provide information about advance medical directives, counsel and console the dying, and offer advice on how to achieve a "good death." In addition, self-deliverance methods are readily available to enable rational adults to choose the time, place, and circumstances of a peaceful, painless death, surrounded, if they choose, by family and other loved ones.

Medical advancements have also dramatically changed our quality of life. Some diseases have been eradicated. Faster, better, and cheaper cures have been found for many others. Surgery can fix numerous damaged organs or replace them with donor-provided transplants or mechanical devices. And around the world, life expectancies have lengthened.

But in some cases, unrestrained use of heroic medical practices, coupled with the lack of death-with-dignity laws, has only extended the duration, pain, and agony of dying. And in the less open-minded and more indigent countries, the length of a healthy life and the quality of death remain as poor as they were a half-century ago.

As medical miracles began to profoundly change the definitions of life and death, the right-to-die movement emerged with the intent of adding the word "good" as the antecedent of the word "death." Starting in the mid-1970s, these organizations began to form alliances based upon a common philosophy: "My life. My death. My

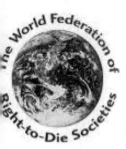

choice." When the Japan Euthanasia Society, now named the Japan Society for Dying with Dignity, was founded in 1976, Dr. Tenrei Ohta called for an international meeting of the existing national right-to-die societies. The 1976 Tokyo conference was attended by representatives from Japan, Australia, the Netherlands, the United Kingdom, and the United States. Attendees quickly recognized the need for vastly improved communication to enable them to benefit from each other's experiences and to obtain a broader international perspective on right-to-die issues. Two years later, a second international conference was hosted in the United States by the Society for the Right to Die, and plans were initiated to form an international organization to further common goals.

The World Federation of Right to Die Societies was founded in 1980 at the third conference of the working group. Held in Oxford, England, and sponsored by Exit, The Society for the Right to Die with Dignity (now known as Dignity in Dying), it brought together twenty-seven groups from eighteen nations. Its member organizations had varying goals and ways to achieve these, but all were dedicated to advancing personal autonomy at the end of life. Collectively, their strategies included both achieving legislative change to allow physician aid-in-dying and promoting individual education to enable rational, well-informed people to end their lives in a peaceful and dignified manner without involving anyone else. Each group, however, was sovereign in choosing which strategies to follow.

Although membership in the world federation has fluctuated over the years, depending upon the evolving views of its member organizations, the group represented the first attempt to bring an international focus to the death-with-dignity movement. It also played a vital role in disseminating information among countries, which eliminates duplication of effort and enables groups to learn from others' successes and failures.

As of this writing, four countries have legalized physician aid-in-dying by statute: Switzerland (1942), the Netherlands (2002), Belgium (2002), and Luxembourg (2009). Colombia decriminalized both assisted suicide and euthanasia by decision of the Colombian Constitutional Court in 1997. Legal euthanasia and assisted suicide (chiefly the former) have been practiced there since then, but no federal law regulating the procedure or reporting it has been passed by the Colombian legislature.

In the United States, two states have legalized assisted suicide by statute: Oregon (1994) and Washington (2008). Montana decriminalized assisted suicide in 2009 by a state supreme court decision, but no state law regulating the procedure or requiring reporting it has so far been passed by its legislature. Most recently, on February 6, 2012, the Georgia Supreme Court unanimously struck down that state's 1994 anti-assisted suicide law on the basis that it did not criminalize assisting a suicide but only forbade advertising the availability of assisted suicide counseling—a violation of the Constitution's First Amendment guarantee of freedom of speech.[1] The drive to decriminalize assisted suicide through the establishment of Oregon-style laws is currently on the front burner in Vermont, Massachusetts, and Hawaii. More state challenges, supported by voter initiatives and the formidable Compassion & Choices legal team, are planned or underway.

The status of an individual's right to die varies enormously by nation. Several country-by-country lists of the legal status of assisted suicide and euthanasia have been published in the last decade. However, none were comprehensively researched or formally documented because a full, accurate study would require massive and costly legal research. Therefore, the information that follows focuses chiefly on countries not already mentioned that have made significant, well-documented changes to their right-to-die laws since 1997.

The Belgians were among the earliest to form a death-with-dignity group. Association pour le Droit de Mourir dans la Dignité (ADMD) Belgique was formed in Brussels in 1981. Two years later, Léon Favyts founded Recht op Waardig Sterven (RWS) to serve the Flemish portion of the country. In 1988, RWS published an explicit, anonymous, thirty-two-page right-to-die manual, *Handleiding voor Vrijwillige Milde Dood* (*Instruction for Voluntary Gentle Death*) in Antwerp. It was available only to members of six months' standing.

In 2002, Belgium became the second European Union country to approve physician aid-in-dying, when it approved three complementary laws. Senator Philippe Mahoux, a member of the Socialist Party, helped draft the patient's rights law. This law embodied the concept that only the dying person should be the judge of his or her quality of life and the dignity of his or her last moments and outlined the text of directives concerning the withholding of medical treatment.[2] The second law addressed palliative care, and the third governed euthanasia.[3]

Belgium's *Act on Euthanasia* went into effect on September 22, 2002. Following the Dutch model, the act defined euthanasia as "intentionally terminating life by someone other than the person concerned, at the latter's request," and stated:

> The physician who performs euthanasia commits no criminal offense when he/she ensures that the patient has attained the age of majority or is an emancipated minor, and is legally competent and conscious at the moment of making the request; [that the request] is voluntary, well-considered, and repeated, and is not the result of any external pressure; and that the patient is in a medically futile condition of constant and unbearable physical or mental suffering that cannot be alleviated, resulting from a serious and incurable disorder caused by illness or accident, and when he/she has respected the conditions and procedures provided in this Act.[4]

The measure was opposed by the Flemish Christian Democrat party and most of Belgium's dwindling number of practicing Catholics. Catholicism had traditionally been Belgium's majority religion, especially in the Flanders region, but the percentage of Belgian religious believers overall has diminished drastically in the last forty years. From 1967 to 2009, for example, attendance at Sunday mass dropped from 42.9 percent to 5 percent.[5]

On September 30, 2002, Mario Verstraete, a thirty-nine-year-old man from Ghent and a long-standing campaigner for assisted suicide who suffered from multiple sclerosis, was the first to take advantage of the law.[6] Between then and December 31, 2007, 1,917 cases of euthanasia were reported.[7] Before and after the law was ratified, Belgian attorney Jacqueline Herremans, past-president of the World Federation of Right to Die Societies, traveled widely throughout Europe and wrote extensively for professional journals and the general media to explain the law and its results.[8]

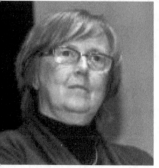

Jacqueline Herremans

The tiny, cosmopolitan, and altogether

charming Grand Duchy of Luxembourg found itself in the middle of a constitutional crisis when its parliament approved its euthanasia law on March 16, 2009.[9] Two primary promoters backed the bill. The first was Jean Huss, a Green Party politician and vice president of Luxembourg's right-to-die group the Association pour le Droit de Mourir dans la Dignité-Leutzebuerg (ADMD-L). The second was Lydie Err, a Socialist lawyer, founding member of ADMD-L, and elected member and former vice president of the Chamber of Deputies for the Luxembourg Socialist Workers' Party. Both had been fighting for the bill for years with heart and commitment, ignoring their opponents' attacks. The Association pour le Droit de Mourir dans la Dignité-Leutzebuerg was founded by Henri Clees, who served as its president for six years until his death.[10]

"This bill is not a permit to kill," said Err. "It's not a law for the parents or the doctors but for the patient and the patient alone to decide if he wants to put an end to his suffering."[11]

When the bill passed in parliament with a 30 to 26 vote, the majority of those who favored it knew the genuine personal anguish that faced Grand Duke Henri Guillaume, Luxembourg's head of state. He ultimately had to choose between his love for his countrymen and women and the doctrine of his Catholic faith. Under Luxembourg's Constitution, a bill passed by parliament does not become law until it is approved by the grand duke. Because he was morally opposed to signing the bill, an impasse seemed certain. Jean-Claude Juncker, Luxembourg's prime minister, also opposed the bill but decided that the grand duke had overstepped the mark in threatening to deny the will of parliament. Juncker noted, "I understand the grand duke's problems of conscience. But I believe that if the parliament votes in a law, it must be brought into force."[12] He declared that in his government, "every parliamentarian should vote on bills according to his personal conscience and conviction."[13]

The impasse was broken when Justice Minister Luc Frieden declared, "The grand duke will no longer participate in the legislative process; he will just sign the law to mark the completion of the procedure."[14] However, the Vatican rewarded the grand duke's religious integrity with the 2009 Cardinal Van Thuan Prize "for his efforts in defending the right to life and freedom of religion." He was also honored with a private audience with Pope Benedict XVI.[15]

Since the 1980s, the French have been among Europe's leaders in producing thoughtful, intellectual books on the peaceful ending of a life. In 1980, Michel L. Landa led the founding of the Association pour le Droit à Mourir dans la Dignité (ADMD-France), which now has over 48,000 members. Landa's forty-page suicide manual, *Autodeliverance* (self-deliverance), written during the last year of his life, was provided free of charge to members of the organization.

In 1982, Claude Guillon and Yves Le Bonniec published *Suicide: Mode d'emploi: Histoire, technique, actualité (Suicide: User's Manual: History, Methods of Use, Reality)*, which was also translated into German and Japanese. A serious, comprehensive work, the book examined historical, social, philosophical, and economic aspects of suicide. The final portion of the book discussed the practical aspects of how to commit suicide, including drug dosage information taken chiefly from Dutch, British, and American publications. It enjoyed huge sales and ample notoriety during its brief lifetime.[16]

France legally banned the sale of all books about euthanasia in 1987. "The new Article 318-1-2 of the French Penal Code introduced a penalty of between two months and three years, or a heavy fine, for the provocation of an attempted or completed suicide. A rider was added to the law making the same penalties applicable to those who 'create propaganda or publicity, regardless of the mode, in favor of products, objects, or methods recognized as ways of bringing about suicide,'" wrote Derek Humphry.[17] "*Final Exit* has been banned since its publication in 1991," he continued, "but few [booksellers] nowadays take any notice of the order."[18]

Technically, France does not have a law specifically banning assisted suicide, but a person could be prosecuted under Section 223-6 of the penal code for failing to assist a person in danger. When this provision has been applied, convictions have been rare and punishments minor, but the law is still on the books.[19] The French have never been bashful about their support for euthanasia, and ADMD-France hosted congresses of the World Federation of Right to Die Societies in Nice in 1984 and in Paris in 2008. I first met the most influential European leaders of the death-with-dignity movement at the Paris conference.

Despite heavy censorship, the French seemed to be well on their way to joining the Dutch as among the most successful death-with-dignity nations in Europe. But the pace slowed. On September 24, 2000, Vincent Humbert, an eighteen-year-old volunteer fireman living in Normandy, suffered a catastrophic car accident that left him quadriplegic, almost blind, and unable to communicate except by moving his right thumb. In 2002, he wrote a letter to French President Jacques Chirac, asking him to waive existing law so that he could be helped to end his life. Chirac commiserated with Humbert and met with his mother, Marie, but refused the request.

The French media took up Humbert's case, generating waves of sympathy for him throughout the country. On September 26, 2003, Humbert's mother injected a lethal dose of barbiturates into his intravenous drip. Instead of killing him, the overdose left him in a coma. Ignoring the furious pleas of Humbert's father to let Vincent die, doctors placed him on life support. However, after determining that keeping him alive would only, at best, restore him to the condition in which he had lived for three years, the physicians withdrew his oxygen and intravenous drip.

Dr. Frédéric Chaussoy, the head of the intensive care unit of the Centre Héliomarin of Berck-sur-Mer, helped Humbert die and took full responsibility for the decision. In his 2004 book, *I Am Not a Murderer*, he explored the depth of the dilemma that he faced when, in direct contravention of the existing law, he acceded to the wishes of his parents by switching off Humbert's life support. Chaussoy was charged with "poisoning with intent to kill." The charges were later dropped.

In 2005, the French passed the *Loi Leonetti* (Leonetti Law), which now governs French end-of-life issues. It allows doctors to stop providing medical assistance when it has no effect other than maintaining life artificially. It also gives patients the right to refuse further medical treatment for incurable illnesses, but it does not permit euthanasia or assisted suicide, even at the express request of the dying person.

Health Minister Philippe Douste-Blazy was quoted in 2005 as saying, "With this law, the end of life in France will have another face: It will be a moment of choice and no longer a moment of submission." The health minister felt that his countrymen did not support active euthanasia, although an independent poll taken in France proved him wrong. Eighty-eight percent of respondents supported a law allowing physician aid-in-dying for terminally ill French citizens.[20]

Although a majority of the French have recently indicated that they support such a law, they face the same head-in-the-sand legislators who have stonewalled progress in many other developed countries. This was demonstrated by the tragic case of Chantal Sébire.

In 2000, Sébire, a retired teacher who lived near Dijon, France, was diagnosed with esthesioneuroblastoma, a rare form of cancer.

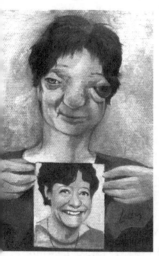

Chantal Sébire

Because of the risks involved, she refused medication and surgery. In time, her face became disfigured, with one eyeball grotesquely enlarged and protruding from her face. She also lost her senses of sight, taste, and smell. She fought unsuccessfully for the right to die by having a French physician provide her with a lethal dose of drugs. In February 2008, she made a public appeal to French President Nicolas Sarkozy asking to be allowed to die through euthanasia, stating, "One would not allow an animal to go through what I have endured."[21] The appeal failed, and a court in Dijon also refused her request. On March 19, 2008, surrounded by her family, she took a lethal dose of barbiturates at home.

In January 2011, the French Senate took a major step towards legalizing physician aid-in-dying. A bill was introduced that would allow "a mature person, in the advanced or terminal phase of an accidental or pathological affliction that is grave or incurable, causing physical or psychological suffering that cannot be relieved, [to] request to receive medical assistance to die."[22] In a vote of the Senate's social affairs committee, twenty-five members supported the bill and nineteen were opposed. Île-de-France regional councillor Jean-Luc Romero, president of ADMD-France, stated, "For the first time in our country's history, the first parliamentary step has been passed in favour of legislation for assisted suicide.[23]"

In response, a group of opposing senators issued a joint statement saying that the law was "regrettable" and parroting the often-raised but threadbare argument that such a law would be a threat to existing legislation that "aims to protect the weakest and most vulnerable and offer to help those who are in a dangerous situation."[24] At a mass rally outside the French parliament building, seven hundred protestors with body bags demonstrated their opposition to the Senate bill. On January 26, 2012, it was defeated by a 172 to 143 vote.

Right-to-die advocates in France's larger neighbor to the east have to struggle with a unique set of ethical circumstances. When it comes to assisted suicide or euthanasia—which the Germans now call *Freitod* (freely chosen death), Germany remains haunted by the ghosts of the Nazi era. During that period, Adolf Hitler carried out a program of racial cleansing, ordering mass executions of millions of Jews, Romani, homosexuals, and physically and mentally disabled persons who did not fit into his vision of a "master race." Many German doctors actively cooperated in the slaughter.

With Hitler's horrific, insane example in mind, modern critics of legalized, safeguarded euthanasia and assisted suicide maintain that adoption of either or both of these will again lead civilization down a slippery slope of moral decay that will inevitably result in the devaluation and neglect of vulnerable classes of people.

Although suicide and assisted suicide have not been illegal in Germany since 1751, German physicians are reluctant to become involved in assisted suicides because of the Nazi atrocities. Direct euthanasia is a crime, but it rarely happens. In 2007, Dr. Christian Arnold pointed out a view of the lingering dilemma that impedes the implementation of modern, humane death-with-dignity laws. As Arnold saw it, "In today's Germany, euthanasia connotes actions that lead to the death of critically ill and incurable persons who indeed wish to die but who would require assistance to implement their wish…. Under Nazism, people were killed against their will, while in present-day Germany, some are kept alive against their freely expressed will." Arnold feels that in both cases, failure to respect the will of the people is a violation of a basic human right and should be seen as such.[25]

The Deutsche Gesellschaft für Humanes Sterben (DGHS)—the German Society for a Humane Death—was formed on November 7, 1980, in Nürnberg. It was the first strong proponent of the death-with-dignity concept in Germany after World War II. Its founding principle held that each person had the unique right, on the grounds of personal autonomy, to end his or her life when, where, and how he or she wished. It currently has over 27,000 members.

Since 1993, the DGHS has focused on providing education and information about the importance of living wills, healthcare proxies, and meeting the challenges of dementia at the end of life, but it does not provide any form of euthanasia or assisted suicide services. Through its own consulting teams, however, it does provide its members with state-of-the-art information on the latest legal techniques of hastened death by self-deliverance.

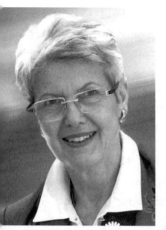

Elke M. Baezner-Sailer, a former high school teacher and now one of the leading right-to-die thinkers and activists in German-speaking Europe, started her human rights work in Switzerland in 1986 as a board member of Exit ADMD Suisse Romande. She later served as president of Exit-Deutsche Schweiz. A veteran right-to-die campaigner and suicide counselor, she became president of the DGHS in 2008. Baezner-Sailer has worked tirelessly for comprehensive legislation in Germany that would respect a patient's rights at the end of

Elke M. Baezner-Sailer

life. She promotes establishing uniform respect for living wills, dealing with end-of-life problems of people who suffer from dementia, and creating conditions to enable voluntary humane death as practiced in Switzerland. She believes that formal education for all levels of end-of-life caregivers is essential and should be widely available.

At the beginning of life, we seek the help of a midwife who serves as a birth attendant . . . who, in French, is known as *'la sage femme,'* meaning the wise [woman] or the one with knowledge. Why should there not be a professional death attendant? This person could either be a man or a woman with a disposition similar to that of a midwife. At a time where 'home births' are becoming increasingly popular, and doctors are not present anymore, dying at home or in the hospital could then be handled as naturally as the act of giving birth. As a counterpart to the gynecologist one could imagine a consultant as a 'thanatologist.' No doubt, at the [outset], the thanatologists would be exposed to the contempt of their colleagues, as were gerontologists twenty years ago, who have now become fully recognized specialists. The course adopted by Exit-Deutsche Schweiz, with its special training programme for assisted suicide attendants, could serve as a model for these new professional areas and could thereby help to ease the relationships between right-to-die societies and the medical profession.[26]

Baezner-Sailer's thanatologist concept is already gaining professional respect and recognition. The Rhode Island University College of Nursing, for example, now offers twelve one-semester undergraduate classes and a respected post-graduate specialization certificate in thanatology.[27]

When an extensive DGHS survey showed that it was no longer possible to grow old with dignity in German nursing homes, the group began to campaign vigorously to obtain better funding for and higher quality of care in such facilities. "The fear of nursing homes among elderly Germans is far greater than the fear of terrorism or the fear of losing your job," noted Eugen Brysch, director of the German Hospice Foundation.[28] Because they lack high-quality eldercare, physician aid-in-dying legislation, and activists who teach self-deliverance methods in their own country, more terminally ill German people travel to the Dignitas and Ex-International facilities in Switzerland than from any other nation.

Roger Kusch, an attorney and a politician representing the Christian Democrat Party, chose not to wait for the German government to clarify its assisted suicide legislation. He decided to facilitate the suicide of seventy-nine-year-old, former X-ray technician Bettina Schardt of Würzburg. Schardt was not terminally ill, but she suffered from diabetes and rheumatism. She contacted Kusch chiefly because she was afraid that she might have to move into a nursing home. Kusch had been an advocate for legalizing assisted suicide for the terminally ill for several years. Just prior to the Schardt case, he established a pro-euthanasia organization, "Dr. Roger Kusch SterbeHilfe e.V." (Roger Kusch Death Assistance), now renamed SterbeHilfe Deutschland e.V.

Kusch told Schardt how to prepare a lethal cocktail that could end her life, and she obtained the relevant drugs and mixed them without his help. Prior to her death, Schardt told Kusch, "If accompanying me until shortly before my death gives you arguments that could persuade politicians to change the law, then my death will have been of some use to other people."[29]

On June 28, 2008, Kusch came to Schardt's apartment, where she was mixing the suicide cocktail of diazepam (Valium) to put her to sleep, and chloroquine, to stop her heart. His video camera was running as she prepared the mixture and took the first sip. He then left the premises, with the video camera running to record her death. When he returned three hours later, Schardt was dead.

Kusch had planned well. Because he did not provide the drugs that killed Schardt, he could not be tried for illegally providing them. And as he was not present when she became unconscious, he could not be charged with failing to act in an emergency to save her.

Shortly after Schardt's death, Kusch called a press conference and played the videotape of

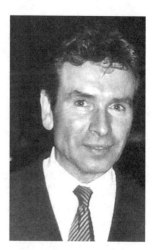

Dr. Roger Kusch

her death, outraging politicians and social workers. The result was an emotional outcry, exemplified by the words of Bavarian Justice Minister Beate Merk. "What Mr. Kusch has done, in my view, is sick and inhuman. Every responsible person would have addressed [Schardt's] fears and given her support. Society shouldn't be moving towards mercy killing but rather improving information about palliative medicine and taking better care of people living alone." [30]

The origin of Kusch's devotion to the death-with-dignity cause was summed up by Jacqueline Jencquel, the secretary general of ADMD-France, who wrote an article about Kusch and his clients. "He is a gentle and kind man," she wrote. "He is acting out of a deep conviction that a person should be able to decide for him/herself when life is not worth living anymore. It was when [Kusch] saw

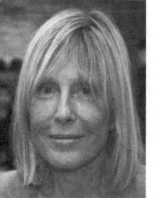

the film, *The Sea Within*, the story of Ramón Sampedro being forced to live for twenty-six years imprisoned in his lifeless body that Roger made up his mind to defend his cause. Roger was very moved by this story and he decided to prevent such cases from happening again and again." [31]

Kusch garnered more attention in March 2008, when he unveiled his Perfusor, a modification of a standard hospital device used to provide long-term intravenous infusions.

Jacqueline Jencquel   Kusch said that he would load it with a dose of sedative, followed by potassium chloride, which would stop the heart. A patient could start the machine by pushing a button. "The machine is simply an option for fatally ill people. Nobody is forced to use it."[32]

The first Perfusor-assisted suicide client was eighty-five-year-old Inge Iassov. After being widowed twice and losing her right breast to cancer, she began to explore the concept of assisted suicide. Her health problems increased when she suffered a stroke. A specialist in neurology and psychiatry examined Iassov and found her desire for assisted suicide to be rational. On September 30, 2008, she ended her life at home, using the Perfusor. The press and the clergy demonized Kusch, but his defenders noted that his assistance in her death was virtually the same as could be obtained across the border in Switzerland, and at a lesser cost.

Max Steinbaur asked Kusch for assistance to end his life in April 2008 and passed a psychiatric examination that October. Just short of ninety-five years of age, he was not terminally ill, but he was incontinent and felt he had nothing to live for. Steinbaur was living in a nursing home with his eighty-nine-year-old wife, who had Alzheimer's disease. He did not feel good about leaving his wife, but he could not bear to watch her getting worse. Steinbaur noted that he and his wife had discussed his desire to die. She said it was his decision and she respected it. He said that she was well and had a nephew who visited her. Steinbaur died at his home on November 12, 2008, after pushing the "start" button on Kusch's Perfusor.

By January 21, 2009, Kusch's website had drawn over one thousand inquiries, and he listed the case histories of five people he helped to die in 2008. That month, he was accused of stepping over the legal line by allegedly providing the drugs used by Inge Iassov to end her life. Violation of the German drug control law could result in a prison sentence of up to three years. That allegation triggered a full-scale police investigation and an injunction to cease his work. Kusch has appealed the order in court, and if he loses his case, he plans to appeal it to Germany's Federal Constitutional Court, which could result in a landmark decision.[33] There is a legal precedent from which Kusch may benefit. In 2000, the Reverend Doctor Rolf Sigg, director of the small Swiss group, Ex-International, traveled to Germany to help a person die. A German appeals court chose not to try him because he had not acted illegally under German law. Although he was convicted of bringing lethal drugs into the country, Sigg was not imprisoned.

Meanwhile, Kusch has continued his work. In his annual report for 2010 (Weißbuch 2011), he stated that SterbeHilfeDeutschland e.V. started the year with 218 members, aged twenty to ninety-four. Their average age was seventy-three, and 57 percent were female. During the year, membership dropped by thirty-six. Four left because they decided not to end their lives prematurely. Two left on other grounds. Nine were dropped from the rolls because they died natural deaths, and twenty-one died via accompanied suicides facilitated by Kusch's group.[34]

German physicians are still conflicted over their official position on physician-hastened death. In February 2011, the German Bundesärztekammer (BAK, or national medical association) announced that it would change its position that medical assistance with suicide is unethical and, therefore, not compatible with professional behavior. The BAK then supported the belief that "such assistance does not belong in the medical repertoire." On June 1, 2011, contrary to what was expected, the majority of delegates voted against changing their code of conduct from "doctors should not actively shorten the lives of dying persons" to "doctors are not allowed to assist in a suicide."[35]

"So," said Elke Baezner-Sailer, "a private medical organization arrogantly tries to supersede existing laws that allow everybody, including physicians, to help legally in self-deliverances under certain circumstances."[36] She added, "The most important criterion making the difference between suicide and mercy killing is the concept of Tatherrschaft (self-empowerment), which means that the person who wants to die acts by himself or herself, is able to take the drugs unaided, and is able to understand the consequences."[37]

Unquenchable memories of the Holocaust also have a chilling effect on the likelihood of passing right-to-die laws in Israel. Orthodox Jews, who hold great power in Israel's parliament, the Knesset, have flatly refused to consider enacting laws that legalize any form of euthanasia or assisted suicide. However, on December 15, 2006, after eight years of discussion, the Terminally Ill Patients Law went into effect, recognizing the right of Israelis to create binding advance healthcare directives. "Active euthanasia will continue to be forbidden," wrote Judy Siegel-Itzkovich in *The Jerusalem Post.*

"However, individuals will be able to set down in advance that they do not want to be attached to a respirator when they are dying or that, if a respirator is attached, it would include a delayed-response timer that can turn itself off automatically at a pre-set time."[38]

Veteran Israeli actress Orna Porat has signed a living will and now carries a special card in her wallet. It declares, "To my doctors, my family, and all hospitals: In the event of an accident or illness from which there is no chance of recovery, I hereby instruct you not to prolong my life by artificial means, and to allow me to die with dignity." It is the standard text on the cards issued by Lilach, the Israel Society for the Right to Live and Die with Dignity.[39]

On November 1, 2009, the nine-thousand-member group sponsored the first Israeli conference to discuss active euthanasia. Held at the Jerusalem Ethics Center, the topic was "Death by Prescription: Ethical Questions in View of Death Approaching." At the same time, a private members' bill, modeled on the Oregon law, was being introduced in the Knesset to allow physicians to help terminal patients die. The bill had the strong support of Professor Avinoam Reches, head of the Israel Medical Association's ethics committee, but it was defeated by a 48 to 16 vote.[40]

In Islamic states, such as Iran, Iraq, and Saudi Arabia, Sharia (Koran-based) law does not tolerate hastening the end of life, and the extent or duration of end-of-life pain is not a factor in determining the matter. In a 2010 fatwah (a religious ruling based upon a scholarly knowledge of the Koran), Dr. Muzammil Siddiqi, of the Fiqh Council of North America, responded to the query, "Is euthanasia allowed in Islam?"

> Islam considers human life sacred. Life is to be protected and promoted as much as possible. It is neither permissible in Islam to kill another human being, nor even to kill one's own self (suicide).... There is no provision in Islam for killing a person to reduce his pain or suffering from sickness. It is the duty of the doctors, patient's relatives, and the state to take care of the sick and to do their best to reduce the pain and suffering of the sick, but they are not allowed under any circumstances to kill the sick person. If, however, a number of medical experts determine that a patient is in a terminal condition and there is no hope for his/her recovery, then it could be permissible for

them to stop the medication. If the patient is on life support, it may be permissible, with due consultation and care, to decide to switch off the life support machine and let the nature take its own time. Under no condition it is permissible to induce death to a patient.[41]

Prior to the implosion and breakup of the former Soviet Union in 1990-1991, the Communist government held an iron grip on all public rights, and both assisted suicide and euthanasia were banned. In present-day Russia, euthanasia and assisted suicide are still illegal. "In the Council of Europe, some of the fiercest opposition against anything dealing with hastened death comes from eastern European states, such as Poland and those of the Communist bloc," said Dr. Rob Jonquière.[42] "Nevertheless, there are sometimes exceptions in the case of 'mercy killings.' In some instances, courts have been sympathetic to people who were charged with helping others to die. In 2004 in Russia, for example, two women were found guilty of manslaughter for ending the life of a paralyzed woman who had asked them to do so. The court nevertheless gave them unexpectedly light sentences."[43]

There is a fundamental difference between how intimate life decisions are made in the West and in the East, and the Japanese approach to the right-to-die issue is a good example. For Westerners, the individual is the center of the universe, and personal autonomy is the lodestar of the decision-making process. For those in Asian countries however, the extended family and the community play a strong role when moral decisions must be made by or for an individual. Dr. Rihito Kimura, a bioethicist and president of Keisen University, Tokyo, wrote:

> At present, a majority of Japanese feel that modern biomedical and medico-technological innovations affecting human life and death have effected a change in our common understanding of the process of death and dying. Historically, death was a natural event, and the criteria for death—cessation of heart beat and respiration—[were] unquestioned. This is no longer the case. An individual's death should be a personal and private matter as well as a familial, communal, and social one. It has been so regarded for many thousands of years in Japanese society and culture. It is well understood that our traditional

socio-cultural understanding of human life admits the natural process of death as a positive event marking of the end of life. The ideas expressed in Zen Buddhist phrases such as 'accept death as it is' and 'life-death as one phenomenon' have been a key motif totally integrated in our traditional understanding of life.[44]

The legal status of euthanasia is unclear in Japan, where several laws and court rulings conflict. A Nagoya High Court decision of 1962, known as the Yamaguchi case, ruled that one can legally end a suffering person's life if specific conditions are fulfilled. Dr. Kimura described the case as follows:

> A son killed his terminally ill father, was charged with homicide, and was prosecuted. The father, a farmer and head of a household, became completely paralyzed. Because of his very severe pain and suffering, the father repeatedly expressed his wish to die, saying, 'Please let me die, please let me go. I want to go to the other world.' The physician informed the family that the farmer's situation was worsening and that his death would probably occur within ten days. The man's son, a kind person, thought that his last filial duty required him to save his father from his severe pain and suffering by killing him, based on his father's verbally articulated 'directive.' The son prepared milk mixed with an agricultural pesticide to which he had ready access at his home. The glass was given to the man by his wife who did not know its poisonous content, and the man died.[45]

In determining the accused son's fate, the Nagoya High Court established six conditions that might mitigate the sentence:

1. The patient's situation should be regarded as incurable with no hope of recovery, and death should be imminent.
2. The patient should be suffering from unbearable and severe pain that cannot be relieved.
3. The act of killing should be undertaken with the intention of alleviating the patient's pain.
4. The act should be done only if the patient makes an explicit request.
5. The euthanasia should be carried out by a physician, although

if that is not possible, special situations shall be admitted for receiving some other person's assistance.

6. Euthanasia must be carried out using ethically acceptable methods.

The court ruled that, although the first four criteria had been met, the final two conditions had not. The son was sentenced to four years in prison with three years suspended.[46]

In 2009, the Japanese Supreme Court found Dr. Setsuko Suda guilty of murder for hastening a patient's death. At the request of the patient's family, she had removed a breathing tube from a fifty-eighty-year-old man whose heart and lungs had stopped functioning. Dr. Suda had then injected him with a muscle relaxant to hasten his death. The court ruled that "the act was not considered a forgivable suspension of treatment," but suspended her eighteen-month sentence. Dr. Suda refused to accept the guilty verdict. "I don't think it's a crime," she said. "In law it may be necessary to specify the life expectancy, but on the medical front we cannot make prim and stiff decisions."[47]

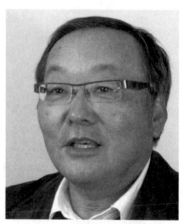

The Japan Society for Dignity in Dying, with over 125,000 members in 2010, is currently tied with the NVVE as the largest right-to-die organization in the world. When I interviewed its vice president, Dr. Soichiro Iwao, in 2010, he explained the traditionally communal nature of Japanese family decision-making when it comes to decisions at the end of life and how modern medical technology has affected this.

Dr. Soichiro Iwao

He commented that fifty years ago, virtually everyone died at home, and both the immediate and extended families were part of the dying process. "When I was young," he said, "usually the father and mother died at their home, and everyone had the opportunity to visit and say their final words to them. It was in some ways a ceremony of emotional closure.... Now, 85 percent of Japanese people die in hospitals, which limits the traditional degree of family involvement and deliberations with their dying loved ones."[48]

"Modern medical practices as used today are eroding the traditionally close bonds of Japanese expanded family relationships," commented Iwao. "The deaths of family members in hospitals [with] the necessities of invasive medical treatments interfere with the final moments between family members. If death is inevitable, we lose that opportunity to be with them as they are set free of their burdens, and of our ability to send the person on in an intimate way. The technological advances which help so many have also weakened the traditional Japanese sense of family bond."[49]

This clash between traditional Japanese family decision-making and the massive invasion of medical technology has also limited the extent to which the Japan Society for Dignity in Dying has been able to promote the usefulness of living wills, DNR orders, and organ donation cards. In these cases, a written document is still not fully enforceable without the family's consent.

"Currently, the society feels it wise to campaign only for passive euthanasia—good advance directives about terminal care, and no futile treatment. Voluntary euthanasia and assisted suicide are rarely talked about," wrote Derek Humphry.[50]

In China, where doctors serve the state, the right to die does not exist. The case of Mr. Wang Mingcheng, a resident of Shaanxi province, is an example. The former factory worker, then forty-nine, triggered China's first recorded euthanasia in 1986, when he asked a doctor to end the life of his mother, who suffered from cirrhosis of the liver. He and Dr. Pu Liansheng, who helped carry out the act, were arrested and tried for murder. In 1992, the court found both not guilty. But in July 2003, when Mr. Wang, who was dying from a combination of lung cancer, heart disease, and asthma, asked for euthanasia for himself, he was emphatically told that it was not permissible.[51]

Four years after Mr. Wang's death, twenty-nine-year-old Li Yan, a resident of Yinchuan, was thrust into the spotlight after pleading with the Chinese government for euthanasia. Diagnosed with muscular dystrophy at the age of six, Li was confined to a rusty wheelchair, unable to control her muscles below her neck. Faced with the prospect of their daughter's bleak, short life of pain, Li's parents borrowed $500—three months' wages—to buy her a computer so that she could communicate with others.

Using a chopstick held between her teeth, Li taught herself

to type and began to blog about her condition. "Fearing that her disease will eventually leave her in a helpless state, she used her blog…to ask the National People's Congress to legalize her right to die," wrote David Pearson of the *Los Angeles Times*.[52] Four weeks after Li's plea for euthanasia was copied to the message board of a prominent national television reporter, her blog had received ninety thousand hits, with many people leaving words of encouragement and support.

Her suffering continues. Li plans to dedicate the time she has left to gaining the right to die. In the bleak society in which she is trapped, she has few other choices. Her sign-in name on the message board where she talks with hundreds of supporters is a line from a Chinese poem: "The fragrance of a plum is conceived in the bitter cold." To her, this signifies that to suffer is to grow. "I really feel close to this idea," she said. The Chinese government's response to her plea is unknown.[53]

As of 2012, thirty-seven years after the start of the modern death-with-dignity movement, the concept has gained strong majority support in some places and little or none in others. In North America, the United Kingdom, Western Europe, South America, South Africa, Australia, and New Zealand—especially in the more secular societies—right-to-die acceptance and laws based on personal autonomy have flourished. In some parts of Eastern Europe and Asia, the trend has started to gain traction. But in nations ruled by political or religious dictators, there has been little or no progress. Where citizens have the right to choose, the fight for the right to die with dignity gains broader acceptance daily. In other cases, acceptance gains grounds, as does the fight for other civil rights, such as ethnic, racial, gender, and religious equality. But where tyranny reigns, all civil rights remain hostage to the edicts and dogmas of those who hold the chains that deny personal liberty and the freedom of choice.

Ω

Seeker of the Grail Secrets

People who do not ask for euthanasia will not have it. Individuals are autonomous, entitled to equality and justice, and self-determined. The right to choose is theirs and that is a choice that must always be respected.

—Russel D. Ogden, founder, The Farewell Foundation

"Call Car 10 and have him arrested right away!"

Russel D. Ogden, at the time a forty-five year-old, award-winning Canadian criminology professor at Kwantlen Polytechnic University in British Columbia, heard the command come through the mobile phone held by the on-scene coroner. As he stood nearby, she had called her supervisor, the Vancouver Regional Coroner, to ask if Ogden could remove the plastic hood covering the face of the deceased woman in the next room.

"I heard that," he said. Ogden knew that the situation had turned serious, as "Car 10" is the call sign for the inspector on duty and first responder of the Vancouver police department.

"You heard that?" asked the coroner.

"Yes," Ogden stood up and prepared to leave. He knew there was no benefit in waiting for the police. The coroner had already taken his statement and examined the body. "You've got my information," Ogden said calmly. "The police can call me at home if they need any other information. I gave you my address and phone number."

Ogden knew that leaving would defuse the potentially touchy, unprecedented situation. If he stayed, the police would almost certainly focus on him as a "person of interest" rather than on the evidence, even though it was Ogden who reported the death. Nothing he could say would reduce the suspicion that he was involved in some nefarious way and not in his professional role as a researcher in sociology and criminology. If he left, the police would have to focus on examining the death scene, collecting evidence, and later, it is hoped, reaching the proper conclusion: the dead woman had invited Ogden to be with her as she died as part of Ogden's research project, the ethics of which had already been approved by Kwantlen's research ethics board.

"Coroners are precluded from finding fault," Ogden explained to me, quoting from the *British Columbia Coroners' Service Policy and Procedures Manual,* "and must remain neutral, unbiased, factual, and objective, not allowing his/her personal bias to cloud the findings of fact in the complex legal/ethical implications of such situations."[1]

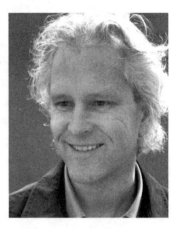

Russel D. Ogden

It was 2007, and the woman, whom he would refer to as Marcie,* was a participant in his research. "Ninety minutes earlier, Marcie had purposefully ended her life in her bed while I sat on a chair nearby and took notes. Marcie had made her peace," Ogden commented, noting that Woody Allen once said, "I am not afraid of death, I just don't want to be there when it happens."[2] "I could agree," said Ogden. "I was changed. There is no pleasure [in] witnessing a self-chosen death, but it is work that must be done if science is to help answer Hamlet's enduring question of the human condition, 'To be or not to be.'"[3]

Marcie died using the helium method of self-deliverance developed by NuTech researchers in 1999. Ogden, who had earned a master's degree in criminology from Simon Fraser University in Vancouver in 1994, had been studying suicides and assisted suicides since 1991.

In 2002, five years before I met him, Ogden had co-authored "Asphyxial Suicide with Helium and a Plastic Bag," the world's first scholarly article on self-deliverance using this system. The article was based on the death of a sixty-year-old South Carolina woman who suffered from adenoid cystic carcinoma and ended her life in September 2002.[4] At the time of her death, I was unaware that she lived five miles from my house and died after diligently following the self-deliverance protocols described in *Final Exit.*

Published in the *American Journal of Forensic Medicine and Pathology*, the article was based on evidence from the scene, but there were no witnesses to interview because the woman was alone when she died. By that time, Ogden had interviewed numerous exit guides who had observed helium exits, but interviewing them and reading their field reports about past events is not the same as directly observing a suicide.

"Marcie had asked me to remove the plastic hood from her head after she died," Ogden said. "It is a common request by those who don't want their friends and family to know that it wasn't a natural death." She had made her hood herself, using a turkey-roasting bag, adhesive tape, and a headband that served as a neck collar. "The turkey bag did not repulse Marcie; indeed, it amused her," Ogden told me. While discussing her plans with Ogden, she told him, "Please take it off so I don't go to the morgue wrapped like a chicken."[5]

"According to Marcie's wishes, I wanted to remove the hood with the coroner present," Ogden said, "because the British Columbia's Coroners Act prohibits interference with a body. The act also requires reporting of unnatural deaths—including suicides—to a coroner, hence my telephone call to report Marcie's death shortly after it happened."[6]

Marcie's self-deliverance was the first time Ogden had watched someone die. Despite the fact that his research had focused on suicide and assisted suicide for years, nothing had prepared him for the reality of it. He had grown fond of Marcie. The morning of her death, she had greeted him on her porch steps with a brilliant smile and a warm hug. "She commented on the fine weather and said she was happy because 'Today I can be free.'" How could someone smiling so beautifully want to die? The answer was simple. Marcie loved life, but progressive physical and mental deterioration and loss of independence were unacceptable to her.

I had first talked with Ogden about assisted suicide shortly after the successful resolution of George Exoo's case in 2007. Exoo told me that he was one of the first exit guides to provide Ogden with detailed reports on the final exits of many anonymous people whom he had counseled in person and accompanied at their chosen times of death.

I met Ogden in person at the 2008 World Federation of Right to Die Societies biennial congress in Paris and filmed his NuTech

presentation. We developed a vigorous professional information exchange. From the long list of peer-reviewed articles and the professional papers he had read at international conferences, it was evident
that Ogden had become the world's foremost authority on the legal
and technical implications of self-deliverance and assisted suicide.

I also learned that the road to his high standing within the
death-with-dignity movement and the scholarly community had
been filled with extensive academic harassment and numerous legal
confrontations over the right to academic freedom. Ogden described
how institutional resistance paradoxically facilitated his research
and maximized his own careful conduct. He conducted extremely
complex research under very difficult conditions, encountered numerous legal and ethical issues, and learned some valuable lessons.

Marcie's case was one of the most important in his quest for
knowledge about suicide, but his aggressive search to learn about
the assisted suicide movement had started much earlier, during the
dreadful early days of the HIV/AIDS explosion. Ogden's seminal
research into self-chosen death began when he enrolled in a master's
program in criminology at Simon Fraser University. He started to
explore the world of underground suicide assistance collectives.
These had evolved spontaneously within the AIDS community because terminally ill sufferers did not have effective medication to
deal with the disease. In addition, doctors, nurses, and hospital
workers were paranoid about the possibility of becoming infected
_____ ___ ¨· ve patients. Scores of people in major
 _a: ;, painful deaths without the benefit of
cause of an unforeseen printing error,   1em, painkillers to help them deal with
t of pages 351-354 were inadvertently   sted dying to minimize the duration of
osed. We apologize for this flaw.

For Ogden, a scholar with strong academic credentials and direct experience with social work and criminology, the workings of
the sub rosa AIDS assisted suicide community were a cutting-edge
research project: one that could have led to better end-of-life care
and gentler deaths for AIDS sufferers. It was also a chance to conduct meaningful, trailblazing research where no other social scien-
tist had ventured.[7]

To gather information, Ogden interviewed about thirty informants who had assisted in the deaths of terminally ill HIV/AIDS patients, an act that was illegal under Canadian law. Ogden found that

and a researcher, invoked in the face of legal pressure to disclose confidential information.

Ogden's lawyer made it clear that without confidentiality, researchers were unlikely to gain information that would improve understanding of the behavior in question and promote better development of policies to respond to social problems. The coroner ultimately backed down and dismissed the contempt of court charge. It was a personal victory for Ogden and a step forward for researchers who needed strategies for protecting confidential information.

His master's thesis, *Euthanasia, Assisted Suicide, and AIDS*, published in 1994, was a revolutionary exploratory study.[10] His findings shocked North America—and branded him as one of Canada's most controversial researchers.[11] Within the death-with-dignity movement, he had strong support. Christopher Docker, director of what is now Exit-Scotland, wrote, "Ogden has put himself on the line and achieved one of the most startling pieces of research that the right-to-die movement has ever seen. He shows the unadorned truth about assisted suicide, as practiced now, and reports it with academic rigour."[12]

Four years later, Simon Fraser's president wrote an apology letter for the university's failure to defend academic freedom and Ogden's right to carry out the research the university had specifically authorized.[13] In October 1998, the university agreed to pay Ogden $10,000 CAD to cover his costs in defending himself in the coroner's court.[14]

"Russel is unusual for many reasons," said criminologist John Lowman, who believes Ogden would not be able to pull off his "brave" and "respectful" research if he did not have great "self-discipline and ruthless professionalism." "[Ogden's] mental strength, determination to go the distance when ethical issues are at stake, and ability to think several moves ahead have served him well when defending academic freedom against the actions of three university administrations. He just hunkers down and deals with it. It's amazing he gets any research done."[15]

Each ethical and legal body that has investigated Ogden's research methods has ultimately vindicated him. The standoff with the coroner showed Ogden to be a man of his word, but the cowardly act by his own university left a bitter taste in his mouth, so he looked elsewhere to pursue his doctorate.

as many as half of the people who tried to kill themselves botched the job, resulting in more serious incapacity and deeper suffering. "Their loved ones, in trying to help them die, sometimes resorted to smothering them with pillows, slitting their wrists, even shooting them, in order to end their pain."[8]

"All research involving human subjects shares a common link," Ogden wrote in 1997. "Whether it be investigation into white-collar crime, child prostitution, or police corruption, subjects won't divulge sensitive information if they risk punishment. For this reason, the professional convention of researchers is to take pains to protect the confidentiality and anonymity of research participants."[9] As is standard practice for researchers exploring such cases, Ogden presented his plan to the Simon Fraser University Research Ethics Board for review and approval. The board authorized him to promise confidentiality to his sources, even under threat of legal pressure.

Most of the assisted deaths that he documented took place without medical supervision. They were clandestine: hidden from the police and court systems. Some of his informants described horrific, prolonged pain during the process of trying to end their suffering. Although *Final Exit* had been published in 1991, few people in the AIDS community knew of it—and their suicide attempts were often ghastly. Many of the dying and their caregivers hoarded and mixed together assortments of powerful drugs, some of which were incompatible or ineffective or created severe medical damage without bringing about the desired hastened deaths. Even worse, some attempts caused tortured, prolonged deaths.

In 1994, Ogden's promise to maintain confidentiality was severely tested when the Vancouver Regional Coroner issued a subpoena and tried to compel him to reveal names and information about two confidential participants. On ethical grounds, Ogden refused to disclose anything. To his complete astonishment, Simon Fraser's administrators, cowering in fear about possible negative publicity for the university, abandoned him to the wolves and refused to support its own requirement that Ogden protect the identities of his informants.

The coroner then told Ogden that he had to find the scholar in contempt of court for refusing to name his sources. Ogden still refused to comply, invoking the Wigmore Criteria, a defense under common law of the right to confidentiality between an informant

He chose to cross the Atlantic Ocean to pursue his Ph.D. at the University of Exeter, England. There, between 1995 and 1998, he continued his research on the underground world of assisted dying. He found that the great distance from home had not improved his hopes for performing life-changing research. The British university turned out to be as devious and ethically bankrupt as Simon Fraser had been.

Exeter had approved Ogden's research into the evolution and practice of "a secret global network conducting assisted suicides" (i.e., the evolving international death-with-dignity movement). Ogden spent two years interviewing more than one hundred people in Canada, Britain, the Netherlands, and the United States who claimed firsthand involvement in helping people with AIDS commit suicide.[16] Prior to conducting an interview, Ogden had to offer respondents absolute confidentiality, particularly if courts ordered him to release their names."[17]

Exeter's ethics committee officially approved this guarantee of confidentiality and gave Ogden a written statement recognizing that "entry into communication of this kind is integral to the pursuit of truth through sociological research, and (we) accept the obligation to support and sustain those who do so."[18]

Exeter did not keep its promise. In 1997, two years into his research, Ogden found out that five days after he received ethical approval for his research, the chair of Exeter's ethics committee had quietly altered the statement, rescinding the committee's support for the confidentiality of his research—without informing Ogden. The change meant Ogden's research participants were unknowingly misled about the true conditions for their "informed consent."

When he learned of the university's ethical treachery, Ogden had only one course of appeal: to petition the university's "visitor" (official sponsor). In Exeter's case, this was Queen Elizabeth II. Ogden's appeal was handled by the Lord Chancellor on her behalf. The Lord Chancellor found that there had been "gross academic malfeasance" and ordered damages for the university's "negligent action." In his ruling, the Lord Chancellor said, "The main consequence of that negligence was that [Ogden] could not use the research he had undertaken in reliance of the university's assurances....Exeter broke its commitment to legally protect him while he conducted his confidential research."[19] He noted that this amounted to "a denial that the university has any responsibility to assist Mr. Ogden in upholding academic freedom."[20] Exeter was ordered to pay Ogden the equivalent of $140,466 USD for the damage done to his career.[21]

In November 2003, the university made a public apology about the affair, but never bothered doing so to the man whose career they had irreparably damaged. Ogden summarized the affair:

> Last week the university apologised …for 'inconveniencing' my Ph.D. studies. I do not know who made the apology, but no communication has been addressed to me personally. Regardless, the apology is morally bankrupt. From start to finish, and at several layers of management, Exeter behaved as if it had little or no moral commitment to free inquiry. It did all it could to crush dissent and resistance. I was scorned and ridiculed. My only two allies on the campus were intimidated—one lost his research fellowship after he supported me at a meeting. When Exeter's senate committee of academic inquiry judged that there were 'inadequacies' and 'incompetence,' the administration appears to have tried to get the committee to change its decision.[22]

In short, his three years of studies at Exeter and his opportunity to earn his doctoral degree there had been flushed down the toilet, not through any lack of competence, diligence, vision, or scholarship but because of behind-the-scenes sabotage by the university.[23] Exeter was simply version 2.0 of Simon Fraser University's total disregard for the ethical treatment of its written obligations to its own scholars. "Years of my life were squandered solely because of Exeter's refusal to keep its written commitments and follow its own policies," Ogden said.[24]

Battered but not even remotely humbled, Ogden returned to Canada in 1997 to teach and resume his suicide studies. In 1999, he was hired as a professor to teach sociology and criminology at Kwantlen Polytechnic University in Vancouver. Kwantlen pledged to set aside funds to defend his promises of confidentiality for the research he was undertaking. Little did he know that Kwantlen was to be the source of yet more academic grief.

Ogden's introduction into the then-secret world of the NuTech development of self-deliverance technologies and techniques came

in 1999, the same year he assumed teaching duties at Kwantlen. The NuTech association was a fortuitous outgrowth of
his acquaintance with John Hofsess, who
had founded the Right to Die Society of
Canada in 1991. Impressed by Ogden's
previous research, Hofsess selected him
to be the first academic allowed full access to all information coming from
NuTech's first and all subsequent working meetings.

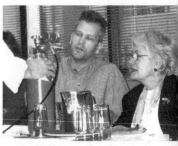

*Ogden and Faye Girsh le
about the nitrogen self-delivera
system at the 1999 Seattle NuT
Conference.*

He wrote to Ogden, "Russel: On Sat/
Sun Nov 13/14 we are holding a conference in Seattle (about 24
people in attendance, hand-picked) devoted to 'new technology' [in-
cluding] (a) demonstrations of equipment (various gas systems, plus
the DeBreather, and other devices; and (b) descriptions of "underground" events and discussions about what took place (various parts
of U.S. mostly).... But first things first... interested?"[25]

Ogden had strong reservations about attending the conference.
Although deeply intrigued with the chance to learn the intimate details of NuTech's secret self-deliverance research, he was reluctant
to get involved because it was clear that confidential information
would be shared within a sizable group. He usually received this
type of information in formal one-to-one encounters, where privacy was easier to manage. If he were to pledge confidentiality to
the NuTech conference participants, it would have to occur without
university oversight—or legal protection. If any legal authorities
demanded the confidential information he had learned, he would not
have the Wigmore Criteria or formal academic legal protection to
shield him from being forced to disclose his sources.

Hofsess persisted. "I think that the conference might be of interest to you as deep background."[26] Ogden ultimately acceded to
Hofsess' appeal. He wrote to me, "Like the fictional Alice in *Through
the Looking-Glass*, I found a world that evoked the power relations
of the game of chess, but the world Hofsess invited me to focused
exclusively on the endgame."[27]

Because of his work with end-stage AIDS sufferers, Ogden
wanted to learn what Hofsess and the renegade physicians, psychologists, technicians, and death-with dignity activists were doing to

offer a gentle death for people experiencing untreatable suffering. He went to the conference as a detached scholarly observer, not a participant or advocate. To paraphrase an old concept, he wanted to learn how clockmakers make clocks to measure time, not how to learn to be a clockmaker himself.

At the conference, he held detailed discussions with virtually all of NuTech's technical and medical founders, inventors, and exit guides and had the unique opportunity to see, handle, and learn about every NuTech deathing device and procedure then in existence or under development. Following that conference, the flow of information and case reports to and from hastened-death counselors and exit guides increased exponentially. Between 1999 and 2005, in his new capacity as NuTech's designated archivist, Ogden accumulated over two hundred firsthand field reports of NuTech self-deliverances in North America.

Since the 1994 publication of his master's thesis, Ogden's prolific authorship of articles in professional journals and popular magazines and his contributions to major end-of-life-related books have greatly broadened the understanding of suicide and assisted suicide and contributed to the rapidly changing views of medical professionals about hastened death.

His subjects include the development of cooperative relationships between palliative care and euthanasia professionals; AIDS, euthanasia, and nursing in both English- and French-speaking Canada; the "open secret" of nurses' and social workers' involvement—or fear of involvement—with hastened death; and the "technological imperative" of the deathing counterculture. Ogden has also written about the role of privacy and confidentiality in research; safeguarding access to euthanasia; the ethical challenges of prenatal testing; and hastened-death practices among the Inuit people. The scourge of his professional accreditation has been the combination of the "yuck factor" of his research topics and academic treachery—not the concrete societal value of his cutting-edge research.

Despite repeated proof that his research was professionally planned, approved in advance by the universities he was affiliated with, and carried out with the highest academic standards, his scholarly ship ran into yet another unmarked shoal in 2006. In December of that year, the administration of Kwantlen Polytechnic University directed him not to engage "in any illegal activity, including attending at an assisted death."[28] The directive came despite the fact that Kwantlen's own ethics review board had previously approved his research in 2005. Furthermore, in 2004, a British Columbia court had acquitted euthanasia activist Evelyn Martens of the charge of allegedly aiding and abetting a suicide in the cases of Monique Charest and Leyanne Burchell. That ruling established that simply being present at an unassisted suicide was not illegal in Canada.

Kwantlen's Faculty Association failed to get Ogden any relief from the "cease and desist" order, and it turned the case over to the Canadian Association of University Teachers, a federation of independent associations and trade unions representing approximately 65,000 teachers, librarians, researchers, and other academic professionals who supported the defense of academic freedom. Their campaign to lift the Kwantlen "stop work" order had failed by 2008, and they appointed a committee to fully investigate whether the university's actions were in violation of Ogden's academic freedom. The university and Ogden reached a compensation settlement, the details of which have not been disclosed.

Ogden is able to easily explain complex concepts to any audience. At the NuTech meeting during the World Federation of Right to Die Societies Congress in Melbourne in 2010, he gave a presentation demonstrating the impossibility of living without oxygen, recreating the classic demonstration of an experiment carried out by Joseph Priestley, who discovered oxygen in 1774.

Priestley's first experiment was to enclose a burning candle in a domed, glass vessel. As the candle flame consumed the fixed supply of oxygen, the flame died out. When he ran the experiment again, he also put a mouse inside the glass dome with the burning candle. When the candle flame went out, the mouse died because all of the oxygen that it needed to live had been consumed.

To demonstrate to the Melbourne audience that life cannot be sustained without oxygen, Ogden recreated Priestley's experiment, using an inverted water glass and helium in addition to a flame. There was only one problem: because of the rushed conference schedule, Ogden had not had time to find the helium for his demonstration. He asked me to find a supply for him on short notice.

We were staying at a conference hotel in the business district of Melbourne, where there was a nearby flower shop. I knew I could find helium party balloons there.

"G'day. How can I help you?" said the smiling young lady behind the counter.

"I need two birthday balloons—you know, the helium ones. Do you have those?"

"Of course!" she answered with a smile and showed me the assortment of designs.

"Two of these will be fine," I said, and she filled the balloons with helium.

"Hope the party's great!" she said.

"It will be," I said and headed back to give Ogden his helium supply for the NuTech presentation.

In front of the international audience of death-with-dignity professionals, Ogden turned the glass upside down and released helium from a balloon into it. Because helium is lighter than air, it immediately filled the glass and replaced all the air. Then he lowered the helium-filled glass over a burning candle. As soon as the flame entered the helium inside the glass, it was immediately extinguished.

Everyone immediately realized the obvious: no oxygen = no possibility of continued life. If a person breathed in only helium, such as in a helium exit bag, consciousness would usually be lost within three or four breaths—ten or fifteen seconds—and total, irreversible brain death would normally follow within three to ten minutes.

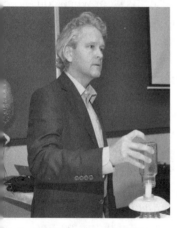
Ogden demonstrates that life can-be sustained without oxygen.

In 2008, Ogden had the opportunity to review the case histories and videotaped assisted suicides of four persons, one of whom was a physician, who died at the Dignitas facility in Switzerland that year. The cases he was interested in were the ones where Dignitas chose to try out the helium method. The organization had helped hundreds of its members die over the years using the standard heavy overdose of Nembutal dissolved in water. But on January 31, 2008, the medical director of the Canton of Zürich took the position that physicians must consult with patients more than once before prescribing the lethal dose.

"Dignitas interpreted this as a signal that the cantonal medical director intended to restrict suicide assistance," Ogden wrote. "It was also viewed as an obstacle to Dignitas' foreign members, especially those who would delay their travel to Switzerland to a point at which return trips for further medical consultations were out of the question."[29]

Therefore, Dignitas explored oxygen deprivation with helium as an alternative to its usual method. The application of a non-drug-related process would help Dignitas establish that medical control over assisted suicide is unnecessary. As a routine legal precaution, a videotape recording is made of each Dignitas-assisted suicide, which is then promptly reviewed by the cantonal police and coroner to assure that the suicides were lawful and no protocols were ignored. The tapes reveal the minute details of each death and are, therefore, extremely valuable to medical, forensic, and police investigators.

To examine how the four Dignitas helium deaths went when compared to the large number of previous cases he had reviewed, Ogden asked Dignitas for copies of the relevant videotapes. The copies of the original tapes given to Dignitas by the police proved to be defective, so Minelli obtained permission for Ogden to visit the Zürich police station and view the tapes there. The police corrected the playback defects and provided good copies to Dignitas and Ogden.

In the helium assisted suicides of the three women and one man in 2008, Dignitas chose to administer the gas through a small, partial face mask instead of using the standard exit bag. This did not prevent the helium system from working painlessly and effectively. However, the duration of the time to unconsciousness was about twice as long, and the involuntary body movements that sometimes occur with the helium method (while the person is totally unconscious and feels nothing) "appeared to concern and confuse the Dignitas attendants."[30]

From close scrutiny of the videotapes, Ogden was able to gain considerable data about the use of face masks with the helium system, making the effort worthwhile and leading to a major scholarly article in the *Journal of Medical Ethics* in 2010. The coauthors of the article were anesthesiologists who knew the material very well. Yet watching videotapes and personally witnessing a self-chosen death were still two significantly different things from a researcher's perspective. Ogden's next opportunity to directly observe—but not participate in—a legal elective death was not long in coming.

In November 2010, he accompanied a dying Canadian woman and several of her family members as she made her one-way trip to Zürich. Her name, illness, and the details of the trip remain private. The profound experience of being with her family as she died cemented once and for all in his mind the idea that dying people in great pain should not have to pay thousands of dollars and endure long, painful, and distressing airplane trips to a distant foreign country in pursuit of gentle elective deaths that could have taken place in their own beds or at a nearby version of Dignitas.[31] After twenty years of studying and analyzing hundreds of self-chosen rational suicides in numerous countries, along with the state and national laws that regulated them, Ogden was convinced that the Swiss model of assisted suicide was superior to any other.

"The Swiss model is a good model from any perspective," he told me. "It's good because it's demedicalized and makes all details immediately available to law enforcement. . . . It calls for immediate reporting and immediate accountability to police coroners and prosecutors. What better safeguards than immediate, official case-by-case review could you ask for? It also provides optimal access to a humane ending of life for those who need it."[32]

"It negates every argument that anti-choice accusers level at the Oregon and Washington models, save for one: the religious objection that 'only God can create a life, and only God can be allowed to end it.'"[33] He noted that adopting this religious view as a required belief system would impose what is solely a personal opinion on all human beings without their choice.

Distressed by the denial of Sue Rodriguez' Canadian Supreme Court challenge in 1993, Ogden decided on a bold course of action. He would found a new organization that would once again confront Canada's prohibition of assisted suicide head-on. The new group's name was the Farewell Foundation for the Right to Die; it would operate under the Swiss model as soon as it could bring about the decriminalization of Canada's anti-assisted suicide law. It accepted its first paying member on February 16, 2011, and four days later, it took legal action to re-ignite the legal battle for the right to die with dignity in Canada.

Ogden's aim was to convince the Canadian Supreme Court to legalize assisted suicide and to have Section 241(b) of the Canadian

Criminal Code struck down. Once the law was abolished, the Farewell Foundation would be free to establish one or more Dignitas-like facilities in Canada. Ogden's original plan was to file a routine request with the British Columbia Registrar of Companies to formally recognize and grant legal standing to the Farewell Foundation as it would to any otherwise ordinary nonprofit organization.

On February 20, 2011, he was one of five applicants to incorporate the Farewell Foundation for the Right to Die as a charitable, nonprofit corporation under British Columbia's Society Act. Ogden knew that the flashpoint would be the organization's stated goal to provide assisted suicides, which were then illegal. The foundation claimed that failure to grant a charter on the basis of the existing criminal code was invalid because assumptions about assisted suicide in Canada had changed drastically since the Rodriguez case in 1993. Therefore, the slender 5 to 4 vote of the supreme court justices against Rodriguez' right to a physician-assisted death could no longer be supported by either fact or reason. The application stated that if the foundation was turned down—as Ogden and his other founding directors assumed it would be—its legal counsel, Jason Gratl, would seek a judicial review in the British Columbia Supreme Court. Implicit in that statement was the understanding that if that court denied the application, its decision would immediately be challenged in the Canadian Supreme Court.

In his initial affidavit to the British Columbia Corporate Registry, Ogden listed many reasons why the Rodriguez decision should be overturned. Chief among them was that the conditions that affected the court's conclusion nearly two decades earlier no longer existed.

"What has been learned since *Rodriguez*," he stated in his affidavit, "demonstrates that the criminal prohibition against assisted suicide is unnecessary, arbitrary and the harms caused by the criminal prohibition grossly outweigh its purported benefits."[34] Based on multiple detailed analyses of nations and states where regulated assisted suicide and euthanasia had been legalized, he stated that it could no longer be concluded that criminalizing assisted suicide is reasonably necessary. He also found that there was no empirical evidence that decriminalizing assisted suicide would result in the notorious slippery slope of moral decay. He stated that his research showed that criminalizing assisted suicide was a strong incentive to hide the fact that thousands of assisted suicides took place both inside and outside the medical community.

Ogden noted that since 1993, a majority of Canadians have believed that those who are suffering in desperate and deteriorating circumstances should have the option of making fully informed, voluntary decisions to die and are entitled to the appropriate information, means, and compassionate assistance to accomplish that end. "Canadians regard those who aid in suicide as altruistic and compassionate, rather than criminal."[35]

In addition, Ogden found that the criminal prohibition of assisted suicide caused immeasurable psychological suffering to rational people who are capable of making informed decisions and who wish to end their own lives to avoid suffering. "This suffering is certain and it is as extreme as any suffering humanity must endure. This case tests whether Parliament is entitled to cause such suffering to the people of Canada," he concluded.[36]

As expected, the request to incorporate the foundation as a nonprofit organization was quickly rejected. The refusal was based on the grounds that the foundation's purposes were "contrary to s. 241(b) of the Criminal Code and thus unlawful."[37] Ogden's organization quickly appealed the decision to the British Columbia Supreme Court on April 8, 2011. It asked the court to rule that the law infringes on the Canadian Charter of Rights and Freedoms (the equivalent of the U.S. Constitution and Bill of Rights); to declare that Section 241(b) was no longer in force or effect; and to rule that the proposed actions of the foundation were, therefore, not contrary to the laws of Canada.

In first year of existence, the foundation welcomed over two hundred new members and raised $46,570 CAD for its operations and the initial legal challenge at the British Columbia Supreme Court level. "I had no idea that we would gain so much support so quickly," Ogden told me. But the legal playing field quickly became more complicated.

In an unexpected move, on April 26, 2011, the British Columbia Civil Liberties Union launched a second attack on the constitutionality of Sections 241(a) and (b). The case, known as *Carter et al. v. Attorney General of Canada and Attorney General of British Columbia*, became the second direct constitutional challenge to abolish Canada's prohibition against aiding or abetting suicide. The chief plaintiff was Lee Carter, a retired flight attendant, who accompanied her eighty-nine-year-old mother, Kathleen (Kay) Carter of North Vancouver, to her death in Switzerland on January 15, 2010. Kay Carter, who was nearly paralyzed by spinal stenosis, desperately wanted to die. She made her journey to Dignitas accompanied by Lee; Lee's husband, Hollis Johnson; and other family members.[38] Under the existing law, the Canadians who accompanied Kay Carter to Switzerland were potentially liable for aiding and abetting a suicide.

A few months after the Carter case was filed, a new plaintiff was added to their roster: Gloria Taylor, who suffered from ALS, as had Sue Rodriguez. Because her health was already deteriorating rapidly, and she could not afford the trip to Dignitas, Taylor would soon need the assistance of a Canadian physician to die. Therefore, Madam Justice Lynn Smith agreed to fast-track the proceedings.

The British Columbia Supreme Court denied the foundation's challenge to Section 241(b) on August 17, 2011, but the judges suggested that it should apply to become an intervener in the Carter case, as both cases had the same ultimate goal. Interveners may submit specialized information directly to the court for consideration, and Ogden wanted to ensure that the court was aware of the unique advantages to Canadians of a Swiss-style assisted suicide model. The foundation was the only right-to-die group participating and the only intervener group to have counsel present every day of the trial.

Two other groups supported Carter's case and two were opposed. One supporter was the Canadian Unitarian Council, representing forty-eight congregations. The council had a long-standing policy that embraced choice in dying. The other group was the Ad Hoc Coalition for People With Disabilities Who Are Supportive of Physician-Assisted Dying, which offers an alternative view about disability to that of the Euthanasia Prevention Coalition (EPC).[39]

In opposition, the EPC, composed chiefly of Catholic and Christian fundamentalists and directed by Alex Schadenberg, has a mandate from its members "to preserve and enforce the laws prohibiting assistance with suicide. It believes that relaxation of the law will harm disabled people, the elderly, and negatively alter the physician-patient relationship."[40]

The second opponent was the Christian Leadership Fellowship (CLF), which opposes death-with-dignity proponents and the liber-

al religious views of the Canadian Unitarian Council. "The CLF...
told the court that it intended to argue that the Constitution has a
positive duty to require the criminal prohibition against assistance
with suicide."[41]

The plaintiffs served sixty-six affidavits and provided a list of
twenty-five expert witnesses. The Attorney General of Canada
and the Attorney General of British Columbia responded with fifteen affidavits and fourteen expert witnesses. Madam Justice Smith
started hearing arguments on November 14, 2011, and these were
wrapped up on December 16, 2011. The parties exchanged further
written submissions until January 25, 2012, mostly to argue matters
about the admissibility of evidence.

Justice Smith's ruling is expected in the spring of 2012, but
whatever her decision, either or both parties may choose to appeal
the ruling to the British Columbia Court of Appeal. If that does not
settle the matter, the case will advance to Canada's highest court.
There, where Sue Rodriguez' case met a narrow defeat, death-with-
dignity supporters worldwide hope that this time the ruling will
make a humane hastened death the right of every Canadian citizen,
once and for all.

The Big Sting

There are many, many people who are doomed to suffer interminably
for years. And why should they not receive our support as well?
—Ted Goodwin, former president, The Final Exit Network

Thursday morning, April 1, 2010, was a beautiful day in Cumming, Georgia, about thirty-five miles northeast of Atlanta. The sun was bright in a luminous blue sky filled with puffy, white clouds. The magnificent mass plantings of pink and white azaleas surrounding the Forsyth County Courthouse were in full bloom. The idyllic setting belied a grim reality. On the previous day, Derek Humphry had flown into Atlanta from his home in Oregon to attend the arraignment hearing of four members of the Final Exit Network.

I had driven for five hours from my South Carolina home to the Atlanta airport to pick up Humphry, act as his taxi driver, observe the proceedings, and discuss some of the legal issues this case had created for the group, which he had helped found. At a local restaurant, Humphry, Thomas E. "Ted" Goodwin, a cofounder and former president of the Network, and I spent the evening discussing the case. After dinner, Humphry and I retired to our hotel, where I interviewed him about his long advocacy career.

The next morning, when the sheriff's deputy unlocked the courthouse door at 9:00, the line of fifty or sixty people emptying their pockets, opening their briefcases, and walking through the metal detector represented a typical day's group of lawyers and people arriving to pay speeding tickets, serve on juries, file forms to force recalcitrant parents to make child support payments, or plead guilty or not guilty to alleged law violations.

The group that Humphry and I accompanied was more focused and serious than those who were trying to evade speeding tickets.

Ted Goodwin, sixty-four; Claire Blehr, seventy-nine; Nicholas A. Sheridan, sixty-two; and Dr. Lawrence D. Egbert, eighty-one, were there to be arraigned and plead not guilty to charges of violating Georgia's assisted suicide law. They had been arrested eight months after providing Network member John Celmer, a cancer victim, with counseling and a bedside presence when he ended his life at his Georgia home on June 20, 2008.

The "Georgia Four," as they came to be known, were arrested as the result of an intensive, expensive "sting" operation—an elaborate deception carried out by the Georgia Bureau of Investigation (GBI) against the Network. On the day of their arrest, exit guides Goodwin and Blehr were at the bedside of a Network member they knew as Richard Arthur Sartain, sixty-one. He had joined the Network several months earlier, claiming that he was dying of advanced pancreatic cancer and wanted to die at home. The explicit medical records he provided made his terminal condition unquestionably clear: he was going to die soon.

Richard Sartain was an imposter. The man who had sought the Network's counseling and deathbed presence was, in fact, extremely healthy and a very convincing actor. His real name was Richard Sells, a special agent for the GBI.[1] Sartain's "home" was the home of another GBI agent, which had been outfitted with a variety of concealed video cameras and microphones to record the sting operation. Sartain's detailed patient medical history and explicit medical records had been fabricated, and a medical timeline of his carefully manufactured dying process was edited by GBI's chief medical examiner, Dr. Kris Sperry, and sent to Sells' field operative colleague, Special Agent in Charge Mitchell M. Posey.[2]

On November 13, 2008, while polishing the script of Sartain's fictional medical disasters, Sperry wrote to Posey, "I made the minor revisions that we discussed on the two reports, which I have attached. Here is the suggested timeline/chronology for Richard Arthur Sartain.... How does that sound? Let me know if you need any clarification of my suggested narrative."[3] When the Network received these documents during the disclosure hearing prior to the trial, they were astonished that Georgia's chief medical officer would so cheerfully create false documents in order to entrap a U.S. citizen who had not been accused or convicted of any crime.

"Under Georgia law, after an arrest, nothing much happens in a case until a grand jury hands down an indictment," said Robert Rivas, the Network's legal advisor.[4] The Georgia Four had been in legal limbo for twenty-one months between the day of their arrest and March 9, 2010, when a Forsyth County grand jury announced on that there was sufficient evidence to try them for evidence tampering and violating both Georgia's assisted suicide act and the federal Racketeer Influenced and Corrupt Organizations (RICO) Act.[5]

The case of the Georgia Four was the latest in a series of attempted entrapments of death-with-dignity groups. In 1993, Cheryl Eckstein, then head of Canada's Euthanasia Prevention Coalition, successfully infiltrated the staff of John Hofsess' Right to Die Society of Canada when he was supporting Sue Rodriguez' attempt to have physician aid-in-dying legalized. In 2011, Neal Nicol, Dr. Jack Kevorkian's closest colleague, posted to the ERGO news list that the anti-euthanasia group run by Rita Marker attempted to entrap Kevorkian in the early 1990s by submitting a fictitious medical history.[6] The sting was uncovered and never caused any damage.

Named after Humphry's book *Final Exit*, the Final Exit Network was the offspring of disenchanted former members of the Hemlock Society, which had been eventually transformed into Compassion & Choices (C&C). After the Hemlock Society had been merged out of existence, C&C abandoned many of the philosophies and practices of Hemlock's Caring Friends Program. To achieve the respectability they felt was needed to effectively promote state physician-assisted-dying laws, C&C cut every tie to what they saw as Hemlock's unruly past and lack of political correctness. Barbara Coombs Lee, C&C's president, repeatedly denounced the Caring Friends Program's recommendation of the helium system to achieve a safe and peaceful self-deliverance. She stated, "[The helium system is] not the way to make it safe. The plastic bag is sort of the end-of-life equivalent of the coat hanger."[7]

Compassion & Choices focuses on the medical model and the vigorous, long-term promotion of state-by-state legislative change. The group, its progenitors, and its allies can rightfully be credited with much of the work that brought about legal physician aid-in-dying in Oregon and Washington and decriminalization of the concept in Montana. It actively supports the future enactment of Oregon-style laws in a number of other states.

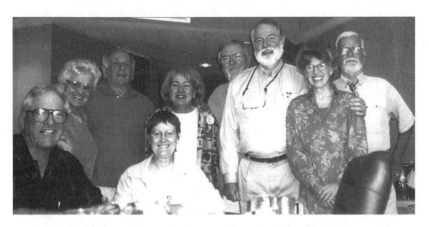

The founding members of The Final Exit Network, August 14, 2004. L-R, front row: Earl Wettstein, Nancy Bedell (standing in for Judith Coats); back row: Ila DeLuca, Derek Humphry, Faye Girsh, Bob Brush, Ted Goodwin, Ruth von Fuchs, Dr. Larry Egbert, and Rosalie Guttman, who took the photo.

The Final Exit Network was formally conceived as a social justice/civil rights movement in a meeting of ten minds at the Four Points by Sheraton hotel in Chicago on August 13 and 14, 2004. All of the founders were motivated, experienced right-to-die activists, chiefly former Hemlock Society members, who were ready to place their careers, professional reputations, life savings, and personal freedom on the line to help their members have dignified, painless deaths at the time of their own choosing. Unlike the Hemlock Society's Caring Friends Program, which operated somewhat clandestinely, the Network decided to "come out of the closet," making its mission public.

One important person was glaringly missing from the organizational meeting—Dr. Dick MacDonald. He was still under contract to retrain Barbara Coombs Lee's C&C guides. "That occupied me for six months, January to June 2005, in six different training sessions in six different states," he told me. "As that was completed, on July 1, Barbara called me to say she no longer wished to have a medical director for the organization. She did tell me the board had met to decide this. I learned from C&C board president, Dr. Robert Brody, two months later, that he had been totally blindsided by her decision and no meeting had been held. Although he kindly urged me to come back, I had decided there was no way to cooperate with

Barbara Coombs Lee. I then quickly became a volunteer with the Final Exit Network, who named me Senior Medical Advisor, in which capacity I serve today."[8]

The Network took off like an Independence Day skyrocket. It was incorporated on September 5, 2004, and its website was active by September 13. The first members joined almost as soon as the website went up. The pace increased greatly as news of this vibrant new group offering comprehensive how-to counseling and a bedside presence at death spread through former Hemlock members and the country. The first exit guide training session was held in St. Louis in November, with eighteen guides in the first graduating class.

After only a few months of existence, the Network was a success. Seventeen members' cases were being evaluated for future exits; fifteen trained, volunteer exit guides were ready to serve them; and the organization had been officially welcomed into the World Federation of Right to Die Societies.[10]

The first Network final exit took place in Atlanta on New Year's Eve 2004. The Network member who wished to die had suffered helplessly as cancer metastasized throughout his body and ravaged it for eighteen months. He chose to end his life with his personal friend, Network cofounder Ted Goodwin, at his side.[9]

The Network focused on providing comprehensive end-of-life education. It specifically included the unassisted use of the helium final exit system and a compassionate, bedside presence, if requested, when a member chose to die. Unlike C&C, the Network chose to concentrate on patients with imminent needs. To serve the 95 percent of dying Americans who do not qualify for physician-hastened death under the Oregon, Washington, or Montana guidelines, it offered counseling and a bedside presence for any mentally competent member with unbearable suffering. No other organization in the United States ever had the courage to make that commitment.

The Network believes that mentally competent adults have a right to end their lives when they suffer from fatal or irreversible illnesses or have a quality of life they can no longer bear. "Such a right shall be an individual choice, including the timing and companion, free of any restriction by the law, clergy, medical profession, even friends and relatives, no matter how well intentioned," wrote psychologist Jerry Dincin, the Network's director from 2008 to 2011.[11] Unlike the majority of right-to-die groups (but similar to their counterparts in the Netherlands and Switzerland), the Network does not limit its membership or provision of services solely to those who are terminally ill and have six months or fewer to live.[12]

In 2004, when the Network was founded, just over 70 percent of Americans believed that a physician should be legally permitted to hasten the death of a cognitively functional person who was experiencing intolerable suffering. The Network's liberal policy of facilitating gentle deaths made it the hero of the medically cursed and the curse of those opposing the right to die with dignity.

The Network was not bashful about its existence and mission. To get the word out that its end-of-life counseling was available, it developed a mission statement, a logo, a professionally designed website, and a newsletter. Network volunteers fanned out throughout the United States to give public talks about its services and answer questions about death and dying. In 2010, after its membership passed the three thousand mark, donors provided funds to erect large highway billboards in California, New Jersey, and Florida proclaiming, "My Life, My Death, My Choice / FinalExitNetwork.org." During the last two weekends in October 2010, the evening sky over Baltimore and Washington, D.C., was lit up by a scrolling message of "Die with Dignity" and the Network's web address, displayed on a giant, lighted grid carried by a helicopter.

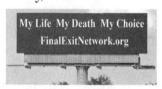

The Network hits the superhighways

No one could ever accuse the Network of being a subtle or covert operation.

The most important activists within the organization were the professionally trained, volunteer exit guides, most of whom had received their instructions from Hemlock's veteran trainer, Dr. Dick MacDonald. "We wanted one and all to know that a highly motivated group of geriatric activists [their average age was seventy-two] intended to bring individual choice-in-dying to the broadest numbers of qualified individuals," commented Goodwin. "Our birth was one which had to happen in order to effect change within the right-to-die movement."[13]

For its first three years, the Network continued to grow and evolve, helping numerous members achieve the peaceful deaths they had chosen. But the inevitable first "bad case" loomed up on April 12, 2007, when a Network final exit went seriously wrong. Jana Van

Voorhis, fifty-eight, was born into a wealthy family. An unmarried resident of Phoenix, Arizona, she had led what often had been a "tortured existence marred by chronic mental illness," family members said. While still in high school, she had been admitted into a psychiatric hospital, and she received mental health treatment for the rest of her life. By the mid-1960s, "she had been increasingly becoming psychotic, claiming roof rats [had] been overtaking her home, sneaking into her house, and attacking her," according to her psychiatrist, Dr. Michael Fermo. On May 7, 2006, Fermo wrote, "She reports having depressed mood swings; periods of irritability; difficulty shutting off her mind, especially at night; erratic sleep; low energy; nervous; socially isolative; and an ongoing feeling that bugs are eating her." [13]

Van Voorhis did not want any member of her family to know of her plans to die, a request the Network honored. If only one family member disapproved, this would deny the Network member a gentle death that the rest of the family had agreed to.

Van Voorhis' case had been reviewed and approved for a final exit accompaniment by Dr. Larry Egbert, the Network's medical director. Roberta Massey, the Network's case coordinator, had assigned Wye Hale-Rowe and Frank Royal Langsner to her case. Eighty-two-year-old Hale-Rowe of Colorado, a retired family therapist, a great-grandmother, and one of the nation's most well-trained, experienced exit guides, was the senior guide for the case. Eighty-five-year-old Langsner, a retired college professor from Scottsdale, Arizona, and a first-time guide, was her assistant. Both had counseled Van Voorhis and were at her side when she died quietly in bed after using the helium method.

After calling several times with no response, Van Voorhis' sister Vicki Thomas and her husband found Van Voorhis' body at home in bed on April 15, 2007. They initially suspected that she had died from a drug overdose because she had a large supply of prescribed painkillers, sleeping pills, and mood stabilizers. But some things looked odd. There were no drugs or pill bottles in sight, and Van Voorhis' body had been neatly tucked under the covers, with her hands on top of the sheets and her hair carefully fanned out on a pillow in a beatific pose.[14] "It looked staged," Vicki Thomas said.[15] It was.

The two Network exit guides had failed to follow some of the rules laid out in their procedures manual, which specifies that "unless the member requested otherwise, the guides rearrange the member as though death had occurred during sleep."[16] Most members do not want anyone to know that the death was a suicide. They want to look as if they had quietly passed away of natural causes.

On the day of Van Voorhis' requested death, Hale-Rowe and Langsner came to her home and had their final conversation with her. She had personally obtained the two critical things she needed: a plastic exit hood, ordered from the Network's recommended source, and two disposable tanks of helium from a nearby store. She then followed the standard procedures, donned the helium hood, lay back on her bed, and turned the knob that started the flow of helium into the hood. With her guides gently holding her hands to provide a human touch—and *not* to make it impossible to remove the hood, as police asserted—Van Voorhis became unconscious in twenty to thirty seconds and died about twelve minutes later. Her guides stayed about fifteen minutes longer to ensure that she was dead. Then, as she had asked, they removed the hood and tanks and put them into plastic bags, which were later discarded in industrial dumpsters.

Unfortunately, the team had failed to ensure that a letter from Van Voorhis to her neighbor was mailed immediately after her death. The letter stated that "Van Voorhis was not feeling well" and wanted her sister to come by to check on her. This would ensure that her body was quickly discovered. That was a firm Network protocol because many members lived relatively secluded lives, and prompt finding of the body was considered an essential courtesy.

Things got worse. After noticing that the letter had not been sent, an unknown female, whose caller ID was traced to Frank Langsner's phone, asked Vicki Thomas to check on her sister. This link between Langsner and Van Voorhis would soon lead to a complicated plague of problems for the Network. Before it was finished, the case, and the one in Georgia, would cover half the country, suck in hundreds of people, and last four years.

On June 7, 2007, police interviewed Langsner at his home. He freely gave them a great deal of information about the Van Voorhis exit. He read from a paper stating that, among other things, Van Voorhis suffered from porphyria, a lesion on the liver, possible breast cancer, head injuries, an enlarged liver and spleen, overexposure to radiation, ingestion of rat poison, and intolerable pain. She was also taking an anti-depressant, a medication to relieve unexpected attacks of extreme fear, and an extremely powerful pain reliever. Langsner believed that she was eager to die and end her pain. She had not volunteered any information or medical records relating to mental illness. Unfortunately, the Network had failed to dig deeply enough into her history. Van Voorhis had severe psychological problems that would have barred her from receiving a final exit if the group had known about them.

On the basis of police interviews with Langsner and Hale-Rowe, warrants were issued to search both of their homes. The subsequent searches turned up extensive documentation of the Network's internal operating principles and the names of hundreds of its members. Included were the names of Roberta Massey and Dr. Larry Egbert, the other two people involved with the Van Voorhis case. All of these data were seized. No one at the Network knew that anything had gone wrong with the Van Voorhis case until Hale-Rowe approached Ted Goodwin at a June 2007 guide training program and told him, "I've got to talk to you. There's something you need to know."[17]

The initial Phoenix police investigation turned up some oddities but nothing to suggest an unusual death, and the county pathologist ruled the death "natural," not a suicide. However, a few days after the funeral, Vicki Thomas and her husband went to clean out her sister's house and found suspicious literature from the Network. They also found a receipt for two helium tanks and could not figure out why Van Voorhis would have needed these. They contacted the police with the puzzling information, and the department reopened the investigation. When they re-interviewed Frank Langsner, he agreed to have his comments taped. The details of Van Voorhis' final exit slowly emerged. Langsner said he had been there as an exit guide when she died and admitted that he had forgotten to take the final letter to the next-door mailbox, where it was supposed to have been left. He then directed the police to a briefcase that contained complete records of the final exit.

The next day, police flew to Denver to serve a search warrant on Wye Hale-Rowe. After a brief phone call to Ted Goodwin, she told the police that she had nothing to say to them. Because of the search warrant, however, the authorities located and seized her records of the Van Voorhis exit. Now Hale-Rowe was a murder suspect—and just one of many operatives in what the police were starting to view as an international death-for-hire network.

The "Arizona Four" —Wye Hale-Rowe, Frank Langsner, Roberta Massey, and Dr. Larry Egbert—were indicted on March 9, 2010, with a trial set to start in Arizona's Maricopa County Superior Court on April 4, 2011. Shortly before the trial, Hale-Rowe, suffering from heart palpitations, was advised by her physician to take a plea bargain if it would keep her out of jail because the trauma of incarceration could be fatal. His advice led her to plead guilty to one count of facilitation to commit manslaughter in an agreement that would ensure little or no jail time if she agreed to testify against her colleagues. Roberta Massey, the case coordinator for the Van Voorhis event, also had severe age-related medical issues and took the same way out, leaving the junior exit guide, Frank Langsner, and the medical director, Dr. Larry Egbert, to face the judge and jury.

Jury selection for the case of *Arizona v. Larry Egbert and Frank Langsner* began on April 4, 2011, in Phoenix. Detailed daily reports were provided by Faye Girsh, a senior member of the Network's advisory board, who sat through every minute of the deliberations. Her reports were published worldwide each evening on the ERGO internet news list, which reached more than two thousand people. Bob Levine, then vice president of the Network, reported, "Larry is in good spirits. Frank seems like he'd rather be anywhere else, but he's OK."[18]

In this first case of its kind in Arizona history, the testimony and questioning of the two remaining defendants was extremely complex. The prosecution sought to portray the Network as "a well-organized, sinister, criminal conspiracy designed to aid (participate in, encourage, and advise) suicide thus violating the laws of Arizona."[19] Girsh commented extensively on the high quality of the eleven-member jury. The testimony was concluded, and three jurors were randomly set aside as alternates to serve only if another juror was unable to do so.

On April 21, 2011, after hearing all of the complicated and conflicting testimony, the jury deliberated for three days before finding Dr. Egbert not guilty of conspiracy to commit manslaughter by aiding the suicide of Jana Van Voorhis. The jury could not reach a unanimous verdict on Frank Langsner's indictment, voting 7 to 1 to acquit him of conspiracy and 4 to 3 (with one abstention) to acquit him of aiding in a suicide. Because a unanimous vote is required for conviction, a retrial was ordered for Langsner. Just before the retrial was scheduled to begin, Langsner agreed to plead guilty to one count of endangerment, and the other charges were dropped. He was sentenced to one year of probation, following which his conviction would be expunged from the public record.

The five years between the death of Jana Van Voorhis in 2007 and the end of the "Big Sting" entrapment case resulting from John Celmer's final exit put a grueling emotional and physical burden on the Network. But its resolve to help the tortured and the terminally ill stayed strong, and the resultant prosecution, persecution, and threats did not shut it down for even one day.

Referring to both the Arizona and Georgia cases, Network President Jerry Dincin said, "Seven members of the Network's leadership were charged with serious crimes for exercising their First-Amendment-protected right to freedom of speech in supporting an individual's right to die, having provided only information, literature, and counseling on how they could safely and effectively terminate their own suffering. It is outrageous that the law enforcement authorities in Phoenix and Atlanta would spend such resources to hunt down and prosecute our geriatric, compassionate volunteers as if they were a threat to society. Don't they have enough real criminals to chase after?"[20] The answer was "no." The GBI was still in the process of prosecuting the four Network members in the alleged assisted suicide of John Celmer.

As described by his wife, Sue, and his closest friends and relatives, fifty-eight-year-old John Celmer of Cumming, Georgia, was a good man who was using his remaining energy to survive cancer that had required two surgeries and left him with chronic pain and a disfiguring hole in his jaw. Although the couple was estranged and living separately after twenty-four years of marriage, the two were in frequent contact and remained close, sharing a car and the love of three children and eight grandchildren.

In September 2006, Celmer had his first mouth surgery. Cancer had appeared as a spot under his tongue, probably caused by a history of smoking. He immediately sought help, which resulted in drastic surgical measures. "They cut the skin along his throat from ear to ear and pulled his face up. They removed the spot from under his tongue and much of the floor of his mouth."[21] That did not solve the problem, and radiation therapy damaged his jawbone. Some cancer remained. By 2007, a hole had appeared in Celmer's lower jaw. He lost teeth. A Christian man who had been positively influenced by his wife's conservative faith, he persevered. He took the prescribed morphine and codeine, and added nicotine and beer, but life had become unbearable. In October 2007, Celmer found the Final Exit Network website.

After contacting the Network and reading *Final Exit*, he decided to proceed with a planned death. At home, "he continued to walk around bandaged up, and everything he ate continued to fall through the hole in his jaw. He brushed his teeth and looked in the mirror and could see the sink through the hole. Working was too difficult, and embarrassing, to continue. He wouldn't let it get any worse."[22]

On June 18, 2008, Celmer was hungry, as always. Before eating, he and his wife had to stop at the drugstore to get more pain-killing drugs. Then it was on to MacDonald's to order a cheeseburger, which Celmer had to eat at home, without the bun, after running it through a blender. Although the doctors had covered the hole in his jaw with a skin graft, his face was still extremely swollen, and he could not chew. The disfiguration and debilitating effects of the cancer surgery were also demoralizing. The cheeseburger would be his last meal.

The following day, his wife called to see how Celmer was doing. He was staying home more now, partly because of the constant pain and partly because of the ruin of his otherwise-handsome face. As usual, he told his wife that he was okay, even if he was not. She phoned him while she was out that night, offering to drop by and help. "Just go home," he said. A short time later, he called to ensure that she was home. He did not want her to drop in unannounced to meet his visitors. Across the Oriental rug from him sat two relative strangers: Ted Goodwin and Claire Blehr.[23]

"On the day of his death, we talked extensively for a couple of hours," noted Goodwin. "He made it clear that he wanted [his wife] left out of his exit, as she would be totally opposed to it. 'There'd be Hell to pay,' he said. And he wasn't kidding…. When he was going through his problems with the cancer and the operations, her reaction was—and this is a direct quote from John, and it will be burned in my memory until I die— John quipped [that] she said, 'Oh, buck up, John. Do what your doctor says.' This was her reaction. He had been operated on at least three times, and he said, 'Every time my doctor operates on me, he'd make money. Every time he operates on me, I'd suffer, and I'm tired of playing this game.'" [24]

He told his story to Goodwin and Blehr sitting in the living room on the night of his final exit. "He was a very gentle man, a very nice man, a considerate man. He didn't want to shoot himself and have his wife or someone else find him with his brains splattered on the wall. 'I have access to a gun. But now that I have found you, I don't have to do that,' he told us. 'Had I not found the Network, that would have been my only option.'"

Sue Celmer had said over and over again that her husband was under the influence of massive doses of medication and that he was not in his right mind. "That wasn't the case," said Goodwin. "The man was depressed, though not clinically depressed because of his condition, which was terrible.... When I met him, three-quarters of his jaw had been removed, about half the soft tissue had been removed from his neck, he drooled, he choked, he had constant pain. His reaction was, 'if I had only known then what I know now, I would have just asked to be put under hospice care and let nature take its course.'"

That evening, John Celmer ended his life using the helium method, with no complications. Shortly after 11 p.m. he, Blehr, and Goodwin went upstairs to his bedroom, where he lay on his bed and began his final journey. Goodwin said, "He just lay there and very peacefully, you know . . . . He knew that we were there for him, and he was happy. I could see his face through the bag, and I know that he was very content." [25]

After finding her former husband dead, Sue Celmer went to the police and got the GBI involved. "That's when they set up a sting," Goodwin said. He and Blehr ran head-on into the sting operation on January 8, 2009. After the two talked with "Richard Arthur Sartain" for about an hour and a half in his supposed home and prepared him for his final exit, GBI agents stormed in and read them their Miranda rights. Goodwin and Blehr were arrested, handcuffed, and taken into custody by the manager of the sting operation, GBI Special Agent Richard Sells.

Sue Celmer said that she and her family were "gratified that the GBI and other law enforcement agencies have pursued this matter vigorously and that their investigation has led to the arrests reported today."[26] She argued for the strongest possible punishment for the Network, based on her deeply conservative beliefs. "God has the power over life and death. God gives life. We can't create life from nothing and we do not have the power to take it. That's not what we have. We were given the job to help. We weren't given the power to decide who's going to live and who's going to die."[27]

Courthouse arraignments are less dramatic and more straightforward than those portrayed on television. The accused must appear at the courthouse, usually with a lawyer, and wait until his or her name is called. While inside the Forsyth County Courthouse, waiting for the Network defendants' names to be called, I looked down the crowded hallway and tried to pick out the "serious criminals." I quickly gave up. The space was filled with people dressed and behaving in the same way as anyone in any public library would on any given Tuesday morning. Except for the attorneys; they stood out. Most wore expensive, tailored suits, and one particularly fashionable lawyer sported a glistening, two-foot-long, braided ponytail. That was Bruce Harvey, Ted Goodwin's criminal defense attorney, thought by many to be the preeminent attorney of his kind in Georgia.

After the defendant's name is called, the accused enters the courtroom, and the charges against him or her are read by the clerk of court. The defendant is asked how he or she pleads: guilty or not guilty. The amount of bail (if any) to be posted has already been set. The presiding judge may or may not even be present at the arraignment because it is generally a formality. As soon as a defendant has signed the plea statement, the brief procedure is over. Unless bail has been denied or cannot be met, the accused person is free until his or her trial starts.

As routine as the events appeared on the surface, the four Final Exit Network defendants and their lawyers were highly focused and totally serious. The accused were Ted Goodwin, a Network co-founder and president from 2005 until 2009 and a veteran of over forty final exits; Claire Blehr, an experienced exit guide who had worked with Goodwin on three previous cases;[28] Nicholas A. "Nick" Sheridan, another veteran exit guide and the Network's southeastern regional coordinator; and the unfortunate Dr. Larry Egbert, the Network's medical director, who was also accused in the Van Voorhis case, which was still underway. The four were charged with assisting a suicide and tampering with evidence in connection with the suicide of John Celmer.

All were charged under Georgia's 1994 assisted suicide law, which was enacted in the wake of Jack Kevorkian's activities to discourage people from emulating the radical activist. At the time, numerous states had pushed hastily drafted laws through their legislatures to put out "no-assisted-suicide-trespassing" signs at their borders.[29]

Robert Rivas, the Network's legal advisor, noted that even Forsyth County District Attorney Penny Penn, who was prosecuting the Network and its volunteers, was clear when she admitted that "physician assisted suicide is legal in Georgia so long as it is done confidentially. She argued that the statute, Section 16-5-5(b) of the Georgia Code, was carefully and intentionally drafted to protect the privacy of a patient's decision, when made in consultation with his doctor, to end his or her life."[30]

Rivas repeated the Network's key policies in 2009. "One of the core principles is that the Network volunteers do not 'assist' in a suicide. Unfortunately, publicity grubbing law enforcement authorities have conned some news media into labeling the Final Exit Network an 'assisted suicide ring.' So much for the truth. The Network's Exit Guides provide education, moral support, and a compassionate presence to competent adults who wish to terminate unbearable suffering. They do not help anyone obtain any of the tools and do not raise a hand or touch anything to help anyone bring about his deliverance."[31]

Each defendant at the arraignment was accompanied by his or her attorney, who normally would speak for the client and plead "not guilty." For Goodwin, it was a point of honor to look the Clerk of Court directly in the eye and personally state, "Not guilty." Each was also required to post a bond of $65,000, after which they were released until the date of their trial.

The Network itself, as a corporate entity, was charged with violating the 1994 RICO act. The act focuses specifically on racketeering, and it allows the leaders of a syndicate to be tried for the crimes which they ordered others to do or assisted them in doing. It is now widely used to provide a legal way to seize large amounts of "laundered" cash and to combat white-collar corporate crime. Georgia used this pretense to freeze $334,786.08 USD of the Network's funds and funds of the World Federation of Right to Die Societies because Goodwin was a signatory on both accounts. The GBI did not offer the banks any evidence that the money came from illicit sources or was intended for illegal use. The banks gave in without a whimper.[32]

The GBI went after the Network's funds because, without the money, the organization would have difficulty paying the high costs of its legal defense. Convinced that they had an airtight case, the GBI never bothered, as required by law, to give evidence in court that the impounded funds had derived from criminal operations under the RICO act. As a result, the Network filed suit, and since the prosecution had not shown any evidence of wrongdoing, the seized funds were returned on October 7, 2009.[33]

What the GBI also did not understand was the depth, breadth, and passion of the Network's members and supporters. Derek Humphry immediately stepped in and formed The Liberty Fund, which quickly raised $130,000 USD through contributions, even though these were not tax deductible. The money came in donations ranging from $5 to $10,000 USD and from individuals and death-with-dignity groups throughout the United States, the Netherlands, Scotland, Australia, Belgium, and New Zealand.[34] The money allowed legal fees to be paid promptly.

Within a week of his arrest, Ted Goodwin had retained Bruce Harvey as his personal defense attorney. Commented Goodwin, "He is quite well known as the best of the best of Georgia's attorneys; highly regarded, brilliant, and wins about 90 percent of his cases. He agreed to my demand that I take the stand in my own defense. After about a week, he told me loud and clear that our defense would be on Constitutional grounds: the First Amendment's guarantee to freedom of speech. He said that in this case, there were issues that the Supremes had never taken into account in 250 years."[35]

Goodwin was familiar with Georgia's anti-assisted suicide law, but he did not see how the law violated the First Amendment and did not realize that it did not specifically outlaw assisted suicide, unless the provider had advertised his or her availability to perform it. To violate the law, someone had to offer active (hands-on) assistance and then provide it. The Network, of course, did neither. Things started to look brighter.

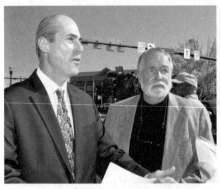

Interview after the arraignment. L-R: Attorney Bruce Harvey and Ted Goodwin

Early in 2011, the defendants moved to have the case dismissed because it violated the First Amendment's guarantee of free speech. The judge denied the request but certified that it could be appealed to the Georgia Supreme Court. On February 6, 2012, the Georgia Supreme Court shocked the prosecution, and thrilled the defense, when it unanimously declared Georgia's 1994 anti-assisted suicide law null and void because it violated the First Amendment by denying freedom of speech. The GBI's case was also declared null and void, and all the defendants were cleared of all charges. The right to die with dignity was now clearly established.

Writing for the court, Justice Hugh Thompson said, "The State has failed to provide any explanation or evidence as to why a public advertisement or offer to assist in an otherwise legal activity is sufficiently problematic to justify an intrusion on protected speech rights. Absent a more particularized State interest and more narrowly tailored statute, we hold the State may not, consistent with the United States and Georgia Constitutions, make the public advertisement or offer to assist in a suicide a criminal offense."[36]

Ted Goodwin was relieved by the ruling but noted, "For years, we all knew that arrests would occur on the journey to our goal of helping liberate suffering people from their misery. This legal assault on our organization and our volunteers was a bumpier ride than I ever imagined, but we knew that at some point, it would happen. For that, we were prepared.[37] This is a bittersweet victory because I'm saddened by what we've been put through.... I'm also sad for all the people who would have benefited from our compassionate presence at their life's bitter end over the last three years."[38]

Despite the great civil rights victory, the investigation and trial left hundreds of victims in its wake. The Maricopa County Sheriff's Department in Arizona had gathered masses of information on the Network from the homes of Langsner and Hale-Rowe. In addition, the GBI had raided the Network's office in Georgia, taking the records of all Final Exit Network members, all forms used to collect data, the case history files of almost every final exit, records of the Network's financial transactions, and copies of its communications with the makers of exit bags and the routine correspondence between Goodwin and the World Federation of Right to Die Societies. Working together, the GBI and the sheriff's office notified police departments in numerous states and dozens of cities about the allegedly menacing "international assisted suicide group" that was instigating unjustified hastened deaths worldwide. The authorities shared thousands of pages of personal information with their colleagues nationwide. Over a period of about six years, police showed up at the doorsteps of hundreds of people, allegedly to see if they had been threatened or endangered by death-with-dignity groups. Hundreds of Final Exit Network members were contacted. Some were harassed or suffered personal losses as a result.

After receiving information from the GBI, the South Carolina Law Enforcement Division (SLED) contacted an exit guide whose identity was revealed in confiscated Network records. Even though there was no evidence that the man had done anything illegal, SLED investigators went directly to the man's employer, the nation's largest federal nuclear weapons construction facility, and interviewed him there. Almost immediately thereafter, the government stripped him of his security clearance and fired him.

Another Network member who paid a high price for his acts of conscience was Dr. Larry Egbert. Prior to the Georgia trial, he had been an assistant professor of anesthesiology at the prestigious Johns Hopkins University, taught an ethics course, conducted interviews with pre-med students, and served as a Unitarian-Universalist minister at the school's chapel. Despite being found not guilty of the charges against him in the Van Voorhis and Celmer cases, he was relieved of all duties at the university and retains only his title as professor.[39]

The authorities consumed vast amounts of time and money to try to piece together a nonexistent menace. In the process, law enforcement agencies nationwide were notified to charge the Network's volunteers with crimes. None did.

On March 7, 2012, in response to the Georgia Supreme Court's nullification of the state's 1994 "anti-Kevorkian" law, Georgia legislators scrambled frantically to replace it. The Georgia House of

Representatives passed a new bill making assisted suicide a felony punishable by a prison sentence of one to ten years.

The bill was sponsored by Ed Setzler, a Republican and a Christian fundamentalist lay minister, who represents the Georgia communities of Kennesaw and Acworth. It passed in the Georgia House of Representatives by a 124 to 45 vote. The forty-five votes all came from Democrats, who were largely conservative Christian African-Americans. The proposed new law defined "assistance" in suicide as "the act of physically helping or physically providing the means to commit suicide." The proposal now goes before the Senate for consideration. If the Senate is to approve the House proposal, it must do so by March 22, the last day of this year's legislative session. Unless a procedural technicality stops it, the bill is almost certain to be passed by the Georgia Senate and signed by Georgia's conservative governor, Nathan Deal.

"In debate on the House floor," said attorney Robert Rivas, "Setzler said the drafters wanted 'to make sure' that one would not be charged with a crime under the bill for giving detailed instructions on how to commit suicide, and even by attending the death, in the absence of a 'physical act' to provide assistance in the suicide."[40]

"The State of Georgia, having found that its old law on assisted suicide was clearly unconstitutional, has crafted new legislation which is designed to outlaw 'assistance' in suicides," said Ted Goodwin. "What they have done is to draw up a law that is explicitly protective of our constitutional rights to free speech—they will not infringe on those rights—and they were most careful to define "assistance" as physical assistance—which the Network does not do. They specifically have said that 'counseling' will not in any way be challenged, as that would constitute prohibition of freedom of speech. We are ecstatic. The law now codifies and protects everything the Final Exit Network *does* and outlaws everything we *do not do*. It could not have been better for us if I had spent three days writing the provisions of the new Georgia assisted suicide law myself."[41]

– 20 –

Seamless Care for a Gentle Death

There is no rational argument for insisting that a person continue to endure pain, indignity, and suffering when they would prefer to die.
—Marshall Perron, former Chief Minister of Australia's
Northern Territory

For nearly four decades, the international death-with-dignity movement has been empowering the dying, and those who care for them, to make rational choices about the end of life. Since 1975, its members have worked to decriminalize altruistic assisted suicide and euthanasia and legalize the options of physician aid-in-dying and self-deliverance. The members of this movement have learned that it is the *quality* of life not the *quantity* that counts, and the quality should be determined by the patient—and no one else. The best end-of-life care does not mean ordering or continuing every medical intervention available but rather having the right care, and the right amount of care, delivered according to the patient's declared wishes.

Should rational adults ever be forced to live when they have expressed their wish to die? Does any nation, state, religion, or professional person have the authority to condemn someone who wants to die to the living hell of a tortured existence? It is the people who demand a peaceful, gentle death on their own terms—not those who want to live—for whom the international death-with-dignity organizations work.

As Holland's Dr. Rob Jonquière said, "Society is obligated to ensure every suffering person, whether from pain or existence, has the inalienable right to make their own choice from the whole spectrum of end-of-life decisions, be it living it to the end on the one hand, or asking to have your life terminated on the other."[1]

The basic right to die has always existed. People have chosen to end their own lives since prehistory, when the first man or woman made the choice to jump off a high cliff. The most common suicide methods, such as shooting and hanging, are horrible ways to die, born of desperation or depression and producing nightmarish aftereffects for those left behind. In response, the death-with–dignity movement's NuTech Group developed humane, respectful ways for rational adults to end their lives gently, peacefully, and legally because the methods require no assistance.

Today, suicide is no longer a crime in most of the world. Such a law would be hard to enforce. What would be the punishment? *Failed* suicide, however, was another matter until the social revolutions of the 1960s. Prior to that time, someone who attempted suicide and failed might be confined indefinitely in a straitjacket in a mental hospital because any act of self-destruction was considered to be evidence of insanity.

Fast-forward to 2012. Rational adults can now choose and plan a legal "good death." Progress has been made to legalize physician aid-in-dying, assisted suicide, euthanasia, or all three. Switzerland, the Netherlands, Belgium, and Luxembourg and the States of Washington and Oregon have passed enabling legislation. Colombia and the State of Montana have decriminalized assisted suicide, leaving it officially legal but unregulated.

Everywhere else, assisting a suicide is still a serious crime, carrying with it a possible prison sentence of one to twenty years, even if the motive was unadulterated compassion with no chance of personal gain. This leaves us with the Great Conundrum: in most places, when it comes to assisted suicide, it is illegal to help someone commit a legal act.

It is a violation of the right to personal sovereignty to permit anyone else to determine who may elect to die and under what circumstances. Any restrictions beyond being of legal age and of sound mind become grotesque illustrations of the concept of being forced to live against one's will. Of course, having the right to do something also brings responsibility. Society has the moral obligation to protect children, the mentally unsound, the poor, racial minorities, and the handicapped from being pressured to end their lives. But we live in an age when society can, and does, establish safeguards to prevent the abuse of numerous classes of people. A mass of credible evidence compiled from places where physician-hastened death is legal clearly shows that "vulnerable groups" are not discriminated against by well-written death-with-dignity laws.

And then there is simple logic. The death-with-dignity community notes that it is absurd to have laws requiring a person to be terminally ill, with six or fewer months to live, in order to qualify for a physician-hastened death—and then deny that right to another person in the same condition who is expected to suffer for seven months. Impartial studies have shown that clinicians are "notoriously poor at predicting how many years [never mind months: ed.] their patients have left."[2] What is the overwhelming logic behind choosing "six" in determining the number of months of predicted suffering before someone may seek physician aid-in-dying or euthanasia? How long must a person be forced to suffer before being granted a "gift" that ought to be an absolute civil right?

And why should "terminal illness" be the line in the sand? What about the slowly dying person who shows the predictable signs of dementia that inevitably leads to a severely degraded quality of life long before death? How long should the Alzheimer's patient dare to wait to apply for a physician-hastened death, knowing that if he or she waits too long and loses the mental clarity to make a rational choice, even legalized physician aid-in-dying cannot be invoked?

And what about the man with ALS, the woman with Parkinson's disease, or someone with multiple sclerosis or a similar degenerative condition that is not always fatal? Is their agony less than that of the person with metastasized cancer? What about those who are physically healthy but suffer from untreatable, profound depression?

How should we treat those on the other end of the quality-of-life scale, such as brilliant, highly accomplished, and totally healthy Lisette Nigot in Australia? These people have a "completed life," having fulfilled all their dreams and ambitions, have no further use for life, and want to die before their inevitable decline begins.

The concept of quantifying the dreadfulness of one disease or condition over another is intellectually and morally indefensible. Only the suffering person is capable of determining how much agony is endurable and deciding that the choice of a peaceful, painless death is preferable. The death-with-dignity movement declares that it is an individual's right to decide whether or not to continue living, not the privilege of someone else to require that he or she must live.

Dr. Rodney Syme noted, "A doctor's duty is to relieve suffering.

One could divide suffering into physical or psychological. Doctors easily recognise physical suffering; some, perhaps many, recognise psychological suffering but with more difficulty. They may not understand existential suffering, which is a component of psychological suffering, but a form of suffering which goes beyond 'simple' psychiatric suffering. Unfortunately, many doctors do not see psychological/existential suffering as sufficient for assistance at the end of life. They fail to understand that all suffering ultimately exists in the mind, whether it is physical or psychological."[3]

And then there is the question of the gatekeepers. Who should make the decision to allow or deny someone else's rational, peaceful, elective death? What qualifications should be used to define who should serve on Forced-To-Keep-Living-In-Agony Panels? And who is qualified to determine the qualifications to serve on such a panel? At every turn, the absurdity of denying the right of rational adults to die with dignity when and how they choose becomes progressively greater.

Next is the matter of political jurisdiction. Should a person who lives on the wrong side of a state or national border by only a single step be denied the dignified death available on the other side of the invisible line? The death-with-dignity map of the world should have no lines on it.

The right-to-die movement wants the world to sanction elective death as a humane act by rational adults who are acting legally, either with a physician's assistance or by themselves, with legal methods that are reliable, readily available, inexpensive, easy to use, and do not leave a distressing scene behind. Because this ideal does not yet exist, everyone who wants to prepare for a "good" death needs to plan carefully.

You are the pilot for your final destination. If a pilot does not choose a destination, determine the flight path, and preselect a place to land before leaving the ground, then chance, the fuel supply, and gravity will make all the choices. It is the same with dying. If you want the best possible flight and a soft landing according to your wishes, you must map out a detailed flight plan. The legislation to permit physician aid-in-dying may be many years in the future for most of us, so we must be responsible for ensuring our own good death. There are many ways to do this when life leaves us no other options.

Develop your landing plan

How do you *really* want to die? Passing away peacefully in your sleep always gets the most votes. As a good friend, a widower in his early seventies, said to me recently, "I'm not in the active dying stage at all. In fact, I'm quite mobile and can take care of myself with just a little help for certain things. But I am facing conditions that may well make life intolerable for me. I want to know my options. I want to know what I can afford. I want to check out whenever *I* want to. That's what I call true freedom."

Start planning now. With good planning, how we die can be largely a matter of personal choice. The body usually takes about six weeks to die once decline becomes irreversible. This leaves years prior to this final glide path to buy medical insurance, arrange for in-home assistance or residential eldercare, and prepare for hospice care. How do you want to spend that period of active dying, and where? How much intervention do you want versus how much comfort care? Where do you want to die?

Organized medicine and pharmaceutical companies will never be the leaders in offering the dying individual the widest range of choices at the end of life. On any given day, the medical industry can make more money keeping a person alive in a hospital, surrounded by medical staff and expensive machines, than by letting him or her die in peace at home, with hospice palliative care and pain-control medication, surrounded by friends and family.

Prepare your advance healthcare directives

In 2011, a survey of 1,669 adult Californians found that 82 percent agreed it is important to have end-of-life wishes in writing, but only 23 percent had done so. When asked, about 70 percent of Americans say that they have, or plan to have, a living will. This document states the care that you want or do not want to receive and is often accompanied by a durable healthcare power of attorney, which gives a person you trust the authority to speak for you if you are unable to do so. This person will be your healthcare proxy. In actuality, only one in five people has both a living will and a healthcare power of attorney in place before dying. Regardless of your age or current health status, no one can predict when a future event might leave you unable to speak for yourself.

Discuss your end-of-life plan with your primary care physician and your designated healthcare proxy. Provide them with a list of your doctors, other caregivers, and close family members. Discuss your plan with family members. Notify your healthcare proxy in writing if there are family members that you do *not* want to be consulted about your end-of-life decisions or who do not agree with your plans.

Communication about your final wishes is vital. "One of the best ways to initiate the end-of-life discussion is to start with 'Five Wishes,'" said Mario Garrett, Ph.D., a professor of gerontology at San Diego State University. The discussion starts with five simple questions.

- Who is the person I want to make care decisions for me when I cannot?
- What kind of medical treatment do I want or not want?
- How comfortable do I want to be?
- How do I want people to treat me?
- What do I want my loved ones to know?[4]

"Dying quickly and painlessly means that we are willing to discuss these final details with those around us," added Dr. Garrett. "This level of dignity implores us to communicate about our eventual death and to design a course of action that reflects our wishes and desires. This is a difficult and uncomfortable topic. But no one said that aging is for sissies."[5]

Ensure in advance that facilities that may take part in your end-of-life care will follow your written directives. This includes complying with DNR orders and accepting a patient's voluntary refusal of feeding tubes or stopping eating and drinking. It is also important to make sure that the facilities will honor your healthcare proxy's request to follow procedures spelled out in your advance directives or to stop existing artificial respiration, feeding, or hydration.

Catholic hospitals may refuse to honor advance directives that do not conform to their religious beliefs. The U.S. Catholic Conference of Bishops, for example, has ordered Catholic institutions to initiate and maintain artificial feeding in permanently unconscious patients, regardless of their advance directive instructions or family wishes. In the United States, Compassion & Choices has developed a document to ensure that patients can be transferred to another facility if a religious healthcare institution refuses to honor an advance directive that conflicts with its theological beliefs. A free copy of "My Directive Regarding Health Care Institutions Refusing to Honor my Health Care Choices" is available online at www.compassionandchoices.org.

If you plan to die through self-deliverance, work closely with the counselors of a recognized right-to-die group, who may legally be able to be present—but NOT to provide any physical assistance—at your bedside when you have chosen to die. This leads us to our next step.

Join a death-with-dignity group

These organizations keep your data completely confidential and provide large storehouses of guidance about how to deal with end-of-life issues. Most have extremely informative, public websites and members-only end-of-life counselors to talk to one-on-one about any aspect of the end of life. Annual membership costs are generally low ($50 USD per year or less). If no such group exists in your country, the websites of the larger, well-established, right-to-die groups in other countries will have most of the information you need.

Get accurate information about the diagnosis and typical progression of your condition(s)

When the time comes to consider using the landing portion of your personal flight plan, you need to get a complete and unambiguous diagnosis of your condition. You also need a detailed prognosis and description of the likely progression of your illness. Physicians are often wary of giving the straight facts to a patient. They do not want to unnecessarily scare the person into assuming that his or her condition is untreatable or terminal. Also, since the day they started medical school, doctors were taught that triumph over disease is always the goal, leading to the concept that having a patient die without a fight constitutes professional failure. Barbara Coombs Lee noted, "To doctors, death is the enemy; suffering is not. Suffering is a heroic contribution to the advance of science, or the worthy price of living one more day in a hospital."[6]

Threatening information is often downplayed; euphemisms abound. At Home and Hospice Care of Rhode Island, Dr. Joan Teno often encounters patients who are admitted with no clear under-standing of their conditions or prognoses. "The oncologist has told them, 'It's time to take a holiday from chemo,'" she commented. "It's a way not to have a conversation he or she finds hard to do."[7] Every patient has the right to know the best- and worst-case scenarios and the full range of treatment options, from aggressive, throw-everything-available-at-it to comfort care to hospice care to self-de-liverance. The best choice can only be made when the patient knows all the options.

Dr. Atul Gawande explained how "the first impulse of doctors, patients, and family members to 'fight' cancer or other serious ill-nesses makes it very difficult to have honest discussions of what treatment can and cannot do. . . . Our medical system is excellent at trying to stave off death with $8,000-a-month chemotherapy, $3,000-a-day intensive care, and $5,000-an-hour surgery. But, ulti-mately, death comes, and no one is good at knowing when to stop."[8]

"Death is seen as a technological defeat," said Dr. Ann McPher-son, who died in 2011 from pancreatic cancer. "Palliative care spe-cialists see it as a failure if patients want an assisted death. I think that's ridiculous—it should be part of good palliative care. We have got into a terrible mess about keeping people alive when they shouldn't be."[9]

End-of-life discussions do not have to be frightening. As Dr. E. James Lieberman noted, "In the Netherlands, frank talks strength-en family and social ties at a crucial time, and the result is power-fully pro-life in spirit and outcome. Unfortunately, U.S. physicians and nurses (and ordinary folks) are mostly tongue-tied when dying comes up."[10]

The ideal situation for any severely ill person facing a rapidly declining quality of life is seamless care to achieve a gentle death. All medical professionals who participate in the person's care must consider themselves as links in a chain. Their goal must be to work together as a seamless team, each member of which provides the best care according to his or her ability and the patient's needs. And when a specialist has made his or her best contribution, and the pa-tient's needs change, the team member should pass the patient along to the next colleague, one with the skills needed at the moment.

This "patient-centered care" concept is old and noble. But the ugly new reality is that this lofty ideal is often replaced with territorial professional and corporate greed that offers care designed to benefit the provider first and the patient second. Currently, no true continuum of care exists. The control of the patient's treatment often resembles a football game, with each team trying to end up with the ball.

Many doctors may be more concerned with extending the patient's life than caring for his or her comfort or dignity. To suggest that hospice care is the best next step may be anathema to some physicians because it would indicate that they failed to fulfill the role of healer. The hospital management team is usually under pressure from its corporate employers to "give the patient the best possible care, no matter what." Translated into straightforward speech, that often means "use the maximum amount of technology and create the longest hospital stay possible so that the medical bill is maximized." And for a hospice with a patient who is no longer comfortable and whose pain cannot be managed, the concept of working with a death-with-dignity group might seem not only loathsome but possibly criminal.

Just as the medical world must make some fundamental changes to ensure a seamless continuum of end-of-life care, the death-with-dignity movement has some changes of its own to undertake. The main issues involve setting priorities, creating death-with-dignity strategies, and ending ideological turf wars.

Death-with-dignity organizations are nonprofit, social activist groups who seek to make the world a better place by eliminating the need for unnecessary and unwanted agony in the dying process. Virtually all these groups worldwide run on shoestring budgets. They have few, if any, paid staff, no fancy offices, and no training seminars held aboard luxury cruise ships or in exotic resorts, as do many professional medical organizations.[11] With extremely low overhead and no profit motive, these humanitarian groups focus solely on their public service mission.

The early right-to-die groups of the 1970s and 1980s emphasized educating the public about the need to have a living will (advance healthcare directive). That was a worthy and cost-effective mission because awareness could be spread widely with very little money and a relatively small group of volunteers. Modern right-to-die organizations would do well to return to their roots and remember that education is the best and longest lasting cure for ignorance. They would only need to update existing information to include two elements not available until the 1990s: the advent of durable healthcare powers of attorney and of legal, simple methods of de-medicalized self-deliverance, such as those described in *Final Exit* and similar professionally recognized books.

Legal decisions in several countries have firmly established that simply providing information, instruction, and a passive presence when people peacefully end their lives is not a crime. Therefore, right-to-die groups should offer free counseling services to their members, providing relevant information, home visits, and, if requested, a compassionate presence for individuals when they die.

One critical problem currently facing the international movement is the contrasting (but not irreconcilable) philosophies of promoting legislative change versus teaching do-it-yourself self-deliverance methods. If the movement is to bring about the greatest good for humanity, it must promote *both* of these concepts, for two very simple reasons.

First, only the enactment of death-with-dignity laws empowering rational adults to request physician aid-in-dying will liberate people from being forced to suffer against their will. The problem is that international right-to-die groups have been struggling for decades to get such legislation passed. Their achievements, while encouraging, have not yet made any difference to the vast majority of the world's citizens. Given the glacial pace of legal reform, this tragedy will take decades to resolve, leaving millions of unnecessarily agonized deaths in its wake.

Second, the movement's liberal wing advocates educating people on how to peacefully end their own lives on their own terms. The concept has an immediate advantage to a person facing death. After attending a one-day "how-to" seminar and reading several associated books and manuals, anyone can end his or her suffering legally, without assistance. An unexpected advantage of the self-deliverance approach also has emerged. When people know they can control their own destinies, they often choose to increase, rather than decrease, their lifespans. When the means of ending your life is always at hand, it is no longer necessary to die before you are completely ready.

Both the "traditional" and "liberal" viewpoints have merit. The problem is that death-with-dignity groups who solely advocate legislative change are convinced that activists who openly and aggressively promote self-deliverance inflame public opinion against the movement as a whole and make the fight for legal reform more difficult. Open, internecine warfare between these rival ideological groups has been especially apparent in the United Kingdom and Australia. And in the United States, Compassion & Choices has likened the teaching of self-deliverance methods to promoting "coathanger abortions." An interesting result of this rivalry and enmity is that especially in Australia and the United States, many people who are concerned about having to face a potentially "bad death" in the near future cover their bases by being members of both legislative change and do-it-yourself groups.

What many people inside the movement know, however, is that some of the larger, conservative groups that most publicly denounce self-deliverance methods, especially the helium system, quietly counsel their members behind closed doors on how to use these very same methods. Given this obvious hypocrisy, it makes no sense for conservative, legislative-change-promoting groups to actively demonize their do-it-yourself colleagues.

A given group should not be required to advocate both legislative change and self-deliverance. However, no group should castigate those who are willing to do one and not the other. Activists who promote do-it-yourself views in countries where other groups promote only legislative change often come across as hostile and confrontational, rather than collaborative—and vice versa. Both teams must learn how to "play together nicely in the schoolyard" and avoid the contentious name-calling and vociferous rebuttals that are common in some countries.

There are examples of how the two views can coexist. Almost from the start, the Hemlock Society promoted living wills and advance directives *and* generated hundreds of thousands of dollars to promote citizen initiatives and bring about legislative change. In addition, as soon as NuTech became active in the late 1990s, Hemlock funneled money into the development of power-to-the-people, do-it-yourself deathing methods. In the United States, even though the Final Exit Network does not invest its efforts in legislative change, it actively supports its colleagues who do.

The obvious course for the right-to-die groups and the movement as a whole is to embrace both philosophies. The publicity generated by the liberal groups will attract one segment of the population to the cause, and the more conservative segment, whose members generally face less-imminent health threats, will attract another. For both reasons, the logic of self-empowerment will help the movement grow. Because the opposition has no new arguments to add to the debate, it will continue to dwindle.

The challenge now is to convert the existing medical-theological-psychological-ideological-methodological battleground that controls the dying person's fate to an integrated system of seamless, patient-directed care. Visions of this seamless system had made their appearance by 1993, when Dr. Meinhard Schär, of Exit-Deutsche Schweiz, established "Villa Margaritha," an integrated hospice and euthanasia facility near Bern, Switzerland.[12] In 1999, Russel D. Ogden and Dr. Michael G. Young proposed that the medical profession might benefit from an interdisciplinary approach.[13] In 2000, Dr. Timothy E. Quill wrote, "Palliative care, which addresses the multiple physical, psychosocial, and spiritual dimensions of suffering, should be the standard of care for the dying."[14]

In 2007, Lesley Martin, founder of the Dignity New Zealand Trust, proposed the creation of "Dignity Havens," which would be specially equipped, designated facilities within hospices capable of providing voluntary euthanasia in a socially responsible, transparent, and accountable manner.[15] At the time, approximately 70 percent of New Zealanders approved legalized access to end-of-life choices.

By 2008, the positive confluence of palliative care and legalized euthanasia was being widely discussed by Dr. Jan Bernheim and his European and British colleagues. The model they proposed was "encapsulated by the term *integral palliative care*, in which euthanasia is considered as another option at the end of a palliative care pathway and the patient's preferences come first."[16] The concept continued to grow, with Canadian nurses weighing in by defining quality end-of-life care as "best provided through the collaborative practice of an interdisciplinary team to meet the physical, emotional, social and spiritual needs of the person and their family."[17]

In 2011, in conjunction with National Palliative Care Week, YourLastRight.com renewed calls for legislative change to allow access to physician aid-in-dying for rational adults experiencing intolerable, unrelenting suffering from a terminal or incurable illness. Dr. Roger Hunt, a leading palliative care specialist from Adelaide, Australia, commented, "Despite high-quality palliative care, patients experience multiple concurrent symptoms and 5-10 percent explicitly request a hastened demise."[18]

There has never been a more vital personal subject for debate and action than the right to die with dignity at the time and place and under the circumstances of our own choosing. The movement that supports this started as a small, intellectual debating society composed of lofty-minded, altruistic intellectuals in the 1930s. It has since evolved into a grassroots international civil rights movement.

The enormous advances in medical care that have taken place over the last fifty years have not been matched by a proportionate improvement in the quality of life we experience as we die. Even the subject itself hides in the back of the closet. "This is an issue that does not get talked about…. As a society, our persistent refusal to face death is hurting us and causing suffering," explained Dr. Katherine Morris.[19]

Yet people cannot escape their final fate. As the world's population becomes concentrated in older age groups, interest in a gentle death will continue to grow and spark discussions. Based on the history and trajectory of that fateful moment when Jean and Derek Humphry carried out their loving, heartrending pact in 1975, the movement they were instrumental in launching has a powerful future.

Acknowledgments

Through personal interviews, letters, emails, telephone calls, and conference presentations, the following people shared their intimate insights and knowledge of the incredibly complex world of the international death-with-dignity movement with me. Without them, this inside view of the movement and its goals would have been impossible.

First and foremost, I would like to thank Derek Humphry, founder of the Hemlock Society, author of *Final Exit*, and godfather of the modern death-with-dignity movement, for granting me unrestricted access to his vast knowledge and invaluable archives.

In the United States, I am deeply indebted to Margaret Pabst Battin, Ph.D., bioethicist, University of Utah, Salt Lake City; Diane Coleman, J.D., founder and president Not Dead Yet, Rochester, New York; Stephen Drake, research analyst Not Dead Yet, Rochester, New York; Lawrence "Larry" Egbert, M.D., cofounder and former medical director Final Exit Network, Baltimore, Maryland; George Eighmey, former executive director Compassion & Choices of Oregon; Marcela Escobar-Gómez, M.D., Daniel Island, South Carolina; Rev. George D. Exoo, cofounder The Compassionate Chaplaincy Foundation, Beckley, West Virginia; Faye J. Girsh, Ed.D., past president Hemlock Society USA and president World Federation of Right to Die Societies, La Jolla, California; Theodore E. "Ted" Goodwin, former president World Federation of Right to Die Societies and cofounder and past president Final Exit Network, Pennington, New Jersey; Frank Kavanaugh, Ph.D., Punta Gorda, Florida; the late Jack Kevorkian, M.D., pathologist, Detroit, Michigan; Rev. Beverly B. Kinraide, pastor *emerita* New River Unitarian Universalist Fellowship, Beckley, West Virginia; James Lieberman, M.D., George Washington University School of Medicine, Washington, D.C.; Richard MacDonald, M.D., past president World Federation of Right to Die Societies, former medical director Hemlock Society Caring Friends Program, and senior medical advisor Final Exit Network, Chico, California; Cassandra E. Mae (aka Susan Wilson), Ph.D., exit guide, Gastonia, North Carolina; Rita L. Marker, J.D., executive director Patients Rights Council, Steubenville, Ohio; Thomas P. McGurrin, treasurer The Compassionate Chaplaincy Foundation, Beckley, West Virginia; Mary Ann Myers, reference assistant, Kingman Arizona Public Library; Rob Neils, Ph.D., founder Dying Well Network, Spokane, Washington; Neal Nicol, president Nicol Associates, Waterford, Michigan; the late Georgene ("Gigi") V. Sandberg, former southeast director Hemlock Society, Diamondhead, Mississippi; Lois Schafer, former director Hemlock Society Caring Friends Program, Denver, Colorado; Wesley J. Smith, J.D., attorney, author, and senior fellow Discovery Institute, Seattle, Washington, and Alexandria, Virginia; the late Karen Stern, musician and songwriter, Pleasantville, New York; Stanley A. Terman, Ph.D., M.D., founder Caring Advocates, Carlsbad, California; Lindsay Thomas, M.D., chief medical examiner Freeborn County, Minnesota; Bernice Thornhill, manager Silver Queen Motel, Kingman, Arizona; Nancy G. Valko, R.N., president Missouri Nurses for Life, St. Louis, Missouri; Edward Weis, Esq., U.S. Public Defender's Office, Charleston, West Virginia; Earl Wettstein, cofounder Arizonans for Death With Dignity, Tucson, Arizona, and cofounder Final Exit Network; Charles E. Whitcher, M.D., Stanford University Medical Center, Palo Alto, California.

I also received information and expert guidance from the following international colleagues.

Albania: Gentian Vyshka, M.D., Faculty of Medicine, Tirana.

Australia: Judy Dent, Tiwi, Northern Territory; Neil Francis, director YourLastRight.com, Melbourne, Victoria; Philip Nitschke, Ph.D., M.D., founder Exit International, Darwin, Northern Territory; and Rodney Syme, M.D., president Dying With Dignity–Victoria, Melbourne, Victoria.

Belgium: Nathalie Andrews, secretary-general Right-to-Die Europe and board member ADMD-Belgium, Brussels; Jacqueline Herremans, attorney, past president World Federation of Right to Die Societies, Brussels.

Canada: Themmis Anno, webmaster Right to Die Society of Canada, Toronto, Ontario; Donald Babey, former executive director Dying With Dignity, Toronto, Ontario; Michael Dawson, former editor *EuthaNEWsia,* Right to Die Society of Canada, Toronto, Ontario; Cheryl M. Eckstein, founder Compassionate Healthcare Network, Surrey, British Columbia; John L. Hofsess, founder Right to Die Society of Canada, Victoria, British Columbia; Alain Jarry, director of communications Association Québécoise pour le Droit de Mourir dans la Dignité, Quebec; the late Evelyn M. Martens, former membership director Right to Die Society of Canada, Victoria, British Columbia; Andy McKay and Andy Anderson, Cundari Group, Ltd.,Toronto, Ontario; Wanda Morris, executive director Dying With Dignity, Toronto, Ontario; Russel D. Ogden, M.A., criminologist Kwantlen Polytechnic University, Surrey, British Columbia; and Ruth von Fuchs, president Right to Die Society of Canada, Toronto, Ontario.

Colombia: Andres Castellana,* medical student, Cali; Camilo Escobar-Jimenez, M.D., Bogotá; Jaime A. Escobar-Triana, M.D., Ph.D., founder and dean Universidad El Bosque, Bogotá; Juan Mendoza-Vega, M.D., past president World Federation of Right to Die Societies and past president Fundación Por Derecho a Morir Dignamente, Bogotá; and Gustavo Alfonso Quintana R., M.D., Bogotá.

England: Michael Irwin, M.D., past president World Federation of Right to Die Societies, London, and founder Society For Old Age Rational Suicide; and Jon Ronson, producer *Rev. Death,* London.

France: Jacqueline Jencquel, secretary-general ADMD-France, Paris.

Germany: Elke Baezner-Sailer, teacher, president Deutsche Gesellschaft für Humanes Sterben (DGHS), Berlin.

Ireland: Denis Staunton, Washington correspondent for *The Irish Times.*

Japan: Soichiro Iwao, M.D., Ph.D., vice chairman Japan Society for Dying With Dignity, Tokyo.

The Netherlands: Boudewijn Chabot, M.D., former director NVVE, Amsterdam; and Rob Jonquière, M.D., past president World Federation of Right to Die Societies and former CEO NVVE, Amsterdam.

New Zealand: Scott Armstrong, detective sergeant North Shore Criminal Investigation Branch, New Zealand Police, Auckland; and Lesley Martin, R.N., trustee Dignity New Zealand Trust, Palmerston North.

Scotland: Christopher Docker, executive director EXIT (Scotland), Edinburgh; Elizabeth "Libby" Wilson, M.D., cofounder Friends at the End, Glasgow; and Hugh T. Wynne, Dr. Ing., past president World Federation of Right to Die Societies, Glasgow.

Switzerland: Ludwig A. Minelli, L.L.M., founder Dignitas, Zürich.

As with my previous books, I am grateful to my long-suffering wife, Nancy Betancourt, who put up with me for five years while I wrote this one.

This book is the product of a complex intellectual collective. At Corinthian Books, Diane Anderson and Elizabeth "Betty" Burnett, Ph.D., my senior editors, contributed invaluable insights and unwavering support, as they have for my other books. Rob Johnson, of Toprotype, in Mt. Pleasant, South Carolina, was the masterful cover designer for this book and all of the others produced by Corinthian Books. My editorial and research assistants, including Sallie J.S. Carrier, Myrtle A. Staples, Rose Tomlin, and a small army of cheerful, hard-working, brilliant interns—Cammie Amacher, Monica Biddix, Maranda Christy, Melanie Creech, Elizabeth E. Estochen, Allyson D. Field, Amanda Harris, Marielle Hartmann, Brittany Hyland, Katherine Lastrapes, Ambar Mendez, Amy McLaren, Tiffany Nichols, and Thomas Pavia, all from the College of Charleston, and Laura Strout from Clemson University—provided an enormous amount of extraordinary support during the book's evolution. Thanks also to our loyal proofreader, J.K. Kelley, who caught some crucial glitches.

Ω

Source Notes

Chapter 1: The Parallel Universe

1 Sharon Voas, "A Dance With Death," Pittsburgh *Post-Gazette*, May 25, 1997.
2 Voas, "A Dance with Death."
3 Voas, "A Dance With Death."
4 West Virginia Application for Registration Certificate, Compassionate Chaplaincy Foundation. Non-profit. April 1, 1997.
5 George D. Exoo (hereafter cited as GDE), interview with Richard N. Côté (hereafter cited as RNC), Jan. 27, 2010.
6 Anya Foos-Graber, *Deathing: An Intelligent Alternative for the Final Moments of Life* (New York: Addison-Wesley, 1984), flyleaf.
7 Ken Foxe and John Mooney, "Seven Years of Battling Depression," *Ireland on Sunday*, Feb. 3, 2002.
8 Liam Ferrie, ed., "No Plans to Return to Ireland," *The Irish Immigrant*, Feb. 11, 2002; Andrew Alderson and Nicola Byrne, "Americans face extradition after 'assisted suicide,'" London *Telegraph*, Feb. 2, 2003.
9 *Republic of Ireland vs. George David Exoo*. Case 5:07-mc-00059.
10 "Ireland probes former WQED 'Church Man' in suicide case," Pittsburgh *Post-Gazette*, Feb. 5, 2002.
11 Gary Bauslaugh, "An Interview with Evelyn Martens," *Humanist Perspectives*, 152, at www.humanistperspectives.org/issue 152/interview_evelyn.html.
12 *Ireland v. Exoo*. Document 3-4, 20 of 24.
13 *Ireland v. Exoo*, Document 3-4, 21 of 24.
14 The need for barbiturates in a helium hood exit was later found to be unnecessary, as the helium alone was found to be entirely sufficient for a swift and certain death.
15 Liz Townsend, "Pro-Life News in Brief," *Sunday Observer*, n.d., at www.nrlc.org/news/2003/NRL01/news.html.
16 Will of Rosemary Toole, Jan. 10, 2002. GDE papers. Private collection.
17 Mairead Carey, "Right to Die Woman Loses Case," *Irish Voice*, Dublin, June 22, 2005.
18 GDE, interview with RNC, Feb. 10, 2008.
19 Declan White, "The Angels of Death," *Ireland on Sunday*, Feb. 3, 2002.
20 *Ireland v. Exoo*, Document 3-3, page 7 of 17.
21 Evelyn Martens, interview with RNC, March 30, 2009.
22 Tara Tuckwiller, "'No Forward Movement' in Suicide Case; Minister Says Exoo Extradition Does Not Seem To Be Imminent," *The Sunday Gazette Mail*, Jan. 14, 2007; also GDE interview with RNC, March 9, 2007.
23 GDE, telephone call to RNC, Aug. 4, 2007.
24 Cassandra E. Mae (speaking as "Susan Wilson") videotaped interview by Jon Ronson, producer, "Reverend Death" (London: World of Wonder, 2008).
25 "Seoige & O'She" on RTÉ One, Dublin, Dec. 12, 2007, at http://www.rte.ie/tv/seoigeand-oshea/today11012007.html
26 Ireland v. Exoo, Document 31, 31-32.
27 GDE, "Compassion 'Evaluated,'" March 20, 2009. GDE Papers.

Chapter 2: Good-bye, My Love

1 "Anti-Christ of the Month…To the End Times in a Flash!" http://web.archive.org/web/20000412145348/http://www.newsminute.com/achristf2000.htm.
2 Warren Allen Smith, *Who's Who in Hell* (New York: Barricade Books, 2000), 556-557; Derek Humphry (DH), interview with RNC, Sept. 4, 2008.
3 "Playboy Interview: Derek Humphry," *Playboy*, August 1992, 56.
4 Derek Humphry, *Good Life, Good Death: Memoir of a writer who became a euthanasia advocate* (Junction City, Ore.: Norris Lane Press, 2008), 52; Humphry, *"The 11ᵗʰ Hour,"* a video autobiography recorded in Denver by KDI-TV for the PBS series, *Frontline*, 2003.
5 DH to RNC, May 23, 2009.

6 Humphry, *Good Life, Good Death,* 155.

7 Humpry, *Good Life, Good Death,* 180.

8 Derek Humphry, with Ann Wickett: *Jean's Way* (London: Quartet Books, 1976; New York: Dell, 1978), 113. The pagination of the 1978 Dell softcover edition is cited throughout.

9 Humphry, *Jean's Way,* 114.

10 Humphry, *Jean's Way,* 115.

11 Humphry, *Jean's Way,* 129.

12 Humphry, *Jean's Way,* 185.

13 Humphry, *Jean's Way,* 191.

14 Humphry, *Jean's Way,* 193.

15 DH interviewed by Paul Connolly and Allison O'Reilly on "The Inbox," Dublin, Ireland radio station 98FM, Sept. 27, 2007.

16 Humphry, *Jean's Way,* 194.

17 Humphry, *Jean's Way,* 194.

18 Humphry, *Jean's Way,* 199.

19 Humphry, *Good Life, Good Death,* 243.

20 Rita Marker, *Deadly Compassion: The Death of Ann Humphry and the Truth About Euthanasia* (New York: William Morrow, 1993), 31.

21 Humphry, *Good Life, Good Death,* 294; Marker, *Deadly Compassion,* 28-30.

22 Marker, *Deadly Compassion,* 34-35.

23 DH to RNC, May 12, 2009.

24 Russel Ogden, "Choosing Not to Be: Christian Beliefs and Modern Canadian Law," *Humanist in Canada,* 58:1 (Spring 2005), 24.

25 Humphry, *Good Life, Good Death,* 208.

26 Marker, *Deadly Compassion,* 38.

27 Humphry, *Good Life, Good Death,* 210.

28 DH to RNC, March 13, 2009.

29 An organization named the Hemlock Society was conceptualized in 1975 by Dr. Arthur W. Anderson, a psychiatrist of Los Gatos, Calif., but he never launched it. Learning of Humphry's formation of the 1980 group, Anderson wrote him to say, "it simply proves that good ideas, like weeds, will spring up in one area if they are eradicated elsewhere." Anderson then joined Humphry's new organization. *Hemlock Quarterly,* January 1981, 2.

30 DH to RNC, March 7, 2009.

31 DH to RNC, March 8, 2008.

32 DH interview with RNC, May 1, 2010.

33 Gerald A. Larue to DH, Aug. 11, 2000; DH to RNC, March 7, 2009.

34 *Hemlock Quarterly,* October 1988, 2.

35 DH to RNC, March 8, 2008.

36 DH to RNC, March 8, 2009; obituary of Richard Scott, *Hemlock Quarterly,* October 1992, 5.

37 Marker, *Deadly Compassion,* 44.

38 DH to RNC, May 1, 2009.

39 Hemlock subsequently used Tuesday, August 12, 1980, the date of the announcement at the Los Angeles Press Club, as its official founding date. Humphry, *Good Life, Good Death,* 216; *Hemlock Quarterly,* July 1990, 14.

40 Humphry, *Good Life, Good Death,* 217.

41 Humphry, *Good Life, Good Death,* 217.

42 *Hemlock Quarterly,* October 1980, 5.

43 Humphry, *Good Life, Good Death,* 224.

44 Membership figures: 1980-1984: from Humphry's personal records, in DH to RNC, May 1, 2009; from 1980-2001: *Hemlock Quarterly* and Hemlock *TimeLines* newsletters, *passim.*

45 Christiaan Barnard, *Good Life, Good Death. A Doctor's Case for Euthanasia and Suicide* (Englewood Cliffs, N. J.: Prentice-Hall, 1980), inside dust jacket flaps.

46 *Hemlock Quarterly,* July 1986, 1.

47 Humphry, *Good Life, Good Death,* 251.

48 Humphry, *Good Life, Good Death,* 253.

49 Marker, *Deadly Compassion,* 72.

50 Humphry, *Good Life, Good Death,* 253.

51 Humphry, *Good Life, Good Death,* 282.

52 Humphry, *Good Life, Good Death,* 284.

53 *Hemlock Quarterly,* April 1990, 9.

54 Marker, *Deadly Compassion,* 175.

55 Humphry, *Good Life, Good Death,* 288.

56 Marker, *Deadly Compassion,* 177

57 DH to RNC, June 20, 2009.

58 Marker, *Deadly Compassion,* 230.

59 Ann's death and its aftermath is described in detail in Humphry, *Good Life, Good Death,* 290-298; Marker, *Deadly Compassion,* 221-232; and Trip Gabriel, "A Fight to the Death," *The New York Times,* Dec. 8, 1991.

60 Marker, *Deadly Compassion*, 230. On page 35, Marker stated that "in my conversations with her, Ann implied that Derek had used pillows to smother Jean."

61 Marker, *Deadly Compassion*, 229.

62 Humphry, *Good Life, Good Death*, 224.

63 Humphry, *Good Life, Good Death*, 297-298.

64 Humphry, *Good Life, Good Death*, 297-298.

65 *Hemlock Quarterly*, July 1991, 6.

66 Humphry, *Good Life, Good Death*, 227; *Final Exit*, first edition, 1991, back cover.

67 "*Final Exit*: euthanasia guide sells out," *Nature*, Aug. 15, 1991, 553.

68 *Hemlock Quarterly*, October 1991, 1.

69 DH to RNC, Sept. 4, 2009; Meg Cox, "Suicide Manual for Terminally Ill Stirs Heated Debate," *The Wall Street Journal*, July 12, 1991.

70 DH interview Sept. 19, 1991, by William F. Buckley, Jr., on *Firing Line*.

71 Thomas Mallon, "Parting Words," *The New York Times*, May 3, 2009.

72 *Hemlock Quarterly*, July 1992, 9.

73 Peter M. Marzuk, Charles H. Hirsch, et. al, "Increase in Suicide by Asphyxiation in New York City after the Publication of *Final Exit*," *The New England Journal of Medicine (NEJM)*, Nov. 11, 1993, 1510; Humphry's response, *NEJM* 330: 1017; also Russel D. Ogden and Shereen Hassan, "Suicide by Oxygen Deprivation with Helium: A Preliminary Study of British Columbia Coroner Investigations," *Death Studies*, 35:4, 345-346.

74 Cox, "Suicide Manual."

75 DH to RNC, July 8, 2009.

76 *Hemlock Quarterly*, April 1991, 6.

Chapter 3: Euthanasia's Lightning Rod

1 "The Kevorkian Verdict," Frontline show #1416, May 14, 1996 at http://www.pbs.org/wgbh/pages/frontline/kevorkian/kevorkianscript.html.

2 Neal Nicol and Harry Wylie, *Between the Dying and the Dead: Dr. Jack Kevorkian's Life and the Battle to Legalize Euthanasia* (Madison, Wisc.: Terrace Books / University of Wisconsin Press), 2006, 25.

3 Nicol and Wylie, *Between the Dying and the Dead*, 41.

4 Nicol and Wylie, *Between the Dying and the Dead*, 61.

5 Isabel Wilkerson, "Physician Fulfills a Goal: Aiding a Person in Suicide," *The New York Times*, June 7, 1990.

6 Jack Kevorkian, *Prescription: Medicide. The Goodness of Planned Death* (Buffalo, NY: Prometheus Books, 1991), 188.

7 Nicol and Wylie, *Between the Dying and the Dead*, 63-65.

8 Nicol and Wylie, *Between the Dying and the Dead*, 66.

9 Jack Kevorkian, "The Fundus Oculi and the Determination of Death," *American Journal of Pathology*, 32 (6) [December 1956]: 1253–1269.

10 Nicol and Wylie, *Between the Dying and the Dead*, 67.

11 Nicol and Wylie, *Between the Dying and the Dead*, 67.

12 Michael Cook, "Yelping at the yuck factor," *BioEdge*, March 5, 2010, at http://www.bioedge.org/index.php/bioethics/bioethics_article/yelping_at_the_yuck_factor/

13 Kevorkian, *Prescription: Medicide*, 27.

14 Kevorikian, *Prescription: Medicide*, 31.

15 Kevorkian, *Prescription: Medicide*, 31.

16 Jack Kevorkian and Glenn W. Bylsma, "Transfusion of Postmortem Human Blood, *The American Journal of Clinical Pathology*, 35 (May 1961): 412-419; "Blood from the Dead," *Time*, May 26, 1961, at www.time.com/time/magazine/article/0,9171,872489,00.html.

17 Kevorkian and Bylsma,"Transfusion of Postmortem Human Blood," 412.

18 "Dead Give Blood to the Living," *The Detroit News*, Jan. 18, 1964.

19 "Blood from the Dead."

20 Jack Kevorkian, Neal Nicol, and E. Rea, "Direct Body-to-Body Human Cadaver Blood Transfusion," *Journal of Military Medicine*, 129 (January 1964): 24–27.

21 Nicol and Wylie, *Between the Dying and the Dead*, 112.

22 Jack Kevorkian, in *Kevorkian* (HBO Documentary Films), June 28, 2010.

23 Nicol and Wylie, *Between the Dying and the Dead*, 140.

24 Nicol and Wylie, *Between the Dying and the Dead*, 143.

25 Auction of personal items from the estate of Jack Kevorkian.

26 Derek Humphry, *The Good Euthanasia Guide: Where, What, and Who in Choices in Dying* (Junction City, Ore.: Norris Lane Press, 2004) 59-60.

27 Kevorkian, *Prescription: Medicide*, 208-209.

28 Kevorkian's response to RNC's question, press conference, Kutztown University, Kutztown, Pennsylvania, Sept. 20, 2009.

29 Jack Kevorkian press conference, Sept. 20, 2009, Kutztown University.

30 Jack Kevorkian, "The Last Fearsome Taboo: Medical Aspects of Planned Death," *Medicine and Law* (Israel), 7 (1988): 3.

31 Humphry, *Good Life, Good Death*, 316.

32 Humphry, *Good Life, Good Death*, 316-317.

33 Nicol and Wylie, *Between the Dying and the Dead*, 144–145.

34 Jack Kevorkian, "A Fail-Safe Model for Justifiable Medically-Assisted Suicide," *American Journal of Forensic Psychiatry*, 13 (1992) 1:7-41.

35 Michael Betzold, *Appointment with Doctor Death* (Troy, Michigan: Michael Betzold, 1995), 30.

36 Kevorkian, *Prescription: Medicide*, 194.

37 Kevorkian, *Prescription: Medicide*, 194.

38 Betzold, *Appointment with Doctor Death*, 35.

39 Betzold, *Appointment with Doctor Death*, 36.

40 Donald William Cox, *Hemlock's Cup: The Struggle for Death with Dignity* (Buffalo, N.Y.: Prometheus Books, 1993), 96.

41 Nicol and Wylie, *Between the Dying and the Dead*, 149.

42 Nicol and Wylie, *Between the Dying and the Dead*, 149.

43 Nicol and Wylie, *Between the Dying and the Dead*, 149

44 Nicol and Wylie, *Between the Dying and the Dead*, 149.

45 Betzold, *Appointment with Doctor Death*, 45.

46 Nicol and Wylie, *Between the Dying and the Dead*, 150.

47 Lisa Belkin, "Doctor Tells of First Death Using His Suicide Device," *The New York Times*, June 6, 1990.

48 DH, email to RNC, July 28, 2009.

49 Nicol and Wylie, *Between the Dying and the Dead*, 52.

50 Nicol and Wylie, *Between the Dying and the Dead*, 54.

51 Jack Lessenberry, "Death Becomes Him," *Vanity Fair*, July 1994, 113.

52 Nicol and Wylie, *Between the Dying and the Dead*, 211.

53 Cox, *Hemlock's Cup*, 163.

54 "Frontline: The Kevorkian Verdict." Show #1416. Air date: May 14, 1996. Accessed at http://www.pbs.org/wgbh/pages/frontline/.

55 Neal Nicol (NN), email to RNC, Jan. 29, 2011.

56 Neal Nicol, "Working With Jack Kevorkian," NuTech Conference IX, Melbourne, Australia, Oct. 7, 2010. Filmed by RNC.

57 NN interview with RNC, Oct. 8, 2010.

58 "Kevorkian Begins Ballot Drive for Suicide Measure," *The New York Times*, Jan. 31, 1994.

59 Nicol and Wylie, *Between the Dying and the Dead*, 185.

60 NN, email to RNC, May 12, 2011.

61 The only known copy of this business card was sold for $1,200 by the Kevorkian estate at auction in New York on October 28, 2011. "Kevorkian suicide machine, disputed paintings don't sell in NYC amid museum dispute," *The Washington Post*, Oct. 28, 2011.

62 "Kevorkian Opens Clinic, Attends 24th Death," *Los Angeles Times*, June 27, 1995.

63 "Landlord to shut down Kevorkian's obitorium," *Eugene* (Oregon) *Register-Guard,* June 28, 1995.

64 Jack Lessenberry, "New Assistant to Kevorkian is an Old Hand at Suicides," *The New York Times,* Aug. 11, 1996.

65 Nicol and Wylie, *Between the Dying and the Dead,* following 132.

66 Lessenberry, "Death Becomes Him," 106.

67 Lessenberry, "Death Becomes Him," 111.

68 Humphry, *Good Life, Good Death,* 312-313.

69 *The New York Times,* April 14, 1999.

70 Nicol and Wylie, *Between the Dying and the Dead,* 259.

71 Not Dead Yet media release, Dec. 14, 2006.

72 Mike Wallace, "Engaged and Warm: The Jack Kevorkian I Know," letter to the editor, *New York Times,* June 10, 2007.

73 Daniel Schorr, "Kevorkian will not assist in any more suicides," "60 Minutes," June 3, 2007.

74 RNC question to Dr. Jack Kevorkian, at press conference, Kutztown University, Kutztown, Penn., Sept. 20, 2009.

75 NN, email to RNC, Oct. 8, 2010.

76 NN, email to GDE, July 1, 2010; GDE, email to NN, July 21, 2010.

77 NN to RNC, email, June 3, 2011.

78 Dennis McLellan, "Dr. Jack Kevorkian," *Los Angeles Times,* June 4, 2011.

79 Wesley J. Smith, "Jack Kevorkian: Pariah or Prophet?" The Center for Bioethics and Culture Network, www.cbc-network.org, June 9, 2011.

80 Brian Dickerson, "Contending with Kevorkian," Detroit *Free Press,* June 5, 2011.

81 Tami Abdollah, "Kevorkian helped states pass assisted-suicide laws," Associated Press, June 4, 2011.

82 Marilynne Seguin and Cheryl K. Smith, *A Gentle Death* (Toronto, Canada: Key Porter Books, Ltd., 1994), 209.

83 John Hofsess, email to RNC, Sept. 4, 2010.

84 "How Kevorkian and assisted suicide fit into America's mixed moral landscape," *Christian Science Monitor,* June 3, 2011.

85 Joe Swickard, Patricia Anstett, and L.L. Brasier, "Kevorkian Lightning Rod for Debate, Controversy," *Detroit Free Press,* June 3, 2011.

86 Francis X. Donnelly "Kevorkian remembered as 'true believer' in assisted suicide crusade," *The Detroit News,* June 10, 2011.

87 John Hofsess, email to RNC, April 20, 2010.

88 Jack Lessenberry, "The Meaning of Dr. K.," http://metrotimes.com/columns/the-meaning-of-dr-k-1.1158341, June, 2011.

Chapter 4: The Twilight Zone

1 Joy Hirsch, "Raising Consciousness," *The Journal of Clinical Investigation,* 115 (May 2, 2005):1102.

2 James Murtagh, "Do-not-resuscitate: A Revolution Now 30 years old," May 26, 2008 at www.opednews.com.

3 Luis Kutner, "Due Process of Euthanasia: The Living Will, a Proposal," *Indiana Law Journal,* 44 (1969): 549.

4 "The Living Will Gains Acceptance," *The New York Times,* Sept. 20, 1984.

5 James Leonard Park, "Right to Die Portal," www.tc.umn.edu/~parkx032/P-RTD.html.

6 E. James Lieberman, M.D., "Safeguards," posted to Right-to-Die-Safegards@googlegroups.com, Feb. 16, 2008.

7 Compassion & Choices, http://compassionandchoices.org/page.aspx?pid=492.

8 Compassion and Choices, "My Directive Regarding Health Care Institutions Refusing to Honor my Health Care Choices," http://community.compassionandchoices.org/document.doc?id=484.

9 O.M.O.*, Facebook message to RNC, Aug. 20, 2011.

10 Saira Kirup, "Four women India Forgot," *The Times of India,* http://timesofindia.indiatimes.com/news/sunday-toi/special-report/Four-women-Indiaforgot/articleshow/1519056.cms.

11 "Supreme Court admits Pinki Virani's

plea to end life of brain-dead rape victim Aruna Shanbaug," http://www.dancewithshadows.com/politics/supreme-court-admits-pinki-viranis-plea-to-end-life-of-brain-dead-rape-victim-aruna-shanbaug/, Dec. 17, 2009.

12 Matathy Iler, "Euthanasia plea sparks off debate among docs," *The Times of India*, Dec. 17, 2009.

13 Bachi Karkaria, *The Times of India* / Blogs, Dec. 20, 2009, at http://blogs.timesofindia.indiatimes.com/erratica/entry/the-unnerving-case-of-aruna.

14 Pratibha Masand, "Aruna will live because of hospital staffs' love," *The Times of India*, March 8, 2011.

15 "Pro-life award goes to hospital staff," http://www.ucanews.com/2011/04/27/pro-life-award-goes-to-hospital-staff/, April 27, 2011.

16 "Aruna Shanbaug case: Supreme Court allows passive euthanasia in path-breaking judgment," *The Times of India*, March 7, 2011.

17 Matthew Stonecipher, "The Evolution of Surrogates' Right to Terminate Life-Sustaining Treatment," American Medical Association *Virtual Mentor*, 8 (September 2006), Number 9: 593-598.

18 Pope Pius XII, "The prolongation of life" (Nov. 24, 1957) *The Pope Speaks* 4 (1985): 397.

19 *In re Quinlan*, 355 A2D 647, 652 (New Jersey, 1976).

20 Anthony Lim, "The Right to Die Movement: From Quinlan to Schiavo" (Harvard University Press, 2005), 6.

21 William H. Colby, *Unplugged: Reclaiming the Right to Die in America* (New York: Amacom, 2006), xiii.

22 www.libraryindex.com/pages /590/Court-End-Life-Case-Nancy-Cruzan.html.

23 "Terri Schiavo Case," en.Wikipedia.org/wiki/Terri_Schiavo-case

24 Stephen Drake, "Disabled are Fearful: Who Will Be Next?" *Los Angeles Times*, Oct. 29, 2003.

25 Charles P. Pierce, *Idiot America: How*

Stupidity Became a Virtue in the Land of the Free (New York: Doubleday, 2009), 180.

26 Pierce, *Idiot America*, 182.

27 "Terri Schiavo Case," Wikipedia.

28 Timothy Quill, "Terri Schiavo.: A Tragedy Compounded," *New England Journal of Medicine* 352 (April 1993): 1630-33.

29 Lim, "The Right to Die Movement," 2005, 44, at http://leda.law.harvard.edu/leda/data/732/Lim05.pdf.

30 "Piergiorgio Welby," en.wikipedia.org/wiki/Piergiorgio_Welby.

31 "Il pensiero magico." Piergiorgio Welby. http://calibano.ilcannocchiale.it/?id_blogdoc=4869.

32 Ian Fisher, "A Poet Crusades for the Right to Die His Way," *The New York Times*, Dec. 20, 2006.

33 "Piergiorgio Welby," Wikipedia.

34 "Piergiorgio Welby," Wikipedia.

35 "Piergiorgio Welby," Wikipedia.

36 "Church denies funeral for Italian," BBC News, Dec. 22, 2006.

37 María José Guerra: "Euthanasia in Spain: The Public Debate after Ramon Sampedro's Case," *Bioethics*, 13:5 (October 1999): 427.

38 "Ramon Sampedro," en.wikipedia.org/wiki/Ramon_Sampedro.

Chapter 5: Who Owns My Life?

1 Lisa Hobbs Birnie and Sue Rodriguez, *Uncommon Will: The Death and Life of Sue Rodriguez* (Toronto: Macmillan Canada, 1994), 36.

2 Birnie and Rodriguez, *Uncommon Will*, 27.

3 Birnie and Rodriguez, *Uncommon Will*, 37.

4 DH, email to RNC, April 15, 2008.

5 DH, email to RNC, April 23, 2008.

6 Birnie and Rodriguez, *Uncommon Will*, 39.

7 John Hofsess, "Sue Rodriguez is 42. She has ALS. Who Cares?" *Last Rights*, 6 (October-November 1992): 8.

8 Hofsess, "Sue Rodrigez is 42" 8.

9 Hofsess, "Sue Rodriguez is 42," 8.

10 "John Leonard Hofsess," The *Canadian Who's Who* (Toronto: University of Toronto Press), 18 (1981): 455.

11 "Publications board fights editor ban," *The Ubyssey* (Vancouver, B.C.), Oct. 20, 1966, 11.

12 T. F. Rigelhof, *This is Our Writing* (Erin, Ontario: Porcupine's Quill, 2000), 161.

13 "Hofsess," *Who's Who;* John Hofsess, email to RNC, March 13, 2011.

14 "Canada's right-to-die leader emerges on the Net," 24 Hours in Cyberspace, at http://undertow.arch.gatech.edu/Home-pages/virtualopera/cyber24/SITE/htm2/5_156.htm.

15 DH to RNC, Sept.3, 2011.

16 John Hofsess, report on The Right to Die Society of Canada, *The World Federation of Right to Die Societies Newsletter*, 25 (Fourth Quarter, 1994): 14.

17 "Right-to-die debate continues." *The CBC Digital Archives Website*, at http://archives.cbc.ca/IDC-1-69-1135-6413/life_society/sue_rodriguez/clip1.

18 Birnie and Rodriguez,*Uncommon Will*, 42.

19 Sue Woodman, *Last Rights: The Struggle Over the Right to Die* (Cambridge, Mass.: Perseus Publishing, 2000, 94.

20 Right to Die Society of Canada, *Last Rights*, issue #6 (October-November, 1992), 4.

21 Nick Orocaylo, "The Other Woman in the Story: Surrey's Cheryl Eckstein takes on advocates of euthanasia," *British Columbia Report*, March 22, 1993, 23.

22 Ian Dowbiggin, *A Concise History of Euthanasia. Life, Death, God, and Medicine.* (New York: Rowman & Littlefield, 2005), 147-148.

23 Birnie and Rodriguez,*Uncommon Will*, 50.

24 The Compassionate Healthcare Network website, http://www.chninter-national.com/default.html.

25 Cheryl Eckstein, email to RNC, Jan. 22, 2009.

26 "Life Force: Cheryl Eckstein's Uphill Fight Against Pro-Euthanasia Public Opinion," *British Columbia Report*, March 22, 1993, 20.

27 The Campaign for Life Coalition website, http://www.campaignlifecoalition.com.

28 "Who owns my life?" *The CBC Digital Archives Website*. Canadian Broadcasting Corporation. http://archives.cbc.ca/IDC-1-69-1135-6396/life_society/sue_rodriguez/clip1.

29 Examples include "Jocelyn Downie is planning to spin the truth about euthanasia at McGill University," http://www.lifesitenews.com/blog/jocelyn-downie-is-planning-to-spin-the-truth-at-mcgill-university/, Jan 12, 2011, and "Israel overwhelming rejects assisted suicide law," http://alexschadenberg.blogspot.com/search/label/nazi%20euthanasia%20program, Jan. 20, 2011.

30 "Who owns my life?" *The CBC Digital Archives Website*. Canadian Broadcasting Corporation, at http://archives.cbc.ca/IDC-1-69-1135-6396/life_society/sue_rodriguez/clip1.

31 "Dossier of Cheryl M. Eckstein," at www.chninternational.com/cheryl_e_dossier.htm.

32 Ann Mullens, "Rodriguez angry over letter to Sun penned in her name," *The Vancouver Sun*, Jan. 30, 1993.

33 Rodriguez *v.* British Columbia (Attorney General), [1993] 3 S.C.R. 519.

34 Helma Libick, "Remembering Sue," *Last Rights*, 13 (Fall 1994):15.

35 Sue Rodriguez to Robert Mason Lee in *The Vancouver Sun*, Sept 19, 1992.

36 Birnie and Rodriguez,*Uncommon Will*, 178.

37 John Hofsess, email posting to the Internet newsgroup sci.med.aids, June 25, 1995.

38 John Hofsess, "DeathNET: Educating the World About 'Choices-in-Dying,'" *Last Rights* #14 (Toronto: The Right-to-Die Society of Canada), Winter 1995.

39 David Morrison, "Death Comes to Cyberspace: Computer Users Discover How-to Guide to Euthanasia," *HLI Reports*, (Gaithersburg, MD: Human Life International, October 1995), at http://www.ewtn.org/library/ISSUES/DEATHNET.TXT.

40 John Hofsess, email posting to the

Internet newsgroup sci.med.aids, June 25, 1995.

41 Hazel Biggs, *Euthanasia, Death With Dignity and the Law* (Oxford: Hart Publishing, 2001), 32n26.

42 Seguin and Smith, *A Gentle Death*, 10.

43 "Change of Leadership at DWD, Canada," *World Right to Die Newsletter*, 31 (February 1998), 6.

44 Richard MacDonald, "Death of Long-time Campaigner Marilynne Seguin," *World Right-to-Die Newsletter*, December 1999, 3; Hemlock Society Timelines, Winter 1998,2; Fall 1999, 4.

45 Richard MacDonald, email to RNC, March 6, 2011.

Chapter 6: Robbing Death of Its Sting

1 Sue Woodman, *Last Rights: The Struggle over the Right to Die* (Cambridge, Mass.: Perseus Publishing, 1998), 96.

2 Woodman, *Last Rights*, 97.

3 John Hofsess, (JH) email to RNC, July 7, 2009.

4 Rob Neils, *Death Readiness: A Short Clinical Scale of Rational Suicide.* Formerly online in 2001 as section 8.02 in *Death With Dignity FAQs* at www.bardo.org/DWD.html. A cached version was accessed at http://web.archive.org/web/20010803081236/www.togopeacefully.com/SCISORS.html; also Valerie Snipes: *Final Exit Network Newsletter* #3 (Spring 2005), 2.

5 JH, email to ERGO Right-to-Die mailing list, Nov. 19, 1999.

6 Colin Brewer, "Self-Deliverance With Certainty," *Hemlock Quarterly* special reprint, updated June, 1989 (Eugene, Ore.: The Hemlock Society, 1989).

7 Anonymous source, email to RNC, Oct. 12, 2010.

8 The 1989 Thanatron prototype and the description and technical drawings of it were put up for auction on October 28, 2011. The $70,000 minimum bid was not met and it was withdrawn from sale.

9 JH to NuTech confidential mailing list, "Victoria Manifesto" (Rob's version), April 17, 1998, 3. Page one of this five-page email printout has yet to be located.

10 Rob Neils, email to RNC, Sept. 10, 2008.

11 John Hofsess, "Introducing the Debreather," *The Art & Science of Suicide, Chapter 6* (version 1.1). Ottawa: HC Publications, December 1998, 3.

12 Hofsess, "Introducing the Debreather." (version 1.1)

13 Hemlock Society *Timelines*, Spring 1998, 11; Hofsess, "Introducing the Debreather." (version 1.1), 4.

14 Hofsess, "Victoria Manifesto" (Rob's version), 3.

15 Hofsess, "Victoria Manifesto" (Rob's version), 3.

16 Hofsess, "Victoria Manifesto" (Rob's version), 5.

17 Hofsess, "Introducing the Debreather." (version 1.1), 7.

18 The realm of "dark humor" is not the exclusive preserve of euthanasia proponents. The healing professions, scientists, engineers, and ethicists have their own versions.

19 Hofsess, "Introducing the De-breather." (version 1.1), 15.

20 Hofsess, "Introducing The De-breather." (version 1.1), 2.

21 John Hofsess, "Beyond Physician-assisted Suicide. The Art and Science of Dying Well," in Robert C. Horn, III, ed. (with Gretchen Keeler), *Who's Right? Whose Right?* (Sanford, Fla.: DC Press, 2001), 331.

22 Rob Neils, email to JH, August 13, 1998. Italics are original.

23 Rob Neils, *Death With Dignity FAQs.* Section 8.06 The Expirator. Offline. Cached at http://web.archive.org/web/20010625231645/http://www.togopeacefully.com/DYING.html.

24 Neils, *Death With Dignity FAQs*, Section 6: History. Offline. cached on August 9, 2002 at http://web.archive.org/web/20020809181348/http://www.togopeacefully.com/HISTORY.html.

25 Dr. Betty Noble, Berkeley, Calif., to George Exoo, postmarked March 9, 1999. GDE collection.

26 "Deaths in the Family," *The Hemlock Times*, Fall, 2001, 5.

27 Compassionate Chaplaincy Foundation minutes for 2000. annual meeting of the board, Jan. 31, 2001, Beckley, W. Va. GDE Collection; also West Virginia Application for Registration Certificate, April 1, 1997, GDE Collection. Sylvia Gerhard died in October 2001.

28 GDE, interview with RNC, June 25, 2008.

29 *The Art & Science of Suicide. Chapter Nine. A first-class death: Self-deliverance through new technology* (Victoria, B.C.: Last Rights Publications, June 2000), 22.

30 Compassionate Chaplaincy Foundation Minutes for 1999. annual meeting of the board, Dec. 29, 1999. GDE Collection.

31 The original Hofsess DeBreather, which I have designated as Spartacus IIa, had a hard, black plastic full facemask, which proved to leak air, thereby slowing the deathing. The problem was solved when it was replaced by an inflatable soft vinyl mask. I have designated the soft-mask version as Spartacus IIb.

32 Philip Nitschke, email to RNC, Sept. 14, 2008.

33 Cheryl K. Smith, Chris G. Docker, John Hofsess, and Dr. Bruce Dunn, *Beyond Final Exit: New Research in Self-Deliverance for the Terminally Ill* (Victoria, B.C.: The Right to Die Society of Canada, 1995), 69-70.

34 Smith et al., *Beyond Final Exit*, 70.

35 JH, email to RNC, Aug. 10, 2008; DH, email to RNC, Aug. 10, 2008.

36 "Head right-to-die activists to meet," Knight-Ridder newspapers, Nov. 13, 1999.

37 Carol M. Ostrom, "A Bustling Search for a Way To Die," *The Seattle Times*, Nov. 15, 1999.

38 "Conference on New Ways of Self-deliverance," *World Right To Die Newsletter*, 35 (December 1999): 4.

39 Erin Hoover Bennett, "Right-to-die proponents showcase suicide aids," *The Oregonian*, Nov. 14, 1999.

40 GDE, interview with RNC, July 22, 2008.

41 Jeff Lee, "Canadian helped to develop suicide machine," *The Vancouver Sun*, Nov. 17, 1999.

42 Wesley J. Smith, "Death-lovers unmasked," *The New York Post*, Nov. 26, 1999.

43 Smith, "Death-lovers unmasked."

44 "Exit this way," *The Economist*, Dec. 6, 2001, at www.societyof-control.com/library/_p-t/suicide_technologies.txt on Sept. 10, 2008.

45 Paul A. Spiers, "A person with disabilities speaks out," Hemlock Society *Timelines*, Spring 1999, 5.

46 Photograph in *World Right-to-Die Newsletter* 30 (November 2000), 7.

47 John B. Kelly, "A battle waged in Boston: right to die vs. will to live," Boston *Sunday Globe*, Sept. 3, 2000.

48 Lisa Lipman, "Euthanasia Expert Advocates Death by Helium," Associated Press, Sept. 2, 2000.

49 Ilene Kaplan, email to RNC, Dec. 14, 2008 and interview, March 1, 2009.

50 JH, email to RNC Aug. 13, 2008.

51 JH, email to RNC, Sept. 18, 2008.

52 Georgene V. ("Gigi") Sandberg, interview with RNC, Dec. 27, 2008.

53 Sandberg Obituary in Biloxi, Mississippi *Sun Herald*, February 16, 2009; Richard N. Côté and Glen Sandberg, "In Memoriam: Gigi Sandberg," at www.bookdoctor.com/gigi.html.

54 Philip Nitschke and Fiona Stewart, *The Peaceful Pill Handbook* (Waterford, Mich.: Exit International USA, 2007), 76.

55 Philip Nitschke, interview with RNC, Sept. 16, 2008.

56 JH, email to RNC, March 21, 2011.

57 Corinna Ariane Schon and Thomas Ketterer, "Asphyxial Suicide by

Inhalation Inside a Plastic Bag," *American Journal of Forensic Medicine & Pathology*, 28(4): 364-367 [December 2007].

58 JH, email to RNC, Sept. 10, 2008.

59 JH email to RNC, Aug. 13, 2008.

Chapter 7: Grandma Martens Makes Her Rounds

1 Evelyn Martens, acceptance speech, Canadian Humanist of the Year award, June 25, 2005.

2 Martens, acceptance speech.

3 Martens, acceptance speech.

4 Martens, acceptance speech.

5 Martens, acceptance speech.

6 Martens, acceptance speech.

7 Russel D. Ogden, "Obituary: Evelyn Marie Martens, Canadian Right to Die Activist," posted to ERGO Newslist (right-to-die@lists@lists.opn.org), Jan. 7, 2011.

8 Hanna Gartner, "Giving Death a Hand: Interview with Evelyn Martens," http://www.cbc.ca/fifth/givedeathahand/interview.html.

9 Martens, acceptance speech.

10 Martens, acceptance speech.

11 Martens, acceptance speech.

12 Martens, acceptance speech.

13 Martens, acceptance speech.

14 Martens, acceptance speech.

15 Martens, acceptance speech.

16 Martens, acceptance speech.

17 Evelyn Martens, interview with RNC, March 30, 2009.

18 Ogden, "Obituary: Evelyn Marie Martens."

19 JH, email to RNC, March 28, 2009

20 JH, email to RNC, Aug. 13, 2008.

21 JH, email to RNC, Aug. 13, 2008.

22 JH, email to RNC, Aug. 13, 2008.

23 JH email to RNC, March 11, 2011.

24 Gary Bauslaugh, "The Trial of Evelyn Martens. The Final Day," *Humanist in Canada*, 38, No. 1, issue 152 (Spring 2001), 10.

25 Bauslaugh, "The Trial of Evelyn Martens. The Final Day."

26 Bauslaugh, "The Trial of Evelyn Martens. The Final Day."

27 Paul Zollman, "Evelyn Martens Defence Fund," [Canadian] *Humanist Perspectives*, 153 (Summer 2005) at www.humanistperspectives.org/issue153/evelynmartens_defense_fund.html.

28 Ogden, "Obituary: Evelyn Marie Martens."

29 Charlie Fieldman, "Living With Dignity," *The Montréal Gazette*, Aug. 13, 2010; Henry Aubin, "Euthanasia Advocates are Dead Wrong," *The Montréal Gazette*, July 18, 2009.

30 "Euthanasia debate straying off course": group, http://www.cbc.ca/news/canada/montreal/story/2010/09/08/quebec-euthanasia-hearings-day-two.html, Sept. 8, 2010.

31 "Euthanasia debate straying off course."

32 CBC News, "Most Québecers back euthanasia poll": at www.cbc.ca/news/health/story/2010/11/22/quebec-euthanasia-poll.html.

33 CBC unregulated poll results: see http://www.cbc.ca/news/pointofview/2010/11/euthanasia-should-it-be-legalized.html

34 "Vivre dans la Dignité – Living with Dignity, June 22, 2010, at http://alexschadenberg.blogspot.com/2010/06/vivre-dans-la-dignite-living-with.html

35 Toula Foscolos, "Being allowed a 'Good Death,'" *The West Island Chronicle* (Montréal), Nov. 26, 2008.

Chapter 8: The Search for the Peaceful Pill

1 Philip Nitschke and Fiona Stewart. *Killing Me Softly: Voluntary Euthanasia and the Road to the Peaceful Pill.* (Melbourne, Vic.: The Penguin Group, 2005), 43; Seth Mydans, "Assisted Suicide: Australia Faces a Grim Reality," *New York Times*, Feb. 2, 1997.

2 Northern Territory of Australia.

Rights of the Terminally Ill (ROTI) Act, 1995.

3 Sandra Kanck, "Voluntary Euthanasia." Speech to the South Australian Legislative Council, Aug. 30, 2006.

4 "Part 2–Request for and Giving of Assistance," ROTI Act.

5 Nitschke and Stewart, *Killing Me Softly*, 31.

6 Philip Nitschke on "The Conversation Hour, with Richard Fiedler," ABC Brisbane, July 21, 2008, at www.abc.net. au/reslib/200807/r273586_1153307. mp3.

7 Leon Compton interview with Philip Nitschke on "The Guestroom," ABC local radio, Darwin, Feb. 22, 2010, at http://mpegmedia.abc.net.au/local/darwin/201002/r518849_2860237.mp3.

8 Gail Tulloch, *Euthanasia–Choice and Death* (Edinburgh: Edinburgh University Press, 2005), 126.

9 Richard Fiedler interview.

10 Compton interview; Nitschke and Stewart, *Killing Me Softly*, 30.

11 Sue Woodman, *Last Rights: The Struggle Over the Right to Die* (Cambridge, Mass.: Perseus Publishing, 1998) 89.

12 Kathleen Foley and Herbert Hendin, eds., *The Case Against Assisted Suicide* (Baltimore, Md.: The Johns Hopkins University Press, 2002), 195-197; David W. Kissane, Annette Street, and Philip Nitschke, "Seven Deaths in Darwin: case studies under the Rights of the Terminally Ill Act, Northern Territory, Australia," *The Lancet*, 352 (Oct. 3, 1998): 1098; and RNC telephone interview with Philip Nitschke (PN), April 21, 2010.

13 Kissane et al., "Seven Deaths in Darwin," 1099.

14 Kissane et al., "Seven Deaths in Darwin," 1099.

15 Philip Nitschke, "Max Bell," *Exit News & Forum*, April 8, 2010, at www. euthanasia.net/page/MaxwellBell.

16 Nitschke, "Max Bell."

17 Compton interview.

18 Kissane et al., "Seven Deaths in Darwin," 1099.

19 Nitschke and Stewart, *Killing Me Softly*, 42

20 Compton interview.

21 Compton interview.

22 Woodman, *Last Rights*, 90.

23 PN, email to RNC, Sept. 14, 2008.

24 Frank Devine, "An Interview with Philip Nitschke," *Quadrant*, 2002, at www. life.org.nz/euthanasia/abouteuthanasia/history-euthanasia2/.

25 Judy Dent, interview with RNC, Oct. 6, 2010, Melbourne.

26 Judy Dent interview.

27 Judy Dent interview.

28 Mydans, "Assisted Suicide."

29 Judy Dent interview.

30 Fiedler interview.

31 Judy Dent interview.

32 Compton interview.

33 Nitschke and Stewart, *Killing Me Softly*, 245.

34 PN, interview with RNC, April 20, 2010.

35 *The Age*, Melbourne, Feb. 22, 1997.

36 Tulloch, *Euthanasia-Choice and Death*, 126.

37 Kathryn Jean Lopez, "Euthanasia Sets Sail: An Interview with Philip Nitschke, the other 'Dr. Death." *National Review Online*, June 5, 2001 at www. nationalreview.com/interrogatory/interrogatory060501.shtml.

38 Nitschke and Stewart, *Killing Me Softly*, 117.

39 Sandra Kanck, *Minutes of the South Australia Legislative Council*, Nov. 20, 2002.

40 Nitschke and Stewart, *Killing Me Softly*, 121.

41 Nitschke and Stewart, *Killing Me Softly*, 82-85

42 Woodman, *Last Rights*, 92.

43 Philip Nitschke and Fiona Stewart, *The Peaceful Pill Handbook* (Lake Tahoe, Nevada: Exit International US, Ltd., 2006), 18.

44 Nitschke and Stewart, *The Peaceful Pill Handbook* [U.S edition], 18; Kissane, et al., "Seven Deaths in Darwin," 1099.

45 "My Mother Valerie," *e-Deliverance*

(Exit International), October 2006, 4.

46 Parliament of the Commonwealth of Australia. Senate Legal and Constitutional Legislation Committee…. Rights of the Terminally Ill (Euthanasia Laws Repeal) Bill 1996), 61.

47 Sandra Kanck, Minutes of the South Australia Legislative Council, Nov. 20, 2002.

48 "Machine rekindles euthanasia debate," *The Guardian,* May 20, 1997.

49 "Machine rekindles euthanasia debate."

50 "Machine rekindles euthanasia debate."

51 "Machine rekindles euthanasia debate."

52 Woodman, *Last Rights,* 91.

53 "Killing Me Softly: Dr. Philip Nitschke," interview by Monica Attard, *ABC Sunday Profile,* June 15, 2008.

54 Nitschke and Stewart, *Killing Me Softly,* 8.

55 Compton interview.

56 Compton interview.

57 Compton interview

58 Compton interview.

59 William DeMaria, *Deadly Disclosures: Whistleblowing and the Ethical Meltdown of Australia* (Kent Town, S.A.: Wakefield Press, 1999), 43.

60 DeMaria, *Deadly Disclosures,* 43.

61 De Maria, *Deadly Disclosures,* 61.

62 Obituary of Huibert Drion (1917-2004), *British Medical Journal* 328 (May 15, 2004): 1204.

63 "Dr. Nitschke: A Pioneer in Australia," Hemlock Society *Timelines,* Fall 1999, 4.

64 Philip Nitschke, "Euthanasia: the right to choose," *Australian Rationalist,* 58/59: 25-26.

65 Lopez, "Euthanasia Sets Sail."

66 Nitschke and Stewart, *Killing Me Softly,* 253.

67 Wesley J. Smith, email to RNC, May10, 2010.

68 Lopez, "Euthanasia Sets Sail."

69 Wesley J. Smith, email to RNC, May 10, 2010.

70 Nitschke and Stewart, *Killing Me Softly,* 257.

71 Nitschke and Stewart, *Killing Me Softly,* 262.

72 Tulloch, *Euthanasia-Choice and Death,* 129-130.

73 Tulloch, *Euthanasia-Choice and Death,* 130.

74 Wesley J. Smith, *Forced Exit: Euthanasia, Assisted Suicide, and the New Duty to Die* (New York: Encounter Books, 1997), 36-38.

75 Tulloch, *Euthanasia-Choice and Death,*130.

76 "Handmaiden of Death," *The Sydney Morning Herald,* Nov. 27, 2002.

77 Michael Cook, "In Nitschke's Hands," *Arena: The Australian Magazine of Left Political, Social and Cultural Commentary,* December-January 2005-2006, at www.australianbioethics.org/Media/2005-12-mc-arena-nitschke-1.html.

78 Nitschke and Stewart, *Killing Me Softly,* 157-159.

79 Nitschke and Stewart *The Peaceful Pill Handbook* [U.S. edition], 159.

80 PN interview with RNC, April 20, 2010.

81 Exit International *e-Deliverance Newsletter,* March 2005, 3.

82 Rodney Syme, *A Good Death, An Argument for Voluntary Euthanasia* (Melbourne: Melbourne University Press, 2008), 214.

83 John Sheerhout and Stan Miller, "Coroner Calls for Ban on Suicide Manual," *Manchester Evening News,* Feb. 16, 2009.

84 Derek Humphry to ERGO *World Right-to-Die Newslist,* Feb. 16, 2009.

85 William Lee Adams, "Foolproofing Suicide with Euthanasia Test Kits," *Time* (London), April 13, 2009, at http://www.time.com/time/health/article/0,8599,1890413,00.html#ixzz1XJ6KcU66.

86 Joan Bakewell, "Why Dr Death should have been given a welcome in Britain," *The Times,* May 15, 2009.

87 Wesley J. Smith, "Australia's Dr. Death comes to San Francisco," November 2, 2009 at http://

articles.sfgate.com/2009-11-02/opinion/17179670_1_assisted-suicide-final-exit-network-nitschke

88 Compton interview.

89 Hilary White, Rome Correspondent, "Dublin suicide 'workshop' a bust with twice as many protesters as attendees," http://www.lifesitenews.com/news/twice-as-many-protesters-as-attendees-at-dublin-suicide-workshop/.

Chapter 9: Death Down Under

1 Rodney Syme, *A Good Death: An Argument for Voluntary Euthanasia* (Melbourne: Melbourne University Press, 2008), 1.

2 Russell Smith, *Health Care, Crime, and Regulatory Control* (Annandale, N.S.W.: Hawkins Press, 1998), 151-152.

3 Smith, *Health Care, Crime, and Regulatory Control*, 152.

4 Syme, *A Good Death*, 4.

5 Syme, *A Good Death*, 4.

6 Syme, *A Good Death*, 4.

7 Syme, *A Good Death*, 5.

8 Syme, *A Good Death*, 6.

9 Syme, *A Good Death*, 6.

10 Syme, *A Good Death*, 7.

11 Syme, *A Good Death*, 7-8.

12 Nick Miller, "Fight to the Death," *The Age*, April 26, 2008.

13 Miller, "Fight to the Death."

14 Miller, "Fight to the Death."

15 Syme, *A Good Death*, 11.

16 Dying With Dignity-New South Wales, "An Australian Timeline, June 1, 2010, at http://www.dwdnsw.org.au/ves/index.php/an-australian-timeline.

17 The "founding dates" vary in specificity. Some groups define theirs as the date of the first exploratory meeting; others use the later date of their legal incorporation.

18 "Last Rights: Interview with Dr. Rodney Syme," Dying With Dignity-Victoria *Newsletter*, February 7, 2011, 1.

19 "Last Rights: Interview with Dr. Rodney Syme."

20 Roger Magnusson, "When the pain is too much, pray he's out there," *The Australian*, June 21, 2008.

21 Magnusson, "When the pain is too much."

22 "An Australian Timeline, June 1, 2010."

23 Address by Marshall Perron, April 16, 2008.

24 "About Us," Dying With Dignity Victoria webpage, Sept. 9, 2011, at www.dwdv.org.au/AboutUs.html.

25 Marshall Perron, Keynote Address at the Voluntary Euthanasia Research Foundation Inaugural National Congress, "Dying in Australia – Taking Control," Broken Hill, Australia, August 3, 2001, in VES of New South Wales *Newsletter*, 95 (November 2001), 3-4.

26 Rodney Syme (RS), interview with RNC, July 29, 2011.

27 RS interview with RNC, July 29, 2011.

28 RS interview with RNC, July 29, 2011.

29 RS interview with RNC, July 29, 2011.

30 RS interview with RNC, July 29, 2011.

31 RS interview with RNC, July 29, 2011.

32 Faye Girsh to Lachlan Parker, "Euthanasia debate reignited," Aug. 4, 2001, "AM" radio, ABC transcript.

33 "Win for ACT democracy," ABC News, Nov. 2, 2011, at http://www.abc.net.au/news/2011-11-02/gallagher-on-territory-rights-bill/3614206?section=act.

34 RS interview with RNC, July 29, 2011.

35 Syme, *A Good Death*, 231.

36 Syme, *A Good Death*, 233.

37 Syme, *A Good Death*, 236.

38 "Steve Guest," Exit International, http://www.exitinternational.net/page/SteveGuest.

39 Syme, *A Good Death*, 238.

40 Syme, *A Good Death*, 239.

41 Syme, *A Good Death*, 239.

42 Syme, *A Good Death*, 239.

43 "Steve Guest," *Geelong Advertiser*, July 30, 2007.

44 Clive Dorman, "Doctor not expecting charges over Steve Guest's suicide,

Geelong Advertiser, April 15, 2008.

45 *Brightwater Care Group, Inc. v. Rossiter,* West Australia Supreme Court 229 (2009).

46 "Perth quadriplegic wins landmark right to die," *ABC News* online, Aug. 14, 2009; "Death a 'relief' for right-to-die man," *ABC News* online, September 21, 2009.

47 "Court grants woman right to die," *ABC News* online, June 18, 2010.

48 RS, email to RNC, Nov. 11,2011.

49 "The Lesley Martin Story," at http://www.life.org.nz/euthanasia/abouteuthanasia/nzeuthanasiahistory5/.

50 "The Lesley Martin Story."

51 Kathy Marks, "Euthanasia advocate faces jail for trying to kill mother, " *The Independent* (Sydney), April 1, 2004.

52 Lesley Martin, *To Cry Inside* (New Zealand: Penguin Books, 2006), 325.

53 "The Lesley Martin Story."

54 "Police ponder charges in euthanasia case," http://www.stuff.co.nz/458252/Police-ponder-charges-in-euthanasia-case, May 25, 2008.

55 DH, email to RNC and others, June 10, 2008.

56 Jon Ronson, "Reverend Death," London: World of Wonder, 2008.

57 Ronson, "Reverend Death."

58 Ronson, "Reverend Death."

59 Ronson, "Reverend Death."

60 Audrey Wallis to ERGO newslist, April 30, 2007.

61 Cassandra Mae, telephone conversation with RNC, October 8, 2011.

62 Karen Stern, email to RNC, April 9, 2007.

Chapter 10: Caring Friends and Hemlock's End

1 Hemlock Society USA, "Hemlock Society Introduces New Program for Terminally Ill," media release, Nov. 9, 1998.

2 "Faculty Roster, Caring Friends Training, San Diego, November 6-8, 1998," courtesy of Lois Schafer, Nov. 27, 2010.

3 *Washington v. Glucksberg,* 521 U.S. 702 (1997).

4 "Announcing the Hemlock Patient Advocacy Program," Hemlock *Timelines,* July-September 1997, 4.

5 Thomas A. Preston and Ralph Mero, "Observations Concerning Terminally Ill Patients Who Choose Suicide," in Margaret P. Battin and Arthur G. Lipman, eds. *Drug Use in Assisted Suicide and Euthanasia* (Binghamton, N. Y.: Pharmaceutical Products Press, 1996), 184.

6 Preston and Mero, "Observations Concerning Terminally Ill Patients," 184.

7 Faye J. Girsh (FJG) to RNC, Aug. 31, 2010.

8 FJG to RNC, Aug. 11, 2010.

9 Rob Zaleski, "Advocating for a Death With Dignity," *The Capital Times,* April 18, 2003.

10 Faye J. Girsh, "How the Caring Friends Program Was Started," No date (2004).

11 Girsh, "How the Caring Friends Program Was Started."

12 Girsh, "How the Caring Friends Program Was Started."

13 Girsh, "How the Caring Friends Program Was Started."

14 Girsh, "How the Caring Friends Program Was Started."

15 "Caring Friends Program gets Green Light," Hemlock Society *Timelines,* Spring 1998, 2.

16 FJG to RNC, May 30, 2011.

17 FJG to RNC, Aug. 11, 2010.

18 FJG, "The Hemlock Story in Brief," no date; "Caring Friends Volunteer List, February 1, 2002," courtesy of Lois Schafer, Nov. 27, 2010.

19 "Caring Friends: Many Have Called, Some Have Chosen," Hemlock *Timelines,* Fall, 1999, 1.

20 FJG to RNC, Aug. 11, 2010.

21 Hemlock Society. *Agreement with Volunteers,* revised Jan. 17, 2002, courtesy of Lois Schafer.

22 Lois Schafer (LS) to RNC, Aug. 13, 2010.

23 LS to RNC, Aug. 13, 2010.

24 LS to RNC, Aug. 13, 2010.

25 Richard MacDonald (RMcD) to RNC, July 25, 2010.

26 RMcD to RNC, July 25, 2010.

27 RMcD to RNC, Aug. 28, 2010.

28 Rosoff was elected to the board in the summer, 1992 board meeting. "New Hemlock Board Members," *Hemlock Quarterly*, January 1992, 3.

29 LS to RNC, Aug. 13, 2010.

30 Diane Martindale, "A Culture of Death," *Scientific American*, May 23, 2005.

31 John A. Pridonoff, "The Dialogue Begins: An Interview with Dr. Jack Kevorkian," Hemlock Society *TimeLines*, March-April 1994, 14.

32 RMcD to RNC, Aug. 28, 2010.

33 DH to RNC, Aug. 21, 2010.

34 Faye J. Girsh, interview with RNC, Aug. 31, 2010.

35 Humphry, *Good Life, Good Death*, 306.

36 Ilene Kaplan, "Eyes Light Up When Name Mentioned," ERGO news list, April 30, 2008;

37 "Paul A. Spiers, PhD.," speaker's biography, "15th John K. Friesen Conference – Quality of Life at the End of Life: Decisions and Choices," Simon Fraser University (Vancouver, Canada), 2005, accessed at http://www.sfu.ca/grc/friesen/2005/paul/.

38 FJG to RNC, Aug. 11, 2010.

39 LS to RNC, Aug. 13, 2010.

40 Earl Wettstein, "Not So Fast, C&C," right-to-die at lists.opn.org, June 4, 2010.

41 Rita L. Marker, "Assisted Suicide & Death With Dignity: Past, Present & Future – Part I," at www.internationaltaskforce.org/rpt2005_I.htm.

42 Paul A. Spiers, "From the President," *EOL Choices*, Fall 2004, 1.

43 Faye J. Girsh, "My Leaving," December 10, 2004, and posted on the ERGO newslist, December 22, 2004.

44 RMcD to RNC, Aug. 28, 2010.

45 Wettstein, "Not So Fast, C&C."

Chapter 11: Going Dutch

1 Sanal Edamaruku, "A Yardstick of Civilization," Rationalist International, 57 (December 7, 2000) at www.rationalistinternational.net/archive/rationalist_2000/57.htm.

2 J. H. van der Berg, *Medische macht en Medische Ethiek* (Nijkerk: Uitgevij G.F. Callenbach, 1969, published in English as *Medical Power and Medical Ethics* (New York: W.W. Norton, 1978); John Griffiths, Alex Bood, and Helen Weyers, *Euthanasia and Law in the Netherlands* (Amsterdam: Amsterdam University Press, 1998, 50.

3 Griffiths et al., *Euthanasia and Law in the Netherlands*, 47-48.

4 Griffiths et al., *Euthanasia and Law in the Netherlands*, 47.

5 Paul Sporken, *Voorlopige diagnose. Inleiding tot en medische ethiek [Provisional Diagnosis. Introduction to a Medical Ethic]* (Utrecht: Ambo, 1969), 221-222, in *Euthanasia and Law*, 48-49.

6 *Euthanasia and the Law in the Netherlands*, 48.

7 H.A.H. Van Till-d'Aulnis de Bourouill, *Medish-juridische aspekten van het einde van het menslijk leven [Medico-legal Aspects of the end of Human Life]* (Deventer: Kluwer, 1970), 105, in *Euthanasia and Law*, 48-49.

8 "The Law: Implications of Mercy," *Time*, March 5, 1973.

9 "The Law: Implications of Mercy."

10 "The Law: Implications of Mercy."

11 "The Law: Implications of Mercy."

12 Gregory E. Pence, "Do Not Go Slowly Into That Dark Night: Mercy Killing in Holland," *The American Journal of Medicine*, 84 (January 1988): 139.

13 "A Suitable Case for Killing?" *Radio Times*, in *Rumoaoita*, no publisher listed, c. 1977, at http://www.rumoaoita.com/materiais/ita_resolvidas/in_89_90.pdf.

14 "A Suitable Case for Killing?"

15 "A Suitable Case for Killing?"

16 "About NVVE," NVVE website,

http://www.laatstewilpil.nl/nvve-english/pagina.asp?pagkey=72177.

17 "Legal Matters," ERGO *World Right-to-Die Newsletter*, 1 (July 1981): 4.

18 Stichting Die Einder websitepage, http://deeinder.nl/.

19 Pence, "Do Not Go Slowly Into That Dark Night."

20 Pieter V. Admiraal, "Euthanasia in the Netherlands," *Free Inquiry*, Winter 1996/97, 5.

21 Francis X. Clines, "Dutch are quietly taking the lead in euthanasia," *The New York Times*, Oct. 31, 1986.

22 DH, email to RNC, May 10, 2010.

23 Admiraal, "Euthanasia in the Netherlands," 7.

24 Admiraal, "Euthanasia in the Netherlands," 7.

25 Griffiths et al., *Euthanasia and Law in the Netherlands*, 203-204.

26 Admiraal, "Euthanasia in the Netherlands," 7.

27 Admiraal, "Euthanasia in the Netherlands," 8.

28 Penney Lewis, "Assisted Dying Regimes," briefing paper for the End of Life Assistance (Scotland) Bill Committee, Sept.19, 2010.

29 Boudewijn Chabot, *A Hastened Death by Self-denial of Food And Drink* (Amsterdam: Chabot, 2008).

30 Anastasia Toufexis, James Geary and Alice Park, "Killing the Psychic Pain," *Time*, July 4, 1994.

31 Boudewijn Chabot (BC) to RNC, May 23, 2011.

32 BC to RNC, May 23, 2011.

33 BC to RNC, May 23, 2011.

34 BC to RNC, May 23, 2011.

35 Tony Sheldon, "The doctor who prescribed suicide," *The Independent*, June 30, 1994.

36 Toufexis et al., "Killing the Psychic Pain."

37 Boudewijn E. Chabot, "Auto-Euthanasie" (self-deliverance), Ph.D. dissertation, University of Amsterdam, May 2007.

38 BC to RNC, May 23, 2011.

39 L. Ganzini, E.R. Goy, L.L. Miller, T.A. Jackson, and M.A. Delorit, "Nurses' experiences with hospice patients who refuse food and fluids to hasten death," *New England Journal of Medicine*, July 23, 2004, 349 (4): 359-365.

40 Stanley A. Terman, "About Caring Advocates: The Mission, the Means, and the Professional Staff," at www.caringadvocates.org/about.php.

41 Chabot, *A Hastened Death*, back cover.

42 Compassion & Choices member email, "A New Campaign Starts Today in Colorado," Aug. 17, 2011.

43 Daniel Vance, "Disabilities Week: Stephen Drake," *Atlantic Highlands Herald*, Sept. 15, 2005, at http://ahherald.com/disabilities/2005/dw050915_drake.htm.

44 Henk Jochemsen, "Dutch Court Decisions on Nonvoluntary Euthanasia Critically Reviewed," *Issues in Law and Medicine*, 13 (4, 1998): 4-6.

45 "Dutch Doctor Guilty," World Federation of Right-to-Die Societies *Newsletter* #26 (second quarter, 1995): 10.

46 "Dutch Doctor Guilty."

47 Jochemsen,"Dutch Court Decisions," 12.

48 Bertha A. Manninen, "A case for justified non-voluntary active euthanasia: exploring the ethics of The Groningen Protocol," *Journal of Medical Ethics*, 2006 (32): 643-644.

49 Manninen, "A case for justified non-voluntary active euthanasia."

50 Wesley J. Smith, "Pushing Infanticide From Holland to New Jersey," *"National Review Online* at http://old.nationalreview.com/smithw/smith200503220759.asp.

51 Lewis, "Assisted Dying Regimes."

52 Stephanie Siek, "Dutch Groups Want to Expand Assisted Suicide Rights," Deutsche Welle, May 28, 2010 at http://www.dw-world.de/dw/article/0,,5627515,00.html.

53 Folkert Jensma, "A citizens action group wants to legalise assisted suicide for all people over 70," Radio Netherlands Worldwide, Feb. 9, 2010,

at http://www.rnw.nl/english/article/ right-die-elderly-back-centre-dutch-debate.

54 Theo Meijer, "Euthanasia in The Netherlands," *Humanist Perspectives*, issue 152, at http://www. humanistperspectives.org/issue152/ euthanasia_in_netherlands.html.

55 Panel discussion, "Dutch Euthanasia 'Not Exportable,'" *World Right-to-Die Newsletter*, 37 (November 2000): 8.

56 Lecture synopsis of Dr. Aycke A. O. Smook, "How I Help My Patients That Choose to Die," *The Independent*, April 6, 2006.

57 Rob Jonquière, interview with RNC, May 30, 2011.

58 Jonquière, interview with RNC, May 30, 2011.

59 Panel discussion, "Dutch Euthanasia 'Not Exportable.'"

Chapter 12: The Battleground States

1 Jacob M. Appel, "A Duty to Kill? A Duty to Die? Rethinking the Euthanasia Controversy of 1906," *Bulletin of the History of Medicine*, 78:3 (Fall 2004), 610-634.

2 Derek Humphry, *Lawful Exit: The Limits of Freedom for Help in Dying* (Junction City, Ore.: The Norris Lane Press, 1993), 19.

3 Derek Humphry, "A Charter for the Legalization of Voluntary Euthanasia," The London *Evening Standard*, April 24, 1978.

4 DH interview with RNC, Dec. 8, 2011.

5 "Physician aid-in-dying law," *Hemlock Quarterly*, 22 (January 1986): 81.

6 *Lawful Exit*, 53.

7 DH interview with RNC, Dec. 8, 2011.

8 DH interview with RNC, Dec. 8, 2011.

9 Humphry, *Lawful Exit*, 57.

10 Humphry, *Lawful Exit*, 20.

11 DH to RNC, Feb. 27, 2010.

12 George Eighmey, "Methods in Oregon: Lessons Learned," an address to the NuTech session, World Federation of Right to Die Societies' biennial congress, Melbourne, Oct. 7, 2010.

13 David Orentlicher and Arthur Caplan, "The Pain Relief Promotion Act of 1999: A Serious Threat to Palliative Care," *Journal of the American Medical Association*, 2000, 283 (2):255-258.

14 Death With Dignity National Center, "Legal and Political Timeline in Oregon," www.deathwithdignity.org/ historyfacts/oregontimeline/.

15 Eli D. Stutsman, "Ashcroft's power grab chilling," *Portland Tribune*, Dec. 21, 2001.

16 *Oregon v. Ashcroft*, May 26, 2004.

17 DH interview with RNC, Dec. 8, 2011.

18 Kathryn Smith et al., "Quality of Death and Dying in Patients who Request Physician-Assisted Death," *Journal of Palliative Medicine*, 14:4 (2011), 1.

19 Ann Jackson, "Death With Dignity: Facts of Oregon's Experience," *The Billings Gazette*, July 17, 2010.

20 Trudy Govier, "Practical Philosophy: The Famous, or Infamous Slippery Slope," *Humanist in Canada*, 152 (Spring 2005): 34.

21 For the official Oregon state DWD document, see http://public.health. oregon.gov/providerpartnerresources/ evaluationresearch/deathwithdignityact/ documents/year13.pdfdocument.

22 The full cumulative report for the period 1998-2010 may be found at http:// public.health.oregon.gov/ProviderPart-nerResources/EvaluationResearch/ DeathwithDignityAct/Pages/index.aspx.

23 Margaret P. Battin et al., "Legal physician-assisted dying in Oregon and the Netherlands: evidence concerning the impact on patients in 'vulnerable' groups," *Journal of Medical Ethics 33* (2007): 591–597.

24 Lisa Belkin, "There's No Simple Suicide," *The New York Times*, Nov. 14, 1993.

25 Belkin, "There's No Simple Suicide."

26 Belkin, "There's No Simple Suicide."

27 Belkin, "There's No Simple Suicide."

28 Belkin, "There's No Simple Suicide."

29 Belkin, "There's No Simple Suicide."

30 Belkin, "There's No Simple Suicide."

31 Belkin,"There's No Simple Suicide."

32 Preston and Mero, "Observations Concerning Terminally Ill Patients." 84.

33 Ralph Mero, "A Careful Way to Assist Dying," World Federation of Right-to-Die Societies *Newsletter*, issue 23 (1993): 4–5.

34 Carol M. Ostrom, "Assisting Suicide is Immoral, Say Group's Critics," *The Seattle Times*, May 21, 1993.

35 Ostrom, "Assisting Suicide is Immoral."

36 Ostrom, "Assisting Suicide is Immoral."

37 George Eighmey, "Oregon's Law Withstands the Test of Time," Death With Dignity National Center *Living With Dying* blog, Jan. 19, 2011.

38 Curt Woodward, "Washington Voters Approve Assisted Suicide Initiative," *The Seattle Times*, Nov. 4, 2008.

39 Janet I. Tu, "Death With Dignity Act passes," *The Seattle Times*, Nov. 5, 2008.

40 Bob Oswald, "No One in Pain, No One Dies Alone," Seattle.: *Belltown Messenger* 54, April 28, 2008.

41 Washington Secretary of State. Nov. 4, 2008 General Election, at http://vote.wa.gov/Elections/WEI/ResultsByCounty.aspx?ElectionID=26&RaceID=101369&CountyCode=%20&JurisdictionTypeID=aceTypeCode=M&ViewMode=Results.

42 Washington State Department of Health 2010 Death With Dignity Act Report.

43 Susan Donaldson James, "Families of Dying Say Assisted Suicide is Right," *ABC News*, Sept. 2, 2009.

44 Drew Zahn, "Doctor-assisted suicide ruled 'a patient's right," *WorldNet-Daily*, Dec. 6, 2008, at http://www.wnd.com/?pageId=82928.

45 Jennifer Mesko, "Montana Judge Reaffirms Assisted-Suicide Ruling" *CitizenLink*, www.citizenlink.org/content/A000009035.cfm, Jan. 9, 2009; *Baxter v. Montana*, 2009 MT 449, paragraph 49.

46 "Montana Court Decides Terminally Ill Patients Have Right to Death with Dignity under Montana Constitution," Dec, 6, 2008, at http://blog. compassion-andchoices.org/?p=134.

47 Wesley J. Smith, "Euthanasia comes to Montana," *The Weekly Standard*, Dec. 29, 2008, at http:www.discovery.org/a/8391.

48 Tristan Scott, "Woman pleads for right to die," *The Missoulian*, April 4, 2009.

49 Alex Schadenberg, "Montana Senate Bill 116 – The Elder Abuse Prevention Act," Jan. 14, 2011, at http://alexschadenberg.blogspot.com/2011/01/montana-senate-bill-116-elder-abuse.html.

50 Matt Gouras, "Montana Lawmakers Punt on Physician-assisted Suicide," Helena: AP, Feb. 21, 2011.

51 Kevin B. O'Reilly, "Assisted suicide statute challenged by 2 doctors," Oct. 19, 2009, at http://www.ama-assn.org/amednews/2009/10/19/prsd1019.htm.

Chapter 13: Esta Es Mi Voluntad

1 Father Jacques Pohier, a French Dominican priest, was the first theologian to be disciplined by Pope John Paul II. In 1979, while dean of the theology faculty at the Dominican theological school near Paris, he lost his license to teach theology and was banned from saying Mass or participating in any liturgical gatherings. He left the Dominicans in 1984. Tara Harris, "The List. Catholic theologians and others disciplined by the Vatican during the papacy of John Paul II." *National Catholic Reporter*, Feb. 25, 2005.

2 Gustavo Alfonso Quintana (GAQ), interview with RNC, Oct. 4, 2009, in Cali, Colombia.

3 GAQ interview with RNC, Oct, 4, 2009.

4 GAQ interview with RNC, Oct. 4, 2009

5 GAQ interview with RNC, Oct. 4, 2009

6 GAQ interview with RNC, Oct. 4, 2009.

7 GAQ interview with RNC, Oct. 4, 2009

8 "I have euthanized about 35 people and have no regrets," says Gustavo Alfonso

Quintana, *Diario Medico* blog, (2008), at http://diariomediko.com/?p=149; GAQ interview with RNC, Oct. 4, 2009.

9 GAQ interview with RNC, Oct. 4, 2009.

10 GAQ interview with RNC, Oct. 4, 2009.

11 Mike Ceasar, "Euthanasia in legal limbo in Colombia," *The Lancet*, 371: Jan. 26, 2008.

12 RNC interview with Dr. Jaime Escobar-Triana, Oct. 21, 2011.

13 RNC interview with Dr. Jaime Escobar-Triana; Jaime Escobar-Triana, *Morir como ejercicio final del derecho a una vida digna* [*Death as a Final Exercise in the Right to a Dignified Life*] (Bogotá, Colombia: Colección Bios y Ethos, Ediciones El Bosque, 1998).

14 Juan Mendoza-Vega, "Muerte cerebral, consideraciones en Colombia" ["Brain Death: Considerations in Colombia"]" *Consulta* 4 (6): 5 - 8, June 1977.

15 Juan Mendoza-Vega, interview with RNC, Nov. 17, 2010.

16 Juan Mendoza-Vega, *Caminas de la Bioética en Colombia* [*The Path of Bioethics in Colombia*] (Bogotá, Colombia: Revista Latinoamericana de Bioética, July 2006), 32-33. This history of bioethics in Colombia appears in both Spanish and English at http://www.umng.edu.co/docs/revbioetik/vol11/mendoza-vega.pdf.

17 Mendoza-Vega, *Caminas de la Bioética en Colombia*, 34.

18 For a comprehensive discussion of this law, see Sabine Michalowski, "Legalizing Active Voluntary Euthanasia Through the Courts: Some Lessons from Colombia, *Medical Law Review* (Nov. 1, 2009) 17 (2):183-218.

19 "Legalizing Active Voluntary Euthanasia Through the Courts," *passim*.

20 Jairo R. Moyano and Sofía C. Zambrono, "Ten Years Later, Colombia is Still Confused about Euthanasia," *British Medical Journal* Rapid Response, Jan.18, 2008.

21 Alan D. Ogilvie, "Colombia confused over legislation of euthanasia," *British Medical Journal* 314 (June 28, 1997): 1997.

22 "Legalizing Active Voluntary Euthanasia Through the Courts," 190-191.

23 Inter Press Service English News Wire, Feb. 5, 2001.

24 Rubén Armendáriz, "Euthanasia, a Debate with No Reprieve," Caracas: Inter Press Service, Feb. 4, 2001.

25 Juan Francisco Alonso, "Criminal bill gives green light to euthanasia in Venezuela," *El Universal*, Oct.11, 2010.

26 Rafael Aguiar-Guevara, "Euthanasia: Venezuelan Tendency. Second Report," Aug. 30, 2006, at http://www.ragaso.com/Ingles/indexos2/articles.htm#Euthanasia:_Venezuelan_Tendency._Second Report.

27 Rubén Armendáriz, "Euthanasia, a Debate with No Reprieve."

28 Aguiar-Guevara, "Euthanasia: Venezuelan Tendency. Second Report."

29 Rafael Aguiar-Guevara, "Euthanasia To Be legalized in Venezuela?" *The Latin Americanist*, Oct. 15, 2010, at http://ourlatinamerica.blogspot.com/2010/10/euthanasia-to-be-legalized-in-venezuela.html.

30 P. Przygoda, G. Saimovici, G. Pollán, and S. Figar, "Physician assisted suicide, euthanasia, and withdrawal of treatment," *British Medical Journal*, 1998, 316 (7124): 71-72.

31 Stephanie Garlow, "Argentina mulls allowing euthanasia," *GlobalPost*, Sept. 28, 2011, at http://www.globalpost.com/dispatches/globalpost-blogs/que-pasa/argentina-mulls-allowing-euthanasia.

32 Luciana Pricoli Vilela and Paulo Caramelli, "Knowledge of the definition of euthanasia: study with doctors and caregivers of Alzheimer's disease patients," http://www.angus-reid.com/polls/3495/most_brazilians_reject_euthanasia/.

33 "Euthanasia in Mexico," http://en.wikipedia.org/wiki/Euthanasia_in_Mexico.

34 "Many Mexicans Open to Legal Eu-

thanasia," Angus Reid Global Monitor/ Parametría, May 8, 2008.
35 "Congress on palliative medicine in Paraguay presents alternative to euthanasia," *Catholic News Agency*, http://www.catholicnewsagency.com/news/congress_on_palliative_medicine_in_paraguay_presents_alternative_to_euthanasia/.
36 Andrés Castellana,* interview with RNC, Nov. 22, 2010.

Chapter 14: One-way Tickets to Zürich

1 Jeremy Laurance, "Anne Turner sang songs and joked with her children - then she went to a clinic to die," *The Independent*, Jan. 25, 2006.
2 Dignitas. "Interim Policy for Prosecutors in respect of Cases of Assisted Suicide Issued by The Director of Public Prosecution September 2009. Forch, Switzerland: Dignitas: Dec. 11, 2009.
3 Ludwig A. Minelli (LAM) to RNC, Aug. 6, 2010; Roger Boyes, "Murky truth behind Swiss suicide 'clinic'," *London Times*, Oct. 25, 2008.
4 Dignitas. "Interim Policy for Prosecutors; 3;" also LAM to RNC, July 17, 2007.
5 This statement from Minelli has been conflated for reasons of clarity from three slightly-varying published versions.
6 LAM to RNC, Aug. 6, 2010.
7 Alison Langley, "Suicide Tourists Go to the Swiss for Help in Dying," *The New York Times*, Feb. 4, 2003.
8 Imogen Foulkes, "Switzerland plans new controls on assisted suicide," BBC News, July 2, 2010.
9 Dignitas. "Interim Policy for Prosecutors," 2; 20,000 members: "Fünf Jahre. Exit Deutsche Schweiz," in VESS *Newsletter*, January 1988, 4.
10 Right-to-Die Society of Canada, "A companion for Dignitas," *Free to Go*, 9 (2 – April June 2007), 3.
11 Sascha Tankerville, "Exit hat inen guten Ruf mehr" [Exit

no longer has a good reputation], http://www.grenchen.net/blog/2001/03/19/%c2%abexit-hat-keinen-guten-ruf-mehr%c2%bb#more-12913; Derek Humphry, "Euthanasia in Practice," http://www.finalexit.org/pract-swiss.html.
12 "Interview with Ludwig Minelli," Jan. 22, 2006 by Frontline, "The Suicide Tourist," http://www.pbs.org/wgbh/pages/frontline/suicidetourist/etc/minelli.html.
13 Ludwig A. Minelli, "Dignitas in Switzerland: Its Philosophies, the Legal Situation, Actual Problems, and Possibilities for Britons who wish to End Their Lives," speech given to Friends at the End, London, Dec. 1, 2007.
14 LAM to RNC, Aug. 6, 2010; Bruce Falconer, "Death Becomes Him," *Atlantic Magazine*, March 2010, at http://www.theatlantic.com/magazine/archive/2010/03/death-becomes-him/7916/.
15 "Death tourism remains a draw," May 27, 2008, at http://www.swissinfo.ch/eng/swiss_news/Death_tourism_remains_a_draw.html?cid=6683066.
16 Ludwig A. Minelli, "The European Convention on Human Rights Protects the Right of Suicide," Physician-Assisted Suicide: Medical, Ethical, Legal, and Social Implications International Symposium, Medical Center of the University of Giessen, Germany, March 19-21, 2004.
17 Frontline / PBS interview with Ludwig Minelli, "Why do you believe in assisted suicide?" at http://www.pbs.org/wgbh/pages/frontline/suicidetourist/etc/minelli.html.
18 "Wife changed husband's will before death" *Sydney Morning Herald*, May 9, 2008.
19 LAM to RNC, Aug. 6, 2010.
20 Helena Bachman, "One-Way Ticket," *Time*, Oct. 6, 2002.
21 Imogen Foulkes, "Dignitas boss: Healthy should have right to die," BBC News, July 2, 2010.

22 Jonathan Brown, "After 54 years together, they decided to die together," *The Independent*, July 15, 2009.

23 Foulkes, "Dignitas boss."

24 "Dignitas defends assisted suicide," BBC News, April 2, 2009.

25 David Cohen, "A £45 suicide in a Zurich flat–where's the dignity in that?" *The Evening Standard*, Jan. 26, 2006.

26 Cohen, "A £45 suicide in a Zurich flat."

27 Reader comment from "Zombini," referring to Amelia Gentleman, "Inside the Dignitas House," June 18, 2010, at http://www.guardian.co.uk/society/2009/nov/18/assisted-suicide-dignitas-house.

28 Langley, "'Suicide Tourists' Go to the Swiss for Help in Dying."

29 Michael Leidig, "Suicide 'factory' reopens - next to a brothel," *The Observer*, March 16, 2008.

30 Leidig, "Suicide Factory reopens."

31 LAM to RNC, Aug. 6, 2010.

32 LAM to RNC, Aug. 6, 2010.

33 Russel D. Ogden, William K. Hamilton, and Charles Whitcher, "Assisted suicide by oxygen deprivation with helium at a Swiss right-to-die-organization," *Journal of Medical Ethics* 36 (2010): 174–179.

34 David Lowe, "A yellow floral duvet and a Swiss chocolate to take away the taste of the poison. . . the bed where you never wake up," *The Sun*, Jan. 23, 2010.

35 "Case closed on Lake Zürich urns," *World Radio Switzerland*, http://worldradio.ch/wrs/news/wrsnews/case-closed-on-lake-zurich-urns.shtml?20219.

36 LAM to RNC, Aug. 6, 2010.

37 2010 charges: www.dignitas.ch.

38 LAM to RNC, Aug. 6, 2010.

39 Laurance, "Anne Turner sang songs."

40 Amelia Gentleman, "Inside the Dignitas House," Manchester *Guardian*, Nov. 18, 2009.

41 Falconer, "Death Becomes Him."

42 "Swiss voters reject ban on assisted suicide for foreigners," *The Guardian*, May 15, 2011.

43 "Swiss voters reject ban on assisted suicide for foreigners."

Chapter 15: The Disunited Kingdom

1 "Voluntary Euthanasia," *The British Medical Journal*, Nov. 2, 1935, 856.

2 Joseph Lelyveld, "1936 Secret is Out: Doctor Sped George V's Death," *The New York Times*, Nov. 28, 1986.

3 J.H.R. Ramsay, "A king, a doctor, and a convenient death," *British Medical Journal*, 308 (May 28, 1994):1445.

4 Robert K. Kastenbaum, "Ralph Mero: An Omega Interview," *Omega*, 29 (1994, #1): 16.

5 Angus Reid Public Opinion poll: "Euthanasia," Feb. 2, 2010, 1.

6 BBC Home, "Euthanasia Chief Jailed over Suicides," at http://news.bbc.co.uk/onthisday/hi/dates/stories/october/30/newsid_2465000/2465183.stm.

7 "Attorney-General v. Able and Others," 1982 G. No. 2610, Queen's Bench Division, [1984] QB 795, April 28, 1983.

8 "World Conference," *Hemlock Quarterly*, October 1980, 1:1.

9 "The dignity of Diane Pretty," BBC News, May 12, 2002, at http://news.bbc.co.uk/2/hi/health/1983781.stm.

10 "Diane Pretty: The fight continues," BBC News, November 29, 2001, July 11, 2010 at http://news.bbc.co.uk/2/hi/health/1682321.stm.

11 The Director of Public Prosecutions (DPP), is head of the Crown Prosecution Service (CPS), the approximate equivalents, respectively, of the U.S. Attorney General and the Department of Justice.

12 "Diane Pretty: Timeline," at http://news.bbc.co.uk/2/hi/health/1983562.stm.

13 "Diane Pretty: The fight continues," *BBC News*, Nov. 29, 2001, http://news.bbc.co.uk/2/hi/health/1682321.stm.

14 "Diane Pretty: Timeline."

15 "Diane Pretty dies in hospice," *Scotsman.com*, May 12, 2002, at http://www.scotsman.com/news/diane_pretty_

dies_in_hospice_1_566926.

16 Gail Tulloch, *Euthanasia - Choice and Death* (Edinburgh: Edinburgh University Press, 2005), 90.

17 "Diane Pretty dies," *BBC News*, May 12, 2002, at http://news.bbc.co.uk/2/hi/health/1983457.stm.

18 "Diane Pretty dies."

19 "Diane Pretty dies."

20 "British woman denied right to die," BBC News, April 29, 2002, at http://news.bbc.co.uk/2/hi/health/1957396.stm.

21 Len Dayal and Lesley Dayal, "Why active euthanasia and physician assisted suicide should be legalized," *British Medical Journal*, Nov. 10, 2001, 1079-1080.

22 "Suicide man's 'dignified' death," BBC News, Jan, 24, 2003, at http://news.bbc.co.uk/2/hi/uk_news/england/2688843.stm.

23 Dignity in Dying Annual Report, 2009, 6; "Suicide man's 'dignified' death."

24 "Dying Man plans Swiss suicide, BBC News, Jan. 3, 2003, at http://news.bbc.co.uk/2/hi/health/2621509.stm.

25 "Death Tourism," The World Federation of Right to Die Societies, at http://www.worldrtd.net/node/560. Italics mine.

26 The Lord Joffe, House of Lords Bill 37, 2003.

27 Haroon Siddique, "Man who helped partner die calls for assisted suicide law change," *The Guardian*, June 15, 2009; "'Come arrest me' challenges cancer patient's partner who helped his lover die at Dignitas," *Daily Mail*, June 15, 2009.

28 Andrew Alderson, "Dignitas: British doctor first to face charges under new assisted suicide guidelines," London *Telegraph*, April 25, 2010.

29 Alderson, "Dignitas: British doctor first to face charges."

30 "Tilting at Windmills," London *Sunday Telegraph*, Dec. 14, 2003, 38-39.

31 Coventry *Evening Telegraph*, Sept. 28, 2005.

32 Michael Irwin, email to RNC, July 10, 2010.

33 Michael Irwin, "Britain: The Soci-

ety for Old Age Rational Suicide goes National," Aug. 11, 2010, at http://euthanewsia.posterous.com/.

34 RNC, video interview with Dr. Michael Irwin, Oct. 8, 2010.

35 Both Debbie and Debby Purdy are used in the media.

36 "A Life in the Day: Debbie Purdy," The *Sunday Times*, Nov. 1, 2009, at http://women.timesonline.co.uk/tol/life_and_style/women/article6896134.ece.

37 Debbie Purdy, "Personal Stories," Dignity in Dying, at http://www.dignityindying.org.uk/personal-stories/uk/yorkshire-the-humber/bradford/debbie-purdy-story-7.html.

38 Astvinr, "Pawned?" *LiveJournal*, Dec, 7, 2008, at http://astvinr.livejournal.com/218070.html.

39 Mary Riddell, "It's an unholy mess—people must be allowed to die as they wish," *The Telegraph*, Aug. 3, 2009.

40 Dignity in Dying, "DPP's policy on assisted suicide," at http://www.dignityindying.org.uk/assisted-dying/faqs-dpps-policy-assisted-suicide.html.

41 "Debbie Purdy Reveals She 'Cancelled End of Life Plans,'" at http://samedifference1.com/2011/04/16/debbie-purdy-reveals-she-cancelled-end-of-life-plans/.

42 Sophie Elmhirst, "The NS Interview: Debbie Purdy, assisted suicide campaigner," *The New Statesman*, Sept. 3, 2010.

43 Chris Irvine, "Sir Terry Pratchett: coroner tribunals should be set up for assisted suicide case," *The Telegrap*h, Aug. 2, 2009.

44 Irvine, "Sir Terry Pratchett: coroner tribunals should be set up."

45 Clair Lewis, "At the end of life's tether," *Heresy Corner*, Feb. 3, 2010, at http://heresycorner.blogspot.com/2010/02/at-end-of-lifes-tether.html.

46 "John Hickleton's 100 Months—a fitting finale," *Forbidden Planet International*, March 23, 2010, at http://forbiddenplanet.co.uk/blog/2010/john-hicklenton-passes-away/.

47 Ludwig A. Minelli, "Some

Information About Dignitas," an address to the British Liberal Party Convention, Brighton, September 2006.

48 Sophie Borland, "Don't mention Dignitas: Nurses warned they would be jailed for talking about assisted suicide," *Mail Online*, Oct. 20, 2011.

Chapter 16: Those Feisty Scots

1 The numerous name changes of the voluntary euthanasia groups in Britain and Scotland are often confusing. In 1982, the London-based Exit changed its name back to The Voluntary Euthanasia Society (VES). In 1983, Scottish Exit changed its name to the Voluntary Euthanasia Society of Scotland (VESS, or VES-S). In 2000, the VES-S changed its name back to Exit (Scotland), and in 2006, the VES (London) changed its name to Dying in Dignity. The word "Exit" is also used in the name of several other right-to-die groups around the world, including as Exit International (Australia–Dr. Philip Nitschke), Exit International (Switzerland–Dr. Rolf Sigg), Exit-Deutsche Schweiz (German-speaking Switzerland), Exit-Suisse Allemande (French-speaking Switzerland), adding yet more confusion. Courtesy of Chris Docker, "A way out by any other name…," *Exit Newsletter*, January 2010, 5.

2 Ludovic Kennedy, "Why I Want to Choose My Moment of Death," reprinted from the Sunday *Standard*, Sept. 6, 1981, in Scottish Exit *News*, Autumn 1981, 3-4.

3 "Scotland First," *Scottish Exit News*, Autumn 1981, 6.

4 Kay Carmichael, "Chris Docker," VESS *Newsletter*, January 1997, 18.

5 Chris Docker, *Five Last Acts* (second edition): Edinburgh, Scotland: Exit, 2010), 273.

6 Chris Docker (CD) interview with RNC, Oct. 17, 2010.

7 CD interview with RNC, Oct. 17, 2010.

8 VES-S Press Release, Dec. 28, 1995.

9 VES-S Press Release (response), Dec. 28, 1995.

10 CD interview with RNC, Oct. 17, 2010.

11 CD interview with RNC, Oct. 17, 2010.

12 "Dr. Death holds his first British DIY suicide workshop," *London Daily Mail*, May 5, 2009.

13 CD interview with RNC, Oct. 17, 2010.

14 Libby Wilson, *Sex on the Rates: Memoirs of a Family Planning Doctor* (Argyll: Argyll Publishing, 2004), 165.

15 Interview of Libby Wilson by Muriel Gray on "Mavericks," BBC Radio Scotland, March 30, 2010.

16 Interview of Wilson by Gray.

17 *Sex on the Rates* descriptive flyer, 2004.

18 Libby Wilson, *Unexpected Always Happen: Journal of a Doctor in Sierra-Leone* (Argyll: Argyll Publishing, 1995), *passim*.

19 Wilson, *Unexpected Always Happen*, 190.

20 "Libby Wilson," VESS *Newsletter*, http://www.euthanasia.cc/libby.html.

21 Interview of Wilson by Gray.

22 Libby Wilson interview with RNC, Oct. 8, 2010.

23 Wilson to RNC, Nov. 21, 2010.

24 Wilson interview with RNC, Oct. 8, 2010.

25 Judith Duffy, "Guide to Assisted Suicide slammed by pro-life groups," *Glasgow Sunday Herald*, Feb. 19, 2006.

26 Duffy, "Guide to Assisted Suicide slammed by pro-life groups."

27 Sarah-Kate Templeton, "Disease pioneer's helium suicide," London *Times*, June 21, 2009.

28 Joanna Till, "Retired GP held for 'helping woman kill herself,'" Sept. 28, 2009 at http://www.getsurrey.co.uk/news/s/2057976_retired_gp_held_for_helping_women_kill_herself.

29 Sam Matthew, "MS sufferer took own life to Sinatra song," *The Scotsman*, Dec. 24, 2010.

30 Stephen McGinty, "Interview: Libby Wilson, doctor," in *Scotsman.com News*, at http://news.scotsman.com/euthanasia/Interview-Libby-Wilson-doctor.5697694.

jp.

31 McGinty, "Interview: Libby Wilson, doctor."

32 Jason Allardyce and Sarah-Kate Templeton, "First legal test of rules on suicide," *The Sunday Times*, Sept. 27, 2009.

33 Libby Wilson, posting to ERGO right-to-die newslist (right-to-die@lists. opn.org), Sept. 30, 2009.

34 Caroline Davies, "No charges against three arrested over academic's suicide," at http://www.guardian.co.uk/society/2010/aug/16/caroline-loder-suicide-no-charges.

35 Shân Ross, "Doctor won't face charges after helping woman to die," Aug.17, 2010, at http://news.scotsman. com/euthanasia/Doctor-won39t-face-charges-after.6477909.jp.

36 Interview of Wilson by Gray.

37 Tom Brown, "Denying dignity to the dying is the final insult," http:// scotlandonsunday.scotsman.com/ comment/Tom-Brown-Denying-dignity-to.3928585.jp, March 30, 2008.

38 Margo MacDonald, "I'll Die When I Choose," on "Panorama," BBC One http://news.bbc.co.uk/2/hi/programmes/ panorama/7767171.stm, December 5, 2008.

39 Margo MacDonald, "I'll Die When I Choose."

40 BBC News, "Sick Patients need Right to Die," July 15, 2008.

41 "MSPs Call for Right to End Life, BBC News Channel, http://news.bbc. co.uk/2/hi/uk_news/scotland/7508068. stm, July 15, 2008.

42 James Park to RNC, May 9, 2011.

43 CD to RNC, Dec. 22, 2010.

44 John Cameron, "End of life options," Feb. 3, 2010, at http://jucameron. wordpress.com/category/assisted-death/ page/2/; Shân Ross, "Suicide clinics give patients 'much-needed service,' says Kirk Minister," http://news.scotsman.com/ churchofscotland/Suicide-clinics-give-patients-39muchneeded.5850321.jp, Nov. 24, 2009.

45 Christopher Docker, "Does anyone represent the people?" Exiteuthanasia, Dec. 3, 2020, at http://exiteuthanasia. wordpress.com/2010/12/03/does-anyone-represent-the-people/.

46 Gary Fitzpatrick, "Press website prompts campaigner to lobby MSPs on assisted dying," *Dumferline Press*, Jan. 29, 2009.

47 Brian Currie, "MacDonald to resume assisted suicide fight," *The Herald Scotland*, May 17, 2011.

48 Brian Currie, "MacDonald to resume assisted suicide fight."

49 "Shock waves in UK over an elderly suicide," Assisted-Dying Blog, April 3, 2011, at http://assisted-dying.org/ blog/2011/04/03/shock-waves-in-uk-over-an-elderly-suicide/.

50 Richard Savill, "British woman takes own life at Dignitas because she did not want to die of old age," *The Telegraph*, Nov. 18, 2011.

51 Richard Savill, "British woman takes own life."

52 Sue Brayne, "Nan Maitland, Dignitas, a lesson for us all," April 5, 2011 at http://myhealthtalk.org/profiles/blogs/ nan-maitland-dignitas-a-lesson?xg_source=activity.

Chapter 17: A Rising Tide Raises All Ships

1 *Final Exit Network, Inc., et al. v. State of Georgia*, No. S11A1960, Feb. 06, 2012; Kim Severson, "Georgia Court Rejects Law Aimed at Assisted Suicide," *The New York Times*, Feb. 6, 2012.

2 "Belgium Euthanasia Law in Effect," at www.euthanasia.com/belgiumlaw.html.

3 Rob Jonquière to RNC, Feb, 13, 2012.

4 *The Belgian Act on Euthanasia of May 28th, 2002*, in *Ethical Perspectives* 9 (2002), 2-3: 182.

5 Marc Hooghe, Ellen Quintelier and Tim Reeskens, "Kerkpraktijk in Vlaanderen: Trends en extrapolaties: 1967-2004 ("Church attendance in Flanders: extrapolated trends, 1967-2004"), *Ethische Perspectieven* 16 (2): 115-116.

6 Tinne Smets, Johan Bilsen, Joachim Cohen, Mette L. Rurup and Luc Deliens, "Legal Euthanasia in Belgium. Characteristics of All Reported Cases," *Medical Care* 2010 (48, 2): 187.

7 Rory Watson, "First Belgian to use new euthanasia law provokes storm of protest," *British Medical Journal*, Oct. 19, 2002 (325: 7369), 854.

8 Jacqueline Herremans, "Belgium's Legalization of Euthanasia," *International Humanist and Ethical Union*, Feb. 1, 2003, at http://www.iheu.org/node/1110.

9 *Euthanasia and Assisted Suicide. Law of 16 March 2009. 25 Questions. 25 Answers.* Luxembourg: Ministry of Social Security, 2009.

10 Association pour le droit de mourir dans la dignité – Lëtzebuerg, *www. admdl.lu/en.*

11 "Luxembourg to become third EU country to allow euthanasia," *AFP*, Feb. 20, 2008, at http://afp.google.com/article/ALeqM5j_LY2E4ut3ccEXydLd0C3zlVOXFA

12 "Grand Duke Henri of Luxembourg opposes euthanasia and loses power," *The Times*, Dec. 4, 2008.

13 Jean Huss, *Depenalizing Euthanasia in Luxembourg*, handout at the 2008 World Federation of Right to Die Societies' biennial congress, Paris, November 2008.

14"Grand Duke Henri of Luxembourg opposes euthanasia and loses power."

15 "Grand Duke of Luxembourg receives 2009 Cardinal Van Thuan Prize," *Catholic News Service*, Sept. 17, 2009.

16 Derek Humphry, "How-to Euthanasia books: an annotated bibliography," at http://www.finalexit.org/how_to_books_on_self-deliverance_and_euthanasia.html, 2005.

17 Humphry, "How-to Euthanasia books: an annotated bibliography."

18 Derek Humphry, "Tread Carefully When You Help to Die," *Assisted Suicide*, updated March 1, 2005, at http://www.assistedsuicide.org/suicide_laws.html.

19 Humphry, "Tread Carefully When

You Help to Die."

20 "Les Français très favorables à l'euthanasie; un débat parlementaire réclamé," http://www.psychomedia.qc.ca/pn/modules.php?name=News&file=article&sid=8230, Oct. 13, 2010.

21 "Cancer victim Chantal Sebire found dead at home," *The Daily Telegraph*, March 20, 2008.

22 "France considers euthanasia law," *The Connexion*, Jan. 19, 2011, at http://www.connexionfrance.com/french-senate-euthanasia-assisted-suicide-law-vote-view-article.html.

23 "France considers euthanasia law."

24 "France considers euthanasia law."

25 Christian Arnold, "The ethical situation in Germany on euthanasia," ERGO right-to-die newslist, vol. 13, issue 202, Nov. 26, 2007.

26 Elke M. Baezner-Sailer, "Physician-Assisted Suicide: Narratives From Professional and Personal Experience," in Dieter Birnbacher and Edgar Dahl, eds., *Giving Death a Helping Hand: Physician-Assisted Suicide and Public Policy. An International Perspective* (New York: Springer, 2008), 143 .

27 "Thanatology studies at the University of Rhode Island College of Nursing," at http://www.uri.edu/nursing/thanatology/thanatology.html.

28 Mark Landler, "Assisted Suicide of Healthy 79-Year-Old Renews German Debate on Right to Die," *The New York Times*, July 3, 2008.

29 Roger Boyes, "German politician Roger Kusch helped elderly woman to die," *The Times*, July 2, 2008.

30 Roger Boyes, "German politician Roger Kusch helped elderly woman to die."

31 Jacqueline Jencquel, "Max Steinbaur, Roger Kusch, and assisted suicide in Germany," *ERGO World Right-to-Die News*, Nov. 14, 2008.

32 Keaton Gray, "Inventor's device simplifies suicide," *The Trojan*, April 3, 2008.

33 Carolina Schmidt and Andreas Ulrich,

"Court Expected to Rule on Assisted Suicide Case," *Der Spiegel*, Jan. 21, 2009

34 Roger Kusch and Johann Friedrich Spitttler, *SterbeHilfeDeutschland e.V., Weißbuch 2011*: Books on Demand (Germany), 9.

35 "Unpleasant surprise at German doctors meeting in Kiel," World Federation of Right to Die Societies, June 25, 2011, at http://worldrtd.net/news/unplaesant-surprise-german-doctors-meeting-kiel.

36 Patientenverfügungsgesetz im *Bürgerlichen Gesetzbuch*, § 1901a, 1-4 and § 1904, as well as the Bundesgerichtshof of June 25, 2010.

37 §217 of the *Strafgesetzbuch* (Criminal Code) defines the difference between a suicide and an assisted suicide. Elke Baezner-Sailer, DGHS, email to RNC, February 18, 2012.

38 Judy Siegel-Itzkovich, "Death With Dignity to be allowed from Next Month," *The Jerusalem Post*, Nov. 12, 2006.

39 Nurit Wurgaft, "Condemned to Life," Nov. 6, 2009, at www.haaretz.com/hasen/spages/1126275.html.

40 Ruth Debel, "Lilach Sponsors Forum in Jerusalem on New Assisted Dying Bill," World Right-to-Die Newsletter, Winter, 2010, 3; Roni Sofer, "Knesset rejects euthanasia law proposal," Jan. 19, 2011, at http://www.ynetnews.com/articles/0,7340,L-4016034,00.html.

41 "Is euthanasia allowed in Islam?" Fatwah of Muzammil Siddiqi, posted 4.22.2010 in *Islamopedia Online*, http://islamopediaonline.org/fatwa/dr-siddiqi-fiqh-council-north-america-responds-query-euthanasia-allowed-islam.

42 Rob Jonquière to RNC, Feb. 13, 2012.

43 Peter Ford, "World Divided on Ethics of Terri Schaivo case," *Christian Science Monitor*, March 25, 2005.

44 Rihito Kimura, "Death, Dying, and Advance Directives in Japan: Socio-cultural and Legal Point of View," http://www.bioethics.jp/licht_adv8.html. Section 5.2. Legal Criteria for Active

Euthanasia in Japan.

45 Kimura, "Death, Dying, and Advance Directives in Japan."

46 Kimura, "Death, Dying, and Advance Directives in Japan."

47 Asia One/AFP, "Japan doctor gets suspended jail term for 'mercy killing,'" Dec. 9, 2009, http://www.asiaone.com/News/AsiaOne+News/Crime/Story/A1Story20091209-184947.html.

48 RNC video interview with Dr. Iwao Soichiro, Melbourne, Oct. 8, 2010.

49 RNC interview with Dr. Iwao Soichiro.

50 Derek Humphry, "Tread Carefully When You Help to Die: Assisted Suicide Laws around the World," revised March 1, 2005, at http://www.assistedsuicide.org/suicide_laws.html.

51 Matthew Davis, "Euthanasia debate sweeps the world," BBC World Online, Sept. 26, 2003, at http://news.bbc.co.uk/2/hi/europe/3143112.stm.

52 David Pierson, "Blogging for the right to choose death," *Los Angeles Times*, May 20, 2007.

53 Pierson, "Blogging for the right to choose death."

Chapter 18: Seeker of the Grail Secrets

1 *British Columbia Coroners Service Policy and Procedure Manual, April 21, 1999.* Section 2.2.G.1 Suicide—Euthanasia and Assisted Suicide.

2 Woody Allen, "Death," (a play), *Without Feathers* (New York: Ballantine, 1975).

3 Russel D. Ogden, "Observing a Self-Chosen Death," preliminary manuscript version, 2010, and interview with RNC, Feb. 10, 2012.

4 Russel D. Ogden and Rae H. Wooten, "Asphyxial Suicide with Helium and a Plastic Bag," *The American Journal of Forensic Medicine and Pathology*, 23 (3): 234-237 (2002).

5 Ogden, "Observing a Self-Chosen Death."

6 Ogden, "Observing a Self-Chosen Death." Interview with RNC, Feb. 10, 2012.

7 Diane Martindale, "A Culture of

Death," *Scientific American*, May 23, 2005, at http://www.scientificamerican.com/article.cfm?id=a-culture-of-death.

8 Sue Woodman, referring to Ogden's discoveries, in *Last Rights: The Struggle Over The Right to Die*, 141.

9 Russel D. Ogden, "An Insult to Free Inquiry," *Simon Fraser News*, Oct. 30, 1997.

10 Russel D. Ogden, *Euthanasia, Assisted Suicide, and AIDS*: (New Westminster, British Columbia: Peroglyphics, 1994.) The formal title of his master's thesis, as noted in the published version cited here, was "Euthanasia and Assisted Suicide in Persons with Acquired Immunodeficiency Syndrome (AIDS) or Human Immunodeficiency Virus (HIV)."

11 Martindale, "A Culture of Death."

12 Christopher G. Docker, in Russel D. Ogden, *Euthanasia, Assisted Suicide, and AIDS*, back cover.

13 Jack P. Blaney, president, Simon Fraser University, to Russel D. Ogden, Oct. 20, 1998.

14 "Russel Ogden," Willamette University College of Law: *Recent Developments in Physician-Aided Death*, March 1999, 8, at www.willamette.edu/wucl/pdf/pas/1999-03.pdf.

15 "At death's door: A B.C. sociologist pushes ahead with taboo-breaking research into assisted suicide," Canada.com, Nov. 10, 2008, at http://www.canada.com/story_print.html?id=5dc8ae55-72e7-480e-b148-bdc493146e4e&sponsor=

16 "Exeter Pays Canadian Prof $140K Damages," *CAUT/ACPPU Bulletin Online*, 50 (9), November 2003.

17 "Exeter Pays Canadian Prof $140."

18 "Exeter Pays Canadian Prof $140K."

19 "Exeter Pays Canadian Prof $140K."

20 "Exeter student wins £63,000," *Times Higher Education*, Oct. 31, 2003, at http://www.timeshighereducation.co.uk/ory.asp?storycode=180841

21 "Exeter Pays Canadian Prof $140K."

22 *Times Higher Education*, "No ring of confidence," Nov. 7, 2003, at http://www.timeshighereducation.co.uk/story.

asp?storycode=180996.

23 "CAUT Reviewing Kwantlen's 'Stop Research' Directive," *CAUT/ACCPU Bulletin* online, 59:2 (February 2012).

24 "Exeter Pays Canadian Prof $140K Damages."

25 John L. Hofsess to Russel D. Ogden (RDO), Sept. 24, 1999.

26 John L. Hofsess to RDO, Oct. 19, 1999.

27 RDO to RNC, Feb. 24, 2012.

28 "CAUT Reviewing Kwantlen's 'Stop Research' Directive."

29 Russel D. Ogden, William K. Hamilton, and Charles Whitcher, "Assisted suicide by oxygen deprivation with helium at a Swiss right-to-die organization," *Journal of Medical Ethics* 2010 (36), 174.

30 Ogden, Hamilton, and Whitcher, "Assisted suicide by oxygen deprivation with helium" 177.

31 RDO interview with RNC, Feb. 28, 2012.

32 RDO interview with RNC, Feb. 28, 2012.

33 RDO interview with RNC, Feb. 28, 2012.

34 Affidavit of Russel Ogden 1, sworn February 20, 2011, In the Matter of an Application to Incorporate The Farewell Foundation for the Right to Die pursuant to The Society Act [RSBC 1996] V.433, 1.

35 Affidavit of Russel Ogden 1, 4.

36 "Assisted Suicide Advocates take case to BC Court," *CTV News*, Aug. 2, 2011, at http://m.ctv.ca/topstories/20110802/farewell-foundation-court-case-110802.html

37 Notice of Appeal to the Supreme Court of British Columbia, April 8, 2011, No. S-112305.

38 Ken MacQueen, "On the need to restart the debate on assisted suicide, *Macleans*.ca, Aug. 17, 2011, at http://www2.macleans.ca/tag/dignitas/ .

39 *Farewell Foundation News*, November 2011, 4.

40 *Farewell Foundation News*, November 2011, 4.

41 *Farewell Foundation News*, November 2011, 4.

Chapter 19: The Big Sting

1 Robert Rivas, Network Legal Advisor, "Network Legal Update," Final Exit Network *Newsletter*, Spring 2010, 1.

2 Affidavit and Application for a Search Warrant in the Superior Court of Cobb County, State of Georgia, February [no day specified]2009.

3 Kris Sperry, email to Mitchell Posey, November 13, 2008, Subject: "Sartain case." [Case] 08-0001-01 Exhibit #16.

4 Rivas, "Network Legal Update."

5 Rhonda Cook, "Forsyth County grand jury indicts members of assisted suicide network," Atlanta *Journal-Constitution*, March 9, 2010.

6 Neal Nicol, "Phony medical history sent to Dr Kevorkian," posted Jan. 10, 2011 to ERGO News List right-to-die@lists.opn.org .

7 *The Daily Global*, "Four members of assisted suicide group are arrested," Feb. 26, 2009, http://www.dailyglobal.com/2009/02/4-members-of-assisted-suicide-group-are-arrested/.

8 Richard MacDonald to RNC, Sept. 21, 2011;

9 Ted Goodwin to RNC, March 14, 2012.

10 Final Exit Network, *2004 Year End Report*, Jan. 4, 2005.

11 Jerry Dincin, "Final Exit Network Die with Dignity Billboards Continue in Washington D.C., Baltimore and South Florida," Final Exit Network media release, Oct. 18, 2010.

12 Final Exit Network, "Who Are We and What Can We Do For You?" Informational flyer, undated (c.2005).

13 Paul Rubin, "Death Wish," Phoenix *New Times*, Aug. 23, 2007.

14 Rubin, "Death Wish."

15 Rubin, "Death Wish."

16 "Final Exit Network Exit Guide Instructions," Affidavit and Application for a search warrant, in the Superior Court of Cobb County, State of Georgia, no date (c. February 2009).

17 Ted Goodwin, interview with RNC, March 10, 2012.

18 Faye Girsh, Tuesday, April 19, 2001 trial report via Compassion and Choices of New Jersey, Inc.

19 Girsh, Tuesday, April 19, 2001 trial report.

20 Jerry Dincin, media release, "Final Exit Network Volunteers Found Innocent in Right-to-Die Case," April 21, 2011.

21 Charles Bethea, "Final Exit," http://www.atlantamagazine.com/features/Story.aspx?ID=1425551.

22 Bethea, "Final Exit."

23 Bethea, "Final Exit."

24 Goodwin, interview with RNC, March 10, 2012.

25 Bethea, "Final Exit."

26 "Four arrested in 2 states in assisted-suicide probe," Feb. 26, 2009, CNN.com, http://articles.cnn.com/2009-02-26/justice/assisted.suicide.probe_1_gbi-final-exit-network-suicide?_s=PM:CRIME

27 Bethea, "Final Exit."

28 Thomas E. Goodwin to RNC, March 17, 2012.

29 Kim Severson, "Georgia Court Rejects Law Aimed at Assisted Suicide," the *New York Times*, Feb. 7, 2012.

30 Robert Rivas, "Quietly, Georgia Becomes Fourth State to Legalize Physician Assisted Suicide," *Assisted Dying* blog, Nov. 6, 2011.

31 Robert Rivas, "Network Legal Update," Final Exit Network *Newsletter*, December 2009, 1.

32 Forsyth County Superior Court, Georgia. Motion for Evidentiary Hearing and for Return of Seized Property, July 8, 2009.

33 Kate Brumback, "Ga. To return $330,000 to assisted suicide group," The *San Francisco Examiner*, Oct. 15, 2009.

34 Derek Humphry, "Liberty Fund to the Rescue," Final Exit Network *Newsletter*, December 2009, 1.

35 Goodwin, interview with RNC, March 10, 2012.

36 *Final Exit Network, Inc., et al. v. State of Georgia,* decided Feb. 6, 2012, 6-7.

37 Ted Goodwin to RNC, March 11, 2012.

38 Bill Rankin, "Court strikes down Georgia's assisted-suicide law," Atlanta *Journal-Constitution,* Feb. 6, 2012.

39 Justin Fenton, "Baltimore doctor helps the ill commit suicide," *The Baltimore Sun,* May 21, 2011.

40 Robert Rivas, "Georgia House Passes Bill to Prohibit Assisted Suicide," Message #1, ERGO Right-to-die@lists. opn.org, March 7, 2012.

41 Ted Goodwin, interview with RNC March 9, 2010.

Chapter 20: Seamless Care for a Gentle Death

1 Rob Jonquière, email to RNC, April 3, 2012.

2 Paula Span, "Interactive Tools to Assess the Likelihood of Death," *The New York Times,* January 10, 2012.

3 Rodney Syme, email to RNC, April 2, 2012.

4 Mario Garrett, "Many shy away from planning their exit," San Diego *Union-Tribune,* Nov. 16, 2010.

5 Mario Garrett, "Many shy away from planning their exit."

6 Barbara Coombs Lee, "Different Worlds," Dec. 6, 2010, at blog. compassionandchoices.org/?p=1175.

7 Paula Span, "A Conversation Many Doctors Won't Have," The *New York Times,* Nov. 16, 2011.

8 Atul Gawande, "Letting Go," *The New Yorker,* Aug. 2, 2010.

9 "Dr. Ann McPherson: The GP who believes she should be allowed help to end her life," *The Independent,* Jan. 24, 2011.

10 E. James Lieberman, M.D., in Amazon.com review of *The Maintenance of Life: Preventing Social Death Through Euthanasia Talk and End-of-Life Care - Lessons from the Netherlands,* by Frances Norwood, 2009.

11 Having observed one such medical "professional development" junket as an observer while on a writing assignment, I can verify that the medical professional development component of the cruise was 10 percent and the exotic vacation portion was 90 percent.

12 "EXIT-run hospice opens in Switzerland," *World Right-to-Die Newsletter,* 23 (1993):1.

13 Russel D. Ogden, "Palliative Care and Euthanasia: A Continuum of Care?" *Journal of Palliative Care,* 1994 (10:2): 82-85. See also Russel D. Ogden and Michael G. Young, "Understanding Assisted Death Decisions: An Interdisciplinary Approach," *Mature Medicine* (Canada), September/October 1999, 283.

14 Timothy E. Quill and Ira R. Byock, "Responding to Intractable Terminal Suffering: The Role of Terminal Sedation and Voluntary Refusal of Food and Fluids," *Annals of Internal Medicine,* March 7, 2000 (132:5), 408.

15 Lesley Martin, "Dignity Havens [PowerPoint] presentation, World Federation of Right to Die Societies biennial congress, Paris, October 21, 2008.

16 Jan L. Bernheim et al., "Development of palliative care and legalisation of euthanasia: antagonism or synergy?" *British Medical Journal,* April 19, 2008 (336): 864–867.

17 Canadian Nurses Association, "Providing Nursing Care at the End of Life." *Position Statement,* 2008.

18 "Voluntary euthanasia can compliment palliative care," media release, YourLastRight.com, May 24, 2011.

19 Russell Contreras/AP, "Two Doctors Challenge New Mexico's Decades-old 'right-to-die' law," *The Republic,* Columbus, Indiana, March 15, 2012.

Bibliography

Some sources that were not cited in the source notes also provided a perspective on the topics covered in this book and are included here for the benefit of future researchers. URLs are provided for all internet-hosted content that was accessed by the author between 1997 and 2012. For URLs cited but no longer active ("dead links"), cached copies dating as far back as 1996 may often be located by using the Internet Archive ("The Wayback Machine") at http://www.archive.org/web/web.php. Names marked with an asterisk have been changed to protect the privacy of the person noted.

Interviews conducted by the author

Babey, Donald, former executive director, Dying With Dignity, Toronto, Ontario, Canada

Castellana, Andrés,* medical student, Cali, Colombia

Cathy,* Baltimore, Maryland, USA

Chabot, Boudewijn, M.D., former president, NVVE, Amsterdam, The Netherlands

Clark, Lindsey, M.D., Chief Medical Examiner, Freeborn, Minnesota, USA

Dent, Judy, widow of Bob Dent, Tiwi, Northern Territory, Australia

Docker, Christopher, M. Phil., director, Exit (Scotland), Edinburgh, Scotland

Eighmey, George, LL.D., former executive director, Compassion & Choices, Portland, Oregon, USA

Escobar-Triana, Jaime A., M.D., Universidad El Bosque, Bogotá, Colombia

Exoo, George D., founder, The Compassionate Chaplaincy Foundation, Beckley, West Virginia, USA

Girsh, Faye, Ed.D., past-president, Hemlock Society, USA; co-founder, the Final Exit Network, La Jolla, California, USA

Goodwin, Thomas E. (Ted), cofounder and former president, the Final Exit Network, Pennington, New Jersey, USA

Hofsess, John L., founder, the Right to Die Society of Canada, Victoria, British Columbia, Canada

Humphry, Derek J., founder, Hemlock Society USA; the Euthanasia Research and Guidance Organization; and author of *Final Exit*

Irwin, Michael, M.D., former chairman, Voluntary Euthanasia Society, U.K.) and founder, the Society for Old Age Rational Suicide, Cranleigh, Surrey, England

Iwao, Soichiro, M.D., Ph.D., vice-chairman, Japan Society for Dying with Dignity, Tokyo, Japan

Jonquière, Rob, M.D., CEO, NVVE, Amsterdam, The Netherlands

Kaplan, Ilene, former president, Hemlock of Connecticut, Avon, Connecticut, USA

Kevorkian, Jack, M.D., pathologist, Pontiac, Michigan, USA

MacDonald, Richard, M.D., former Medical Director, Hemlock Society's Caring Friends Program; Senior Medical Advisor, Final Exit Network; Chico, California, USA

Mae, Cassandra E., Ph.D., (aka Susan Wilson), independent exit guide, Gastonia, North Carolina, USA

Martens, Evelyn, exit guide, British Columbia, Canada

McGurrin, Thomas, treasurer, The Compassionate Chaplaincy Foundation, Beckley, West Virginia, USA

Mendoza-Vega, Juan, M.D., Bogotá, Colombia

Metz, Jerry, former president, Final Exit Network, Addison, Maine, USA

Minelli, Ludwig A., LL.D., founder, Dignitas, Forch, Switzerland

Morris, Wanda, executive director, Director, Dying With Dignity, Toronto, Ontario, Canada

Neils, Rob, Ph.D., founder, The Dying Well Network, Spokane, Washington, USA

Nicol, Neal, Nicol Associates, Waterford, Michigan, USA

Nitschke, Philip, Ph.D., M.D., founder, Exit International, Darwin, Northern Territory, Australia

Ogden, Russel D., M.A., criminologist, Kwantlen Polytechnic University, Vancouver, British Columbia, Canada

Quintana-Romero, Gustavo, M.D., former director, DMD, Bogotá, Colombia

Ronson, Jon, film producer, London, England

Sandberg, Georgene ("Gigi"), former Southeast Regional Coordinator, Hemlock Society, Diamondhead, Mississippi, USA

Schaefer, Lois, former director, Hemlock Society USA Caring Friends program; corresponding secretary, NuTech, Denver, Colorado, USA

Stern, Karen, musician, self-delivered in Kingman, Arizona, USA

Syme, Rodney, M.D., president, Dying With Dignity-Victoria, Melbourne, Victoria, Australia

Terman, Stanley A., M.D., Ph.D., Carlsbad, California, USA

von Fuchs, Ruth, president, The Right To Die Society of Canada, Toronto, Ontario, Canada

Whitcher, Charles E., M.D., retired anesthesiologist, Stanford University Medical Center, Palo Alto, California

Wilson, Libby, M.D., director, Friends at the End, Glasgow, Scotland

Wynn, Hugh T., Eur. Ing., Glasgow, Scotland, past president, World Federation of Right to Die Societies

Manuscript Collections

Dore, Margaret. "Choice is a Lie," May 26, 2009. Handout and DVD of her presentation at the Second International Symposium on Euthanasia and Assisted Suicide," Landsdowne, Va., May 29-30, 2008.

Dore, Margaret. "Washington State [I-1000] Postmortem," May 26, 2009. Handout at the Second International Symposium on Euthanasia and Assisted Suicide," Landsdowne, Va., May 29-30, 2008.

Exoo, George David. Personal and professional papers, 1942-2008. Private collection in the possession of the author.

Hofsess, John L. The Victoria Manifesto (Rob [Neils'] version), April 17, 1998.

Kingman, Arizona Police Department. "Death Investigation of Karen Stern," October 29, 2007. Case Number 2007 00026449.

Republic of Ireland v. George David Exoo, 2007.

Sandberg, Georgene V. (1926-2009). Personal and professional papers. Private collection in the possession of the author.

Stern, Karen (1954-2007). "A Medical History," Kingman, Arizona, August 2007. Typescript copy in the possession of the author.

Syme, Rodney. *"Doctors Help Their Patients to Die."* A speech made to Dying With Dignity-Tasmania, Australia, 2009.

Toole, Rosemary. GDE Papers. Private Collection. January 10, 2002.

Books

Note: only books cited as reference material or for background knowledge are listed here. Articles, other printed materials, and online sources are fully cited in the chapter source notes.

Admiraal, Pieter V., Boudewijn Chabot, Russel D. Ogden, Aad Rietveld and Jan Glerum. *Guide to a Humane Self-Chosen Death.* Delft, The Netherlands: WOZZ Foundation, 2006.

Admiraal, Pieter V. *Justifiable Euthanasia: A Manual for the Medical Profession.* Amsterdam: NVVE, 1978.

Aldrich, Robert, and Garry Wotherspoon, eds. *Who's Who in Contemporary Gay and Lesbian History, From World War II to the Present Day.* Florence, Kentucky: Taylor & Francis, Inc., 2000.

Barnard, Christiaan. *Good Life, Good Death: A Doctor's Case for Euthanasia and Suicide.* Englewood Cliffs, N.J: Prentice-Hall, 1980.

Battin, Margaret P. *Ending Life: Ethics and the Way We Die.* Oxford: Oxford University Press, 2005.

Battin, Margaret P. *The Least Worst Death: Essays in Bioethics on the End of Life.* New York: Oxford University Press, 1994.

Batttin, Margaret P. and Arthur G. Lipman, eds. *Drug Use in Assisted Suicide and Euthanasia.* Binghamton, N.Y.: Pharmaceutical Products Press, 1996.

Battin, Margaret P., Rosamond Rhodes, and Anita Silvers. *Physician Assisted Suicide: Expanding the Debate.* New York: Routledge, 1998.

Betzold, Michael. *Appointment with Dr. Death.* Troy, Mich.: Momentum Books, Ltd., 1993.

Biggs, Hazel. *Euthanasia, Death With Dignity and the Law.* Oxford: Hart Publishing, 2001.

Billson, Janet Mancini and Kyra Mancini. *Inuit Women: Their Powerful Spirit in a Century of Change.* Lanham, Md.: Rowman & Littlefield, 2007.

Birnie, Lisa Hobbs and Sue Rodriguez. *Uncommon Will: The Death and Life of Sue Rodriguez.* Toronto: Macmillan of Canada, 1994.

Brewer, Colin. *A Guide to Self-Deliverance.* London: Voluntary Euthanasia Society, 1981.

Brown, David Jay. *Mavericks of Medicine: Conversations on the Frontiers of Medical Research.* Petaluma, Calif.: Smart Publications, 2006.

Chabot, Boudewijn E. *A Hastened Death by Self-denial of Food and Drink.* Amsterdam: Boudewijn Chabot, 2008.

Cohen-Almagor, Raphael. *The Right to Die With Dignity: An Argument in Ethics, Medicine, and Law.* New Brunswick, N.J.: Rutgers University Press, 2001.

Colby, William H. *Unplugged: Reclaiming Our Right to Die in America.* New York: Amacom, 2006.

Colt, George Howe. *November of the Soul: The Enigma of Suicide.* New York: Scribner, 2006.

Cox, Donald W. *Hemlock's Cup: The Struggle for Death With Dignity.* Buffalo, New York: Prometheus Books, 1993.

DeMaria, William. *Deadly Disclosures: Whistleblowing and the Ethical Meltdown of Australia.* Kent Town, S.A., Australia: Wakefield Press, 1999.

Docker, Chris, Cheryl Smith, and the International Drugs Consensus Working Party. *Departing Drugs.* Edinburgh: Exit, 1993.

Docker, Chris, Cheryl Smith, John Hofsess, and Bruce Dunn. *Beyond Final Exit: New Research in Self-Deliverance for the Terminally Ill.* Victoria, B. C.: The Right to Die Society of Canada, 1995.

Dowbiggin, Ian. *A Concise History of Euthanasia: Life, Death, God, and Medicine.* New York: Rowman & Littlefield Publishers, Inc., 2005.

Dowbiggin, Ian. *A Merciful End: The Euthanasia Movement in Modern America.* London and New York: Oxford University Press, 2003.

Dowbiggin, Ian. *Life, Death, God, and Medicine.* New York: Rowman & Littlefield Publishers, Inc., 2007.

Fletcher, Joseph. *Morals and Medicine: The Moral Problems of The Patient's Right to Know the Truth, Contraception, Artificial Insemination, Sterilization, Euthanasia.* 1954; reprinted Boston: Beacon Press, 1963.

Foley, Kathleen and Herbert Hendi. *The Case Against Assisted Suicide.* Baltimore, Md.: Johns Hopkins University Press, 2002.

Foos-Graber, Anya. *Deathing: An Intelligent Alternative for the Final Moments of Life.* York Beach, Maine: Nicholas-Hays, Inc., 1989.

Fox, Elaine, Jeffrey L. Kamakahi and Stella N. Capek. *Come Lovely and Soothing Death: The Right to Die Movement in the United States.* New York: Twayne Publishers, 1999.

Gorsuch, Neil M. *The Future of Assisted Suicide and Euthanasia.* Princeton, N. J.: Princeton University Press, 2006.

Griffiths, John, Alex Bood, and Heleen Weyers. *Euthanasia and Law in The Netherlands.* Amsterdam: Amsterdam University Press, 1998.

Hillyard, Daniel, and John Dombrink. *Dying Right: The Death With Dignity Movement.* New York: Routledge, 2001.

Hofsess, John L. *"Sue Rodriguez is 42. She has ALS. Who Cares?"* Last Rights Publications #6. Toronto: Right to Die Society of Canada, 1992.

Hofsess, John L. *Inner Views: Ten Canadian Film-makers.* Toronto: McGraw-Hill Ryerson Ltd., 1975.

Hofsess, John L. *NuTech Report #1,* May 2000. Victoria, B.C.: Last Rights Publications, 2000.

Hofsess, John L. *NuTech Report #2,* October 2000. Victoria, B.C.: Last Rights Publications, 2000.

Hofsess, John L. *The Art & Science of Suicide. Chapter 1. Self-Deliverance & Plastic Bags: Introducing the Customized Exit Bag.* Version 1.2. Ottawa, Ont: HC Publications,1997.

Hofsess, John L. *The Art & Science of Suicide. Chapter 6. Introducing the Debreather.* Version 1.1. Ottawa, Ont: HC Publications,1998.

Hofsess, John L. *The Art & Science of Suicide. Chapter 8. Helium and the New 'Exit Bag' for Helium.* Version 2. Ottawa, Ont.: Last Rights Publications, 2000.

Hofsess, John L. *The Art & Science of Suicide. Chapter 9. A first-class death: Self-deliverance through new technology.* Version 1. Victoria, B.C.: Last Rights Publications, 2000.

Horn, Robert C. III and Gretchen Keeler. *Who's Right? Whose Right? Seeking Answers in the Debate Over The Right To Die.* Sanford, Fla: DC Press, 2001.

Humphry, Derek. *Good Life, Good Death: A Memoir.* Junction City, Ore.: Norris Lane Press, 2008.

Humphry, Derek. *Final Exit: The Practicalities of Self-Deliverance and Assisted Suicide for the Dying.* New York: Dell Publishing, 2002; third edition, revised, with supplement, 2006-07.

Humphry, Derek. *The Good Euthanasia Guide.* Junction City, Ore.: Norris Lane Press, 2006.

Humphry, Derek. *The Good Euthanasia Guide.* Junction City, Ore.: Norris Lane Press/ERGO, 2005.

Humphry, Derek. *Why I Believe in Voluntary Euthanasia and Assisted Suicide: The Case for a Rational Approach to Freedom of Choice.* Junction City, Ore.: ERGO, 2001.

Humphry, Derek. *Self-deliverance From an End-stage Terminal Illness by Use of a Plastic Bag.* Revised 1999. Junction City, Ore.: ERGO, 1999.

Humphry, Derek. *Lawful Exit: The Limits of Freedom for Help in Dying.* Junction City, Ore.: Norris Lane Press, 1993.

Humphry, Derek. *Euthanasia: Essays and Briefings on the Right to Choose to Die.* Eugene, Ore.: The Hemlock Society, 1991.

Humphry, Derek. *Final Exit: The Practicalities of Self-Deliverance and Assisted Suicide for the Dying.* Eugene, Ore.: The Hemlock Society, 1991. First edition.

Humphry, Derek. *Compassionate Crimes, Broken Taboos (former title: Assisted Suicide: The Compassionate Crime).* Los Angeles: The Hemlock Society, 1986.

Humphry, Derek. *Let Me Die Before I Wake: Hemlock's Book of Self-Deliverance for the Dying.* Los Angeles: The Hemlock Society, 1981.

Humphry, Derek, and Mary Clement. *Freedom to Die: People, Politics, and the Right-To-Die Movement.* New York: St. Martin's Griffin, 2000.

Humphry, Derek, and Ann Wickett. *Jean's Way.* New York: Dell Publishing, 1986.

Humphry, Derek, and Ann Wickett. *The Right to Die: Understanding Euthanasia.* New York: Harper & Row Publishers, 1986.

Humphry, Derek, and Gus John. *Because They're Black.* London: Penguin Books Ltd., 1972.

Hyde, Michael J. *The Call of Conscience: Heidegger and Levinas, Rhetoric and the Euthanasia Debate.* Columbia, S.C.: University of South Carolina Press, 2001.

Ilardo, Joseph A. *As Parents Age: A Psychological and Practical Guide.* Acton, Mass.: Vander Wyck & Burnham, 1998.

Irwin, Michael. *Old Age Rational Suicide.* London: privately printed, 2009.

Jamison, Kay Redfield. *Night Falls Fast: Understanding Suicide.* New York: Alfred A. Knopf, 1999.

Jamison, Stephen. *Final Acts of Love: Families, Friends, and Assisted Dying.* New York: Jeremy P. Tarcher/Putnam, 1995.

Kevorkian, Jack. *Medical Research and the Death Penalty: A Dialogue.* New York: Vantage Press, 1960.

Kevorkian, Jack. *Prescription Medicide: The Goodness of Planned Death.* Buffalo, New York: Prometheus Books, 1991.

Kosma, Joseph L. *Killer Plants: A Poisonous Plant Guide.* N.P.: Milestone Publishing Co., 1969.

Kübler-Ross, Elisabeth. *On Death and Dying.* New York: Macmillan Publishing Co., 1969.

Lamb, David. *Down the Slippery Slope: Arguing in Applied Ethics.* London: Croom Helm, Ltd., 1988.

Larue, Gerald A. *Euthanasia and Religion: Survey of the Attitudes of World Religions to the Right to Die.* Los Angeles, California: The Hemlock Society, 1985.

Larue, Gerald A. *Playing God: Fifty Religions' Views on Your Right to Die.* Wakefield, R. I.: Moyer Bell, 1996.

Magnusson, Roger S. *Angels of Death: Exploring the Euthanasia Underground.* New Haven, Conn.: Yale University Press, 2002.

Mair, George Brown. *Confessions of a Surgeon.* London: William Luscombe Publishers, 1974.

Mair, George Brown. *How To Die With Dignity.* Edinburgh: Scottish Exit, 1980.

Marker, Rita L. *Deadly Compassion: The Death of Ann Humphry and the Truth About Euthanasia.* New York: William Morrow, 1993.

Martin, Lesley. *To Cry Inside: Love, Death, and Prison, The Hidden Face of the Euthanasia Debate.* New Zealand: Penguin New Zealand: 2006.

Martin, Lesley. *To Die Like a Dog: The Personal Face of the Euthanasia Debate.* Wellington, N. Z.: M-Press, Ltd., 2002.

Mendoza-Vega, Juan. *Caminos de la Bioética en Colombia.* Bogotá, Colombia: Revista Latinoamericana de Bioética, 2006.

Mitchell, John B. *Understanding Assisted Suicide: Nine Issues to Consider. A Personal Journey.* Ann Arbor, Mich.: University of Michigan Press, 2007.

Mullins, Anne. *Timely Death.* Toronto: Alfred A. Knopf, 1996.

Nederlandse Vereniging Voor Een Vrijwillig Levenseinde (NVVE). *Choices of the end of Life: Perspectives on Dying With Dignity.* Amsterdam: NVVE, 2008.

Neils, Rob. *Death With Dignity FAQs.* Dubuque, Iowa: Kendall/Hunt Publishing Co., 1997.

Nicol, Neal and Harry Wylie. *Between the Dying and the Dead: Dr. Jack Kevorkian's Life and the Battle to Legalize Euthanasia.* Madison, Wisc.: The University Press, 2006.

Nitschke, Philip. *The Peaceful Pill Handbook.* New Revised International Edition. Waterford, Mich.: Exit International US Ltd., 2007.

Nitschke, Philip, and Fiona Stewart. *Killing Me Softly: Voluntary Euthanasia and the Road to the Peaceful Pill.* Camberwell, Vic.: The Penguin Group, 2005.

Ogden, Russel D. *Euthanasia and assisted suicide in persons with Acquired Immunodeficiency Syndrome (AIDS) or Human Immunodeficiency Virus (HIV).* New Westminster, B. C.: Peroglyphics Publishing, 1994.

Pierce, Charles P. *Idiot America: How Stupidity Became a Virtue in the Land of the Free.* New York: Doubleday, 2009.

Portwood, Doris. *Common Sense Suicide: The Final Right.* New York: Dodd, Mead, 1978.

Putnam, Constance E. *Hospice or Hemlock: Searching for Heroic Compassion.* Westport, Conn.: Praeger Publishers, 2002.

Quill, Timothy E. *Death and Dignity: Making Choices and Taking Charge.* New York: W.W. Norton & Co., 1993.

Rigelhof, T.F. *This is Our Writing.* Erin, Ont.: Porcupine's Quill, 2000.

Rollin, Betty. *Last Wish.* New York: Linden Press, 1985.

Seguin, Marilynne and Cheryl K. Smith. *A Gentle Death.* Toronto: Key Porter Books, 1994.

Singer, Peter. *Practical Ethics.* Cambridge, England: Cambridge University Press, 1979.

Singer, Peter. *Rethinking Life and Death: The Collapse of Our Traditional Ethics.* New York: St. Martin's Press, 1994.

Singer, Peter. *Writings on an Ethical Life.* New York: The Ecco Press, 2000.

Smith, Cheryl K., Christopher G. Docker, John Hofsess and Bruce Dunn. *Beyond Final Exit.* Victoria, B.C.: The Right to Die Society of Canada, 1995.

Smith, Warren Allen. *Who's Who in Hell: A Handbook and International Directory for Humanists, Freethinkers, Naturalists, Rationalists, and Non-Theists.* New York: Barricade Books, 2000.

Smith, Wesley J. *Forced Exit: Euthanasia, Assisted Suicide and the New Duty to Die*. New York: Encounter Books, 2006.

Smith, Wesley J. *The Culture of Death: The Assault on Medical Ethics in America*. San Francisco: Encounter Books, 2000.

Smook, Ayke. *Helping People to Die In Dignity*. Junction City, Ore.: ERGO, 2006.

Somerville, Margaret A. *Death Talk: The Case Against Euthanasia and Physician-Assisted Suicide*. Montreal: McGill-Queen's University Press, 2002.

Stone, Geo. *Suicide and Attempted Suicide: Methods and Consequences*. New York: Carroll & Graf Publishers, 1999.

Syme, Rodney. *A Good Death: An Argument for Voluntary Euthanasia*. Melbourne,: Melbourne University Press, 2008.

Terman, Stanley A. *Peaceful Transitions: Stories of Success and Compassion*. Second Ed. Carlsbad, Calif.: Life Transitions Publishing Co., 2011.

Terman, Stanley A. *The Best Way to Say Goodbye: A Legal Peaceful Choice at the End of Life*. Carlsbad, Calif.: Life Transitions Publications, 2007.

Thomasma, David C. and Thomasine Kushner. *Birth to Death: Science and Bioethics*. New York: Cambridge University Press, 1996.

Tulloch, Gail. *Euthanasia-Choice and Death*. Edinburgh: Edinburgh University Press, 2005.

Warnock, Mary. *Easeful Death: Is There A Case For Assisted Suicide?* Oxford: Oxford University Press, 2008.

Wertenbaker, Lael Tucker. *Death of a Man*. 1957; reprinted by Beacon Press, Boston, 1974.

Wickett, Ann. *Double Exit: When Aging Couples Commit Suicide Together*. Eugene, Ore.: The Hemlock Society, 1989.

Williams, Glanville. *The Sanctity of Life and the Criminal Law*. New York: Alfred A. Knopf, 1957.

Wilson, Libby. *Sex on the Rates: Memoirs of a Family Planning Doctor*. Glendaruel, Argyll, Scotland: Argyll Publishing, 2004.

Wilson, Libby. *Unexpected Always Happen: Journal of a Doctor in Sierra-Leone*. Argyll, Scotland: Argyll Publishing, 1995.

Woodman, Sue. *Last Rights: The Struggle over the Right to Die*. Cambridge, Mass.: Perseus Publishing, 2000.

Film, Video, and Audio Recordings

Euthanasia Prevention Coalition. *Never Again: The Second International Symposium on Euthanasia and Assisted Suicide*, May 29-30, 2009, Landsdowne, Va. 6-DVD set.

Hofsess, John. *Using the DeBreather and Helium Systems.* Victoria, B.C.: Last Rights Publications, 2000 (VHS).

Humphry, Derek. *"The 11th Hour,"* a video autobiography recorded in Denver by KDI-TV for the PBS series, *Frontline*, 2003.

Humphry, Derek. "The Right to Death." *Firing Line* television interview hosted by William F. Buckley, Jr., on September 17, 1991. PDF transcript accessed at http://hoohila.stanford.edu/firingline/programView.php?programID=1301

Humphry, Derek. "The Inbox." Dublin, Ireland, radio program station 98FM, September 27, 2007.

Humphry, Derek. Autobiographical talk for "The Eleventh Hour," for KBDI-TV, Denver Center Media / Front Range Education Media Corporation and the Denver Center for the Performing Arts, 2003.

Kevorkian, Jack. "The Kevorkian Verdict." *Frontline*, May 14, 2006.

Kevorkian, Jack. *Kevorkian.* HBO Documentary Films, June 28, 2010.

McGuiness, Frank (writer) and Simon Curtis (director), "A Short Stay in Switzerland." London: BBC, 2009.

Minelli, Ludwig. "The Suicide Tourist." *Frontline*, Jan. 22, 2006.

Nicol, Neal. "Working with Jack Kevorkian," NuTech Conference IX, Melbourne, Oct. 7, 2010. Filmed by RNC.

Nitschke, Philip. Interview by the Australian Broadcasting Corporation, Brisbane, July 21, 2008. Accessed at http://www.abc.net.au/local/stories/2008/07/21/2309846.htm?site=brisbane

Nitschke, Philip. *Mademoiselle and the Doctor.* Darwin, Northern Territory, Australia: Exit International, 2004. Documentary, Janine Hosking, director.

Ronson, Jon, producer, "Reverend Death." London: World of Wonder, 2008.

Schorr, Daniel. "Kevorkian will not assist in any more suicides," *60 Minutes*, June 3, 2007.

van Dijck, Eveline. *Maj ik Dood* (Please Let Me Die). DVD. Holland: Fonds Psychische Gezondheid (Foundation for Psychological Health), 2008.

Zaritsky, John (producer), "The Suicide Tourist (Craig Ewert)" 2007.

Conferences

2008. World Federation of Right to Die Societies. 17th World Congress, Paris, France, October 30-November 1, 2008; also NuTech Conference IX, same location. Presenter.

2009. Euthanasia Prevention Coalition. "Never Again. Second International Symposium on Euthanasia and Assisted Suicide," Landsdowne, Virginia, May 29-30, 2009. Observer.

2010. World Federation of Right to Die Societies. 18th World Congress, Melbourne, Australia, October 7-10, 2010; also NuTech Conference X, same location. Presenter.

2012. World Federation of Right to Die Societies. 19th World Congress, Zürich, Switzerland, June 14-16, 2012; also NuTech Conference XI, same location. Presenter.

Index